Love
Your
GUT

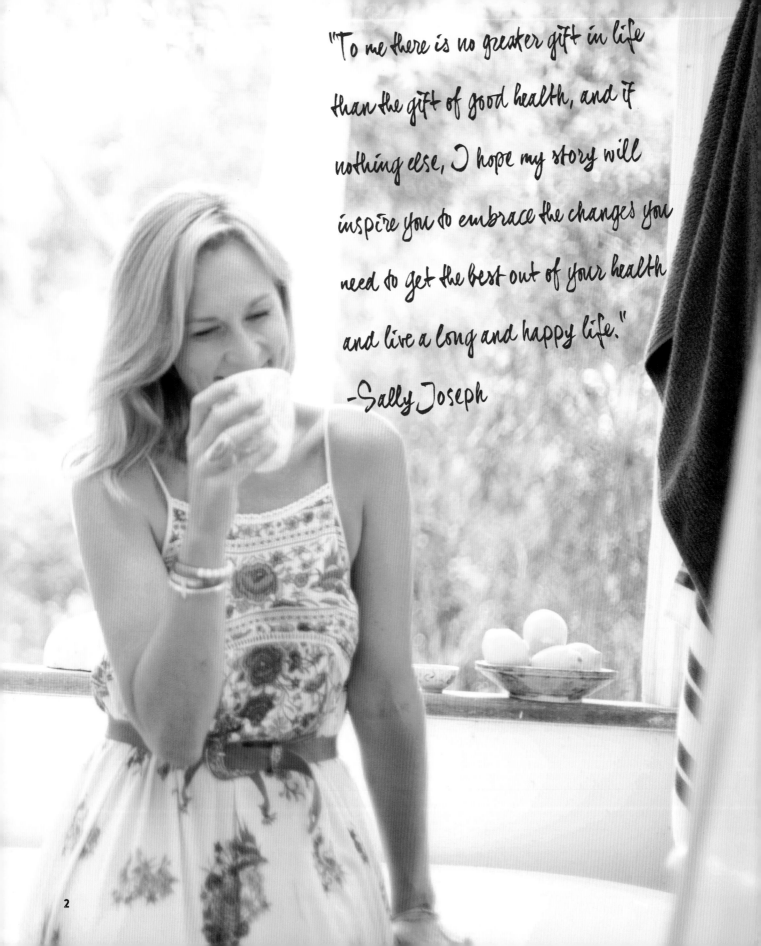

"To me there is no greater gift in life than the gift of good health, and if nothing else, I hope my story will inspire you to embrace the changes you need to get the best out of your health and live a long and happy life."

-Sally Joseph

Love Your GUT

BY

SALLY JOSEPH C.N.

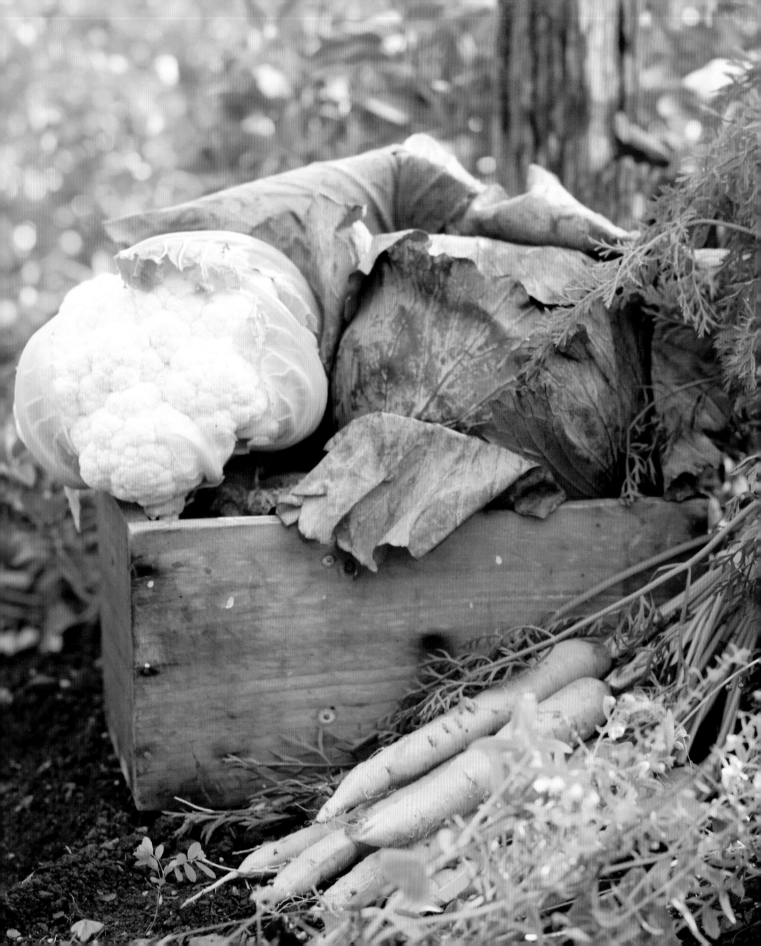

Contents

Dedication

This book is dedicated to all those people who have struggled to find answers to their health. Know that with the right approach to your diet, your lifestyle, yourself and your environment, your body has the skill and ability to heal itself, all you have to do is make the necessary changes and create an environment conducive to healing. I also dedicate this book to my patients who I have travelled the journey with over the years, you have been a constant source of inspiration and motivation to continuously dig deeper in search of answers, even when it seems like there aren't any. But most importantly I dedicate this book to my incredible Mum and Dad and those friends who have constantly supported me throughout my journey. As the saying goes… the race is not always to the swift, but to those who keep on going. Thank you from my "heart's bottom" x

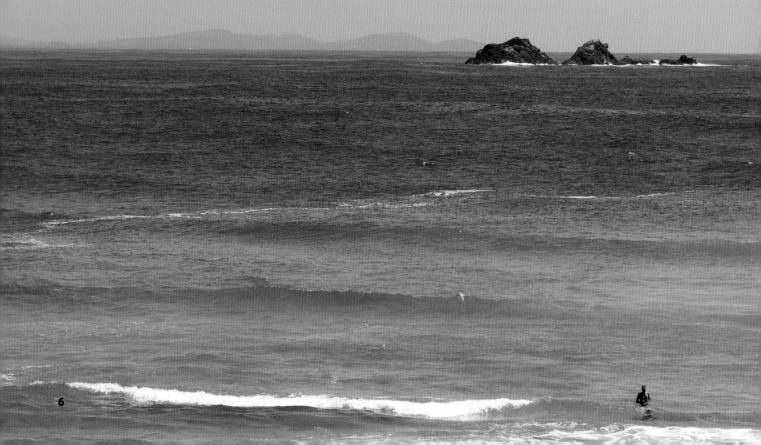

Foreword by
Layne Beachley

Having a Leaky Gut is far from sexy. Reflecting on my childhood, with the wealth of information currently available to us, I now understand why I was so sick all of the time.

Due to being adopted at birth I was unable to be breast fed, so my gut health was already off to a bad start. I truly believe my poor diet and gut health contributed to the depression and myriad of health challenges I developed later in life.

A diet rich in refined carbohydrates, processed foods, sugar and dairy products was the norm back in the 1970s and 80s. Vegemite sandwiches, white buttered toast, hot chips, hamburgers, chocolate milkshakes and pizza crusts were my go-to staples well into my teenage years, frustrating my Dad to tears as he attempted to have me eat anything with any nutritional value. My crocodile tears and stubborn defiance ensured I always got what I wanted. When friends invited me over for a sleepover, their parents would always panic because they had no idea what to feed me. As long as Vegemite was in the pantry I was sorted! Fortunately, I was a hyperactive kid, so I was lucky enough to avoid obesity. However, misdiagnosed lactose intolerance was always treated with multiple courses of antibiotics for my "flu like" symptoms.

Considering this precarious start to life, combined with my lack of culinary skills and understanding of basic nutrition, it's obvious why my immune system and gut health were compromised from the start. Twenty-twenty hindsight is a luxury, especially when you can reflect on a time in your life, learn from it, be grateful for it, let it go and move on.

I realized my health is my wealth back in 1993 when I was diagnosed with my first bout of Chronic Fatigue Syndrome. Being diagnosed with CFS provided me with some comfort once I took the time to understand what contributed to my continuous feeling of dis-ease. Poor diet, mental and physical stress, an intense competition schedule, onerous physical training and a lack of quality sleep sabotaged my immune system, resulting in my body demanding I give it a break.

At the time my symptoms were pretty mild: bloated stomach, poor concentration, abysmal memory and a general feeling of fatigue. I was uncomfortable enough to get a food allergy test. The results revealed I had become intolerant to much of what I was eating, including gluten, red meat, green apples and even raw almonds! Now what was I going to eat? There was no such thing as a gluten-free menu in the 90s! Fortunately, I was still living at home with my Dad, who is a master chef in the kitchen and he whipped up some meals that fitted in with my new dietary guidelines. Weekly Vitamin B shots, self-administered vitamin C injections and hundreds of dollars worth of nutritional supplements, supported by proper hydration, consistent sleep patterns and reduced physical output enabled me to overcome this health challenge in a matter of months. Crisis averted due to rapid action... well, so I thought. What I failed to understand is that, after experiencing CFS, I would be forever susceptible to the effects, unless I adopted the right eating habits and continually maintained my gut health.

Two years later I relapsed, only this time it was more intense: memory loss, horrendous tinea between my toes, extreme sugar cravings, bloating and a lack of confidence, not to mention the extreme fatigue I felt upon trying to get out of bed in the morning. I was trapped in a foggy haze of negativity, depression and fear, unable to acknowledge, identify or accept this was happening all over again. 'What you resist persists' and my reluctance to own and recognize my suffering ensured every other aspect of my life suffered, including my professional surfing career, health and friendships. Trapped in a negative vortex of despair and hopelessness, I began to have suicidal thoughts fuelled by the unrealistic amount of pressure, expectation and judgment I was living under. You can't change what you can't see, and after 18 months of living in denial, it was time to take action.

Similar to the original diagnosis two years prior, my life was restricted to supplements, injections, and a diet free of yeast, gluten, dairy, red meat, mushrooms, fruit, alcohol, sugar and anything processed. I was advised to sleep 12-14 hours per day, increase my water intake, stop all exercise, including surfing and to take on no work. Two years later I was given the all clear and won my first of seven world titles eight months later. What doesn't kill you makes you stronger!

Lessoned learned. Having overcome two bouts of Chronic Fatigue, numerous injuries and depression, I was still plagued by ongoing gut problems and an insatiable addiction to sugar! It was at this point I found Sally. As she had experienced CFS herself, I trusted in a practitioner who had lived through the health challenges she had spent her life diagnosing and treating. Sally was the first practitioner to truly put me and my gut under the microscope, assessing every inch of my digestive function, from the balance of my gut flora colonies, my digestion and absorption of nutrients, through to identifying and treating unwanted pathogens that had taken up residence within my gut. Her approach was the most informative and comprehensive I had ever experienced. This thorough treatment plan gave me greater mental clarity and a sense of vitality, enabling me to go on and claim my seventh world title at an age where most athletes are considering retirement.

CFS was (and to a degree, still is) a mysterious illness, with an array of conflicting evidence, treatments and steps to retaining and maintaining a normal, healthy life. I now understand it's all about balance and learning to listen to your body, , and most of all, I now understand, it's about looking after your gut!

To this day I am still sensitive to yeast, gluten, red meat, mushrooms and dairy, and, quite honestly, I don't miss any of these foods and my body loves me for it. Being susceptible to fatigue and depression, I am now on high alert to the symptoms, preventing me from falling victim to the pain and suffering I once endured, whilst encouraging me to maintain a conscientious commitment to my long term health and wellbeing. A regime of a daily surf, fresh seasonal produce and the occasional sweet treat is my recipe for good health and happiness.

I am extremely grateful for Sally's empathy, professional knowledge and diversity of treatment options. Surrounding myself with professional and knowledgeable practitioners like her provided me with the confidence to reach out and ask for help. Sharing your fears and challenges with people gives you strength and understanding to realise there are other people out there like you, dealing with similar challenges and you are not alone in your fight. When we experience challenges, we naturally isolate ourselves, but this is the time when you must put your hand up, ask for help and acknowledge that you can't fight this battle on your own. You are as successful as the people you surround yourself with so do your research and never take your health for granted.

FOREWORD BY

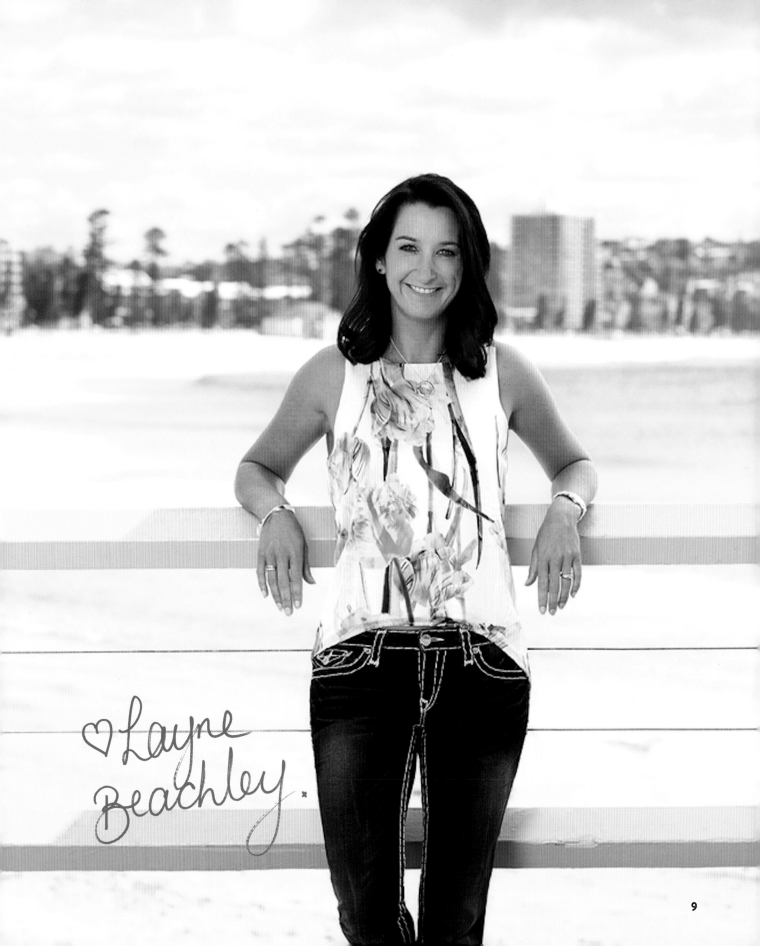

♡ Layne Beachley.

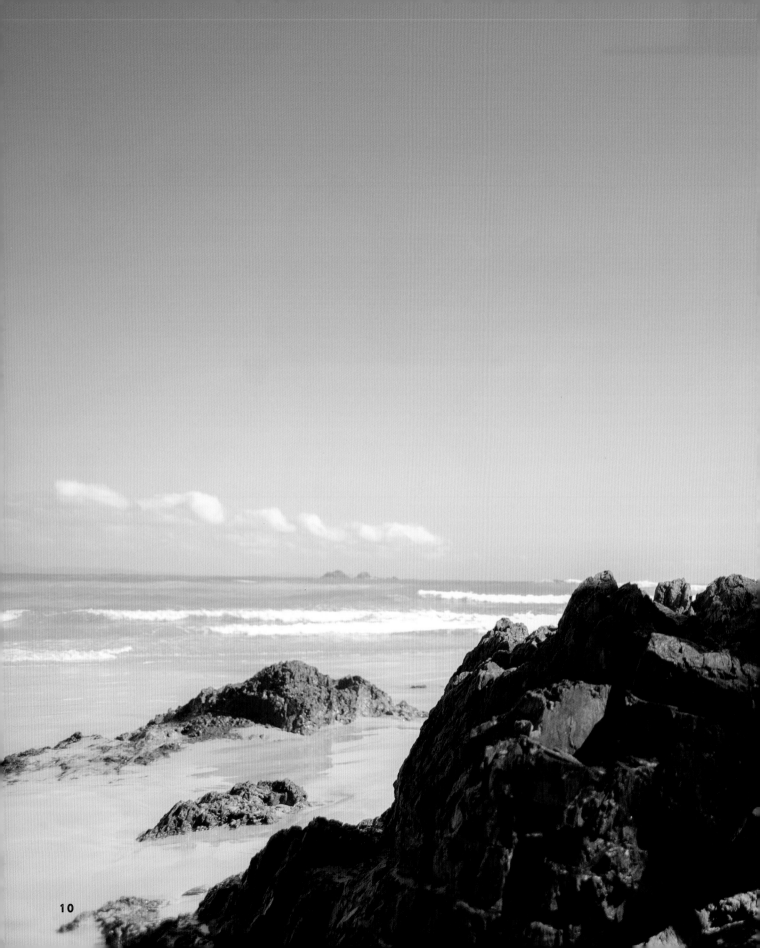

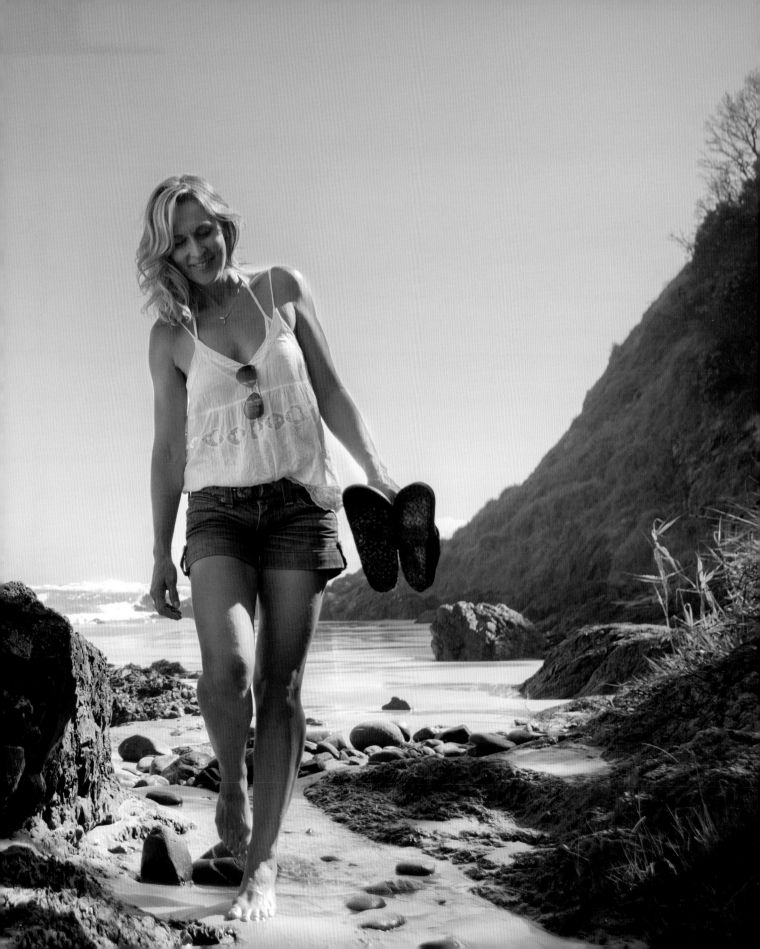

Love your gut,
love your life

What if I told you there was a simple and easy answer to your weight and health problems, beyond just diet and exercise? Or, better still, what if I told you there was a way to unlock your full health potential, maintain a feeling of boundless energy and vitality, and a healthy weight and appearance, simply by adopting a few daily habits into your everyday life? Would you want to know more?

Some 2000 years ago the Ancient Greek Physician, Hippocrates, considered the father of Western medicine, claimed that, 'All diseases begin in the gut.' As a Clinical Nutritionist who has treated thousands of patients over the past 17 years, as well as having suffered and recovered from a number of chronic and supposedly 'incurable' illnesses myself, I can safely say I subscribe to this same philosophy!

The word 'gut' has acquired some rather unappealing associations — 'muffin top', 'spare tyre', 'beer belly', or that most unsavoury of expressions ... 'dropping one's guts', often used to describe passing wind. However, I intend to use the term 'gut' to refer to a vast and intricate eco-system within your body, also referred to as the gastrointestinal tract, rather than any excess flab you may be carrying around your girth.

You could say that the gut is king of the castle when it comes to the power and influence it has over the other body systems. This claim to fame stems from the sheer size of the human gut and the occupants that live within it. Imagine this: if you were to take your gastrointestinal tract and flatten it out, the surface area would equate in size to an entire tennis court! But it's what lives inside your gut that holds the key to influencing your overall health, and that's trillions and trillions of microbes or microorganisms, including bacteria, fungi, parasites and viruses, that make up what's known as the human 'microbiome'. Recent research has established that about 90 percent of all cells and all genetic material within our body are bacterial, fungal or otherwise non-human cells - the majority of which live in our bowel or large intestine. Put simply, our microbial cells outnumber our human cells by a ratio of 10:1, which makes us 90 percent microbial and only 10 percent human! You may also be interested to know that you're carrying around 1.5 kg (nearly 3.5 pounds) of microorganisms inside your gut which are responsible for a wide range of essential functions, including the production of around 30 percent of your energy, the digestion and absorption of your food, the synthesis of many vitamins and nutrients, the production of anti-inflammatory compounds to help regulate your immune system and the production of hormones, such as serotonin. Now like all things in life, when it comes to the microbes living within your gut, there are 'good' guys and 'bad' guys. The trick to managing your overall health and wellbeing lies predominantly in maintaining a healthy balance between the 'good' and the 'bad' – ideally 85 percent 'good' microbes to 15 percent 'bad', and I'll explain more on how to do just that in the following chapters.

The Australian Gut Foundation claims that 40 percent of people in the Western world experience digestive-related problems at some point in their life, and I would argue this statistic is even higher in my clinical experience. If you consider the typical ailments that people complain of – bloating, flatulence, constipation and diarrhoea, heartburn and reflux, fatigue, depression, anxiety, obesity, PMS, arthritic pain, high cholesterol and blood pressure, it may surprise you to learn that the majority of these conditions have their origin in the gut!

These everyday health problems have undeniably reached epidemic proportions. The questions we'll explore in this book are: why these problems occur; what you can do about it; how you can solve your health and weight problems through fixing your gut.

In my experience, it doesn't matter what your specific health complaint, ailment or disease may be. The most important way to start to heal your body and achieve a long-term and hopefully permanent resolution, is to repair your gut. This book is going to help you to do just that!

I'm also going to open your eyes to perhaps the most common and lethal condition suffered in the world today – chronic inflammation. The gut is the very place where all chronic inflammation begins, and I'll be explaining exactly how you can switch this inflammation off, and keep it off, in an effort to avoid the many associated illnesses and diseases.

Love Your Gut is not just about how to get rid of the spare tyre around your girth, nor is it just 'another fad diet' to get you all hyped up, only to fall off the bandwagon a few weeks in. In fact, this book isn't about a diet at all, but rather a way of eating for life that has the power to unlock your full health potential and provide you with the level of wellbeing you desire. By maintaining the health of your gut, you will be working to preserve your physical, mental and emotional health, and that means preventing illness and disease.

So whether you're after a beautiful, clear complexion, or you want more energy and vitality, or you want to crank up your metabolism and turn your body into a fat burning machine for life, then … yep, you guessed it … you need to start with your gut! And perhaps most importantly, if you want to improve the way your brain functions, and your mental or emotional state, then your gut is the most important starting point by a country mile. By simply turning your focus to this amazing organ called 'The Gut', and showing it a bit of love, you'll be well on your way to solving your health problems.

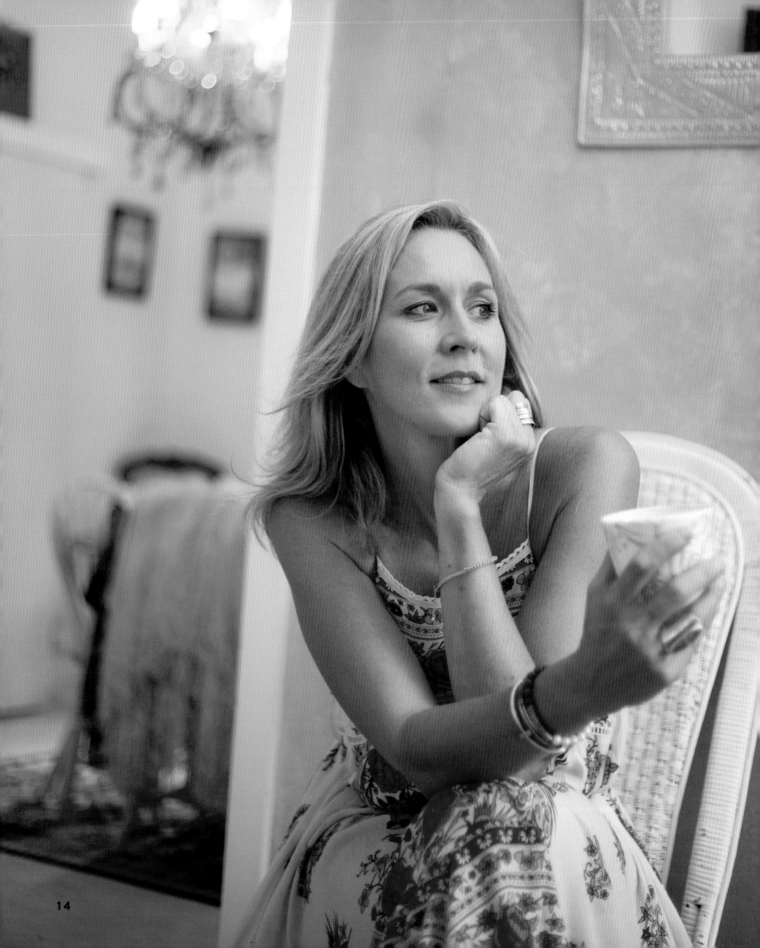

How I came
to tell this story

My journey towards understanding and learning about the gut didn't begin with my study to become a Clinical Nutritionist, but several years prior, when I was just twenty one and training for a marathon and studying for a communications degree, whilst holding down a rather demanding job in advertising. My life was pretty jam-packed, and you could say I was running on all cylinders and feeling invincible, until it became clear that life had another plan in store for me.

After coming down with two nasty viral infections, Glandular Fever and Cytomegalovirus, I found myself struggling to get back on track. I even tried returning to my running training, in the hope it would somehow reignite my energy, but something wasn't right. Weeks and still months later I wasn't getting any better and my GP was prescribing me ongoing courses of antibiotics and penicillin in an attempt to overcome the recurrent ear, throat and kidney infections that had plagued me since falling ill. Little did I know back then that these medications were actually decimating my immune system and driving my health further into a downward spiral.

Less than 3 months down the track, I was so fatigued that by 9am each day I would find myself falling asleep at my computer and had resorted to setting an alarm on my watch to wake me from the lunchtime kip I needed to take in the park each day.

Eventually I was forced to quit my job and take what I thought would be a few months off, but instead it was nearly four years before I would fully recover. I discovered I was suffering from Chronic Fatigue Syndrome (CFS), an illness conventional medicine knew little about back then, and struggled to acknowledge, and that society viewed as just the 'yuppy flu'.

Further testing revealed I had also developed 'multiple chemical sensitivity disorder', (resulting from compromised immune function), an unusually severe sensitivity to common chemicals, many of which were being emitted from devices within my office like printers, computers and photocopiers.

After countless courses of antibiotics failed to combat the multiple infections I was fighting, I was placed under the care of a leading immunologist who delivered the news I had gone on to develop Systemic Lupus, an autoimmune disease similar to Rheumatoid Arthritis. For those of you who aren't familiar with the effects of CFS or

Lupus, life is spent pretty well sleeping for much of the day – for me, it was up to 21 out of 24 hours at my worst, and not because I was lazy or couldn't be bothered to get out of bed, but because my body was flat-out broke! At one point, a good day meant I was able to un-stack the dishwasher, or walk across the road to post a letter; a bad day meant I was unable to get out of bed, except to go to the toilet, and that often involved crawling backwards up the stairs on my bottom because of the severe pain in my joints and muscle weakness. Then there was the heat that would exude from my body, which made me feel unbearably hot causing me to scratch my skin to the point that it would become red raw and bleed. But the only treatment option I was offered was a cocktail of pharmaceutical medications, many of which carried additional and very unpleasant side effects.

You could say I was a pretty sick chick, and for someone used to being super fit and active, I felt like I was experiencing hell on earth - being stuck in bed all day, unable to do all the things I wanted. I felt imprisoned in my own body and couldn't understand what I had done for it to let me down so badly and why I couldn't get better. I was angry with myself, with my body and with the doctors, and longed to be like my friends who were leading 'normal', active lives.

But the turning point in my health came after a visit to my immunologist when he informed me of the long term prognosis I faced with Lupus and that there was 'no cure', no known cause, and the only treatment option was to take strong steroid medications and powerful painkillers to manage the symptoms - which would likely get progressively worse over the course of my life.

Wow! What a fantastic life I have ahead of me, I thought. Where do I sign up? More to the point, where did this all go so horribly wrong?

But then something inside me stirred as the words 'no cure', and 'no explanation for this disease' rang loud in my ears. I knew what he was saying made no sense. If I had once been fit and healthy, then surely there had to be a way to get back to that place, it just seemed logical to me. So I asked the specialist doctor if there was anything I could change in my diet that might help improve my immune function and stop it from attacking itself, and his reply was quite simply, 'No.' As it turned out, that was exactly the answer I needed to hear to stir me into action. Tell me it's not possible and I'll find a way to make it happen! And so, as the doctor pushed the prescription for steroid drugs across his desk towards me and said, 'If you don't start these medications, you will only get worse,' I stood up, thanked him for his time, muttered the words, 'We'll see,' under my breath and walked out.

Those scripts were never filled and I never relied on another painkiller or course of antibiotics to get me through the CFS or Systemic Lupus again. Instead I turned my focus to reading and researching everything I could on the immune system, nutrition and diet. What I discovered was that 80 percent of our immune system is contained within our gut, so it made perfect sense to me that if the gut is where your food ends up and this is where the bulk of our immune activity stems from, then surely the answer to my problems with my immune system lay in the food I was putting into my body, and the function of my digestive system.

So how did my story end? Well, in a nutshell, I was eventually able to overcome the Lupus and CFS. I did this by repairing the damage to my gut, and eliminating the pro-inflammatory foods from my diet that were wreaking havoc on my immune system.

I also learnt how to adopt certain practices into my daily routine to reduce stress in my life. Now I'm excited to be able to share with you so much of what I learnt in the course of that journey throughout the rest of this book. I am confident that you can incorporate these methods to improve your health too, no matter where it is at.

But like all good stories, mine had a twist. Several years after overcoming the Lupus and CFS, I was diagnosed with yet another AI immune disease, known as Hashimoto's, which affects the function of the thyroid gland and caused my weight to balloon by 10 kilograms (22 pounds), in 10 weeks! To add insult to injury, an angry red rash developed across my face and I was retaining so much fluid (thanks to the myxedema associated with the Hashimoto's) that I resembled something like a six months pregnant, pimply pineapple! You could say I was pretty damn distressed by what was going on with my body, especially as I was a qualified Clinical Nutritionist by this stage, eating a super healthy diet and running six laps of soft sand at Bondi beach each morning. I put the reason for my relapse down to that lethal six-letter word - STRESS - following a traumatic relationship break up.

But before I was given a full diagnosis, I consulted with five different endocrinologists, but none of them were able to offer any effective long-term solution other than to prescribe Oroxine, the standard medication for treating an underactive thyroid, which I failed to respond to. Once more I found myself at a crisis point with my health and feeling extremely disheartened that this could be happening all over again.

So there I was, back at the drawing board trying to unravel my health conundrum. I decided to take a step back and ask myself, 'If I was my own patient, what would I do?' My reply: 'I'd go straight to the gut!' So that's exactly what I did and once again I set about restoring optimal function to my gut.

The whole journey to recovery took a lot of hard work and persistence to improve my adrenal function from the debilitating effects of chronic stress, as well as regulate my low thyroid hormone levels, using a combination thyroid hormone treatment (prescribed by a doctor) and various nutritional supplements.

I now look upon these experiences with my health as a gift, because they have shaped who I am today. Best of all, they have provided me with the knowledge and insight to help others who have consulted me about their health over the years, especially those who had been told there was nothing they could do but to rely on pharmaceutical medications for the rest of their life.

Perhaps this is one of the main reasons I decided to become a Clinical Nutritionist. If there was a way I could help others avoid going through the same long and arduous journey that I had endured in my quest for good health, then it would all be worthwhile.

There is no doubt that conventional medicine and certain pharmaceutical drugs play a valuable role in aspects of supporting human health. However, if the underlying cause of an illness is not accurately identified, some treatments can actually exacerbate the condition or progress of an illness, which is what occurred in my case and with many people I have treated over the years.

I have spent the past 17 years working with people from all walks of life - from super models to elite athletes and rock stars, through to everyday people like you and me - treating them for a wide range of common and complex health conditions, and I can honestly say that in all the people I have treated over the years, there wasn't a single one who did not suffer some form of digestive problem. No matter how simple or complex their presenting health condition, the common denominator with each and every patient I have treated, is the function of their digestive system.

If nothing else, this observation supports the notion that the gut really is the gate way to our overall health and the gatekeeper for the optimal function of all body systems. It is my belief that not only by feeding your body with nutritious food, but also through healing your gut, you will achieve optimal health, and experience what it's like to look and feel your best, for life.

Today, I maintain the same eating habits that I recommend you do on the LYG program, but you don't need to suffer from a chronic illness to reap the benefits. No matter what your current level of health, or even if you enjoy good health, I strongly believe you will feel even better by following this program. Best of all, you should enjoy a far more functional and energetic life and hopefully greater longevity when you finally glide gracefully into old(er) age.

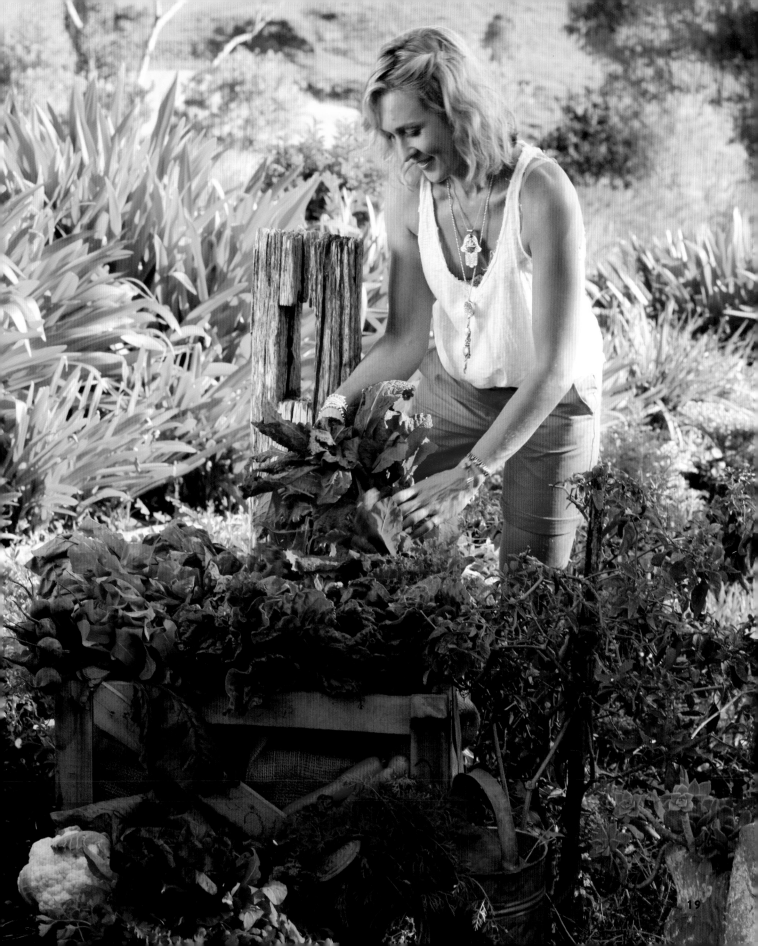

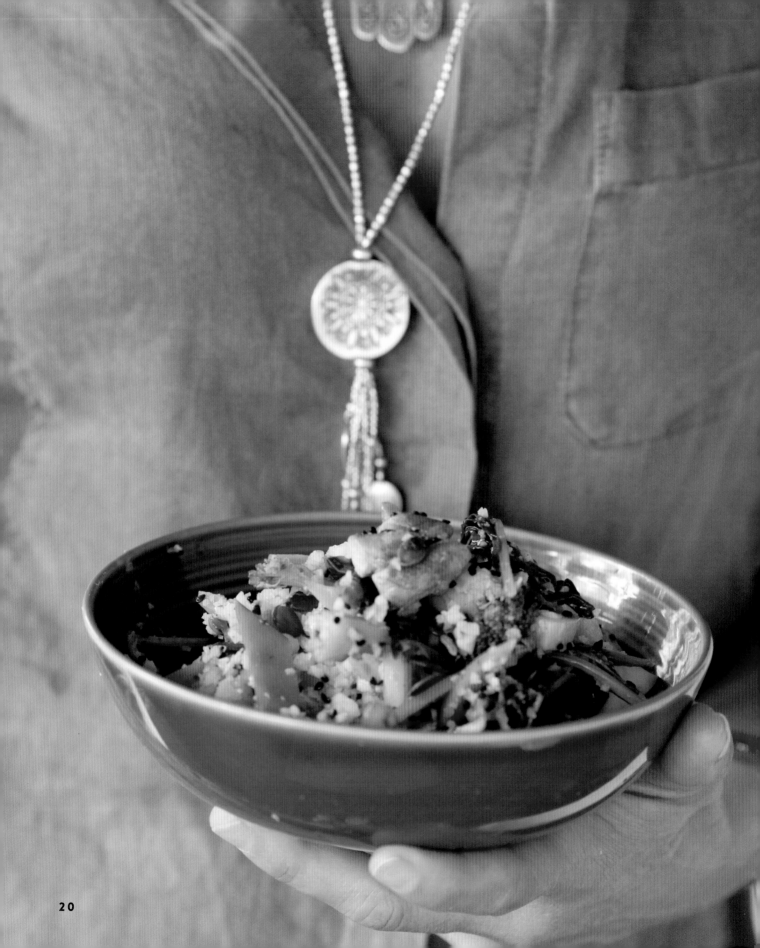

Your health
is in your hands

Human health has reached a crisis point, with lifestyle and degenerative diseases reaching epidemic proportions, in many cases thanks to a diet that no longer resembles anything like what our grandparents ate, or what the human body was designed to consume. The modern Western diet, in combination with excess exposure to toxins found in our food and environment, along with chronic stress, is pushing the human body to the limit.

By the time a patient suffering a chronic illness would consult me, they had usually seen a handful of doctors, taken countless prescription medications and been tested for everything under the sun - and often told there was either no known explanation for their health problem, or nothing more that could be done, beyond surgery or managing symptoms with pharmaceutical medications. But, in reality, there was a whole other side to their health that had not been explored. In many cases, no one bothered to ask some of the most basic questions, such as: 'How often do you have a bowel motion each day?'; 'How much water do you drink in a day?"; Is your sleep restful?' ; 'What are you feeding your body each day?'; 'How is your home life?'; 'What are your relationships like?'; 'Are you happy?' These simple questions can reveal so much about a person and the contributing factors to their health problems.

When I see a patient for the first time, I typically spend around an hour and a half with them, sometimes more if necessary, but let's be honest, we're lucky if our doctor spends more than 15 minutes with us before we leave with a script or two in hand. So rather than wait for the system to change, I encourage you to take responsibility for your own health, because nobody can care for your body better, or knows it better, than YOU!

You may not be suffering a disease right now, but this doesn't necessarily mean your body is functioning at its optimal best. A disease may take 10, 20, 30 years or a lifetime to develop, and your risk factors are largely determined by the dietary and lifestyle choices you make each and every day.

I know it can be easier to put off your health until tomorrow, thinking it's just all too hard, or you don't have time right now, but in reality, what's far harder and more inconvenient is being sick or developing a disease that takes away your freedom to do the things in life you enjoy, with the people you love.

Picture your body a little like an onion, made up of layer-upon-layer of cellular information that has accumulated over the course of your life, based on the foods you have fed it, the lifestyle choices you've made and the physical and emotional environment to which you have exposed it. If you aspire to be healthy, and to feel and look as good as you can, for as long as you can, then you need to be conscious that each and every food choice you make, every day, may be either creating a disease, or preventing one.

Let me put this theory into more practical terms for you. Think of your body like a bank account for a minute. When you deposit money into your account, the balance goes into surplus. When you make a withdrawal from your account, the balance goes into deficit. If you make more withdrawals than deposits, you will go into debt. Go too far into debt and the bank manager will freeze your account and you'll lose your freedom of choice. Say you take out a loan to pay back that debt, but then you start spending the money you have borrowed: you will find it harder and harder to repay that loan and get your bank balance back into a state of surplus. Well this is similar to the way your body works. Depending on your food and lifestyle choices, the environment you live in and the state of your relationships, you will either be making more 'withdrawals' or more 'deposits' towards your health. If you go into debt with your health because you've made too many unhealthy choices over time, your body will allow you to borrow from its reserves to a certain point ... borrowing that comes in the form of stress hormones, adrenalin and cortisol. But run on these for too long, and eventually the body can't sustain the pace, leaving you susceptible to illness or disease.

This was exactly the case with my body when I literally 'ran it into the ground' by over training. I kept spending 'energy dollars' I didn't have, and tried to get by on borrowed energy from adrenalin, caffeine and sugar to keep myself afloat. My health was able to return to a state of 'surplus' only when I was able to repay the debt, through feeding it with nutritious food and nutritional supplements to heal my gut, as well as changing my physical and emotional environment.

Over the page you will see a list of examples for typical 'deposits' versus 'withdrawals' relating to our health. Read through each list and identify which ones relate to you, then add up how many you score from each list and see on which side you score higher. This will provide some indication of how your health is tracking, or is likely to in the future

- based on your current diet and lifestyle choices. I believe our health is determined by 'the sum of all parts', not just the presence of one or two factors, meaning your health is a product of each and every choice you make day-to-day. Over time, these choices add up to influence how your inherent DNA is either 'expressed' or 'repressed'. In other words, if you have a family history of say, heart attack or stroke, or even depression, the food and lifestyle choices you make throughout your life, as well as environmental factors, have the power to influence the extent your inherent predisposition to certain diseases is expressed – meaning your genetics are not set in stone.

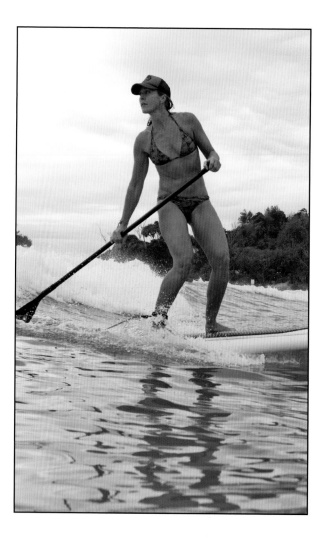

DEPOSITS

Deep, restful sleep

2 - 3 litres of water each day

Plenty of healthy fats each day

Low sugar diet

2–3 servings green leafy vegetables each day

Fresh organic foods daily

Exercise 4–7 days p/wk

Regular Meditation

Stretching and moving daily

Minim alcohol

Live and work in a smoke free environment

Chemical free cleaning & personal care products

WITHDRAWALS

Less than 7 hrs. sleep /broken sleep

2 plus coffees per day

Margarine and processed vegetable oils

Processed sugar or fruit juice each day

Fast food 1+ times p/wk

Processed packaged foods daily

Exercise less than 1 time p/wk

Experience daily stress

Sitting for 6-8 hrs + p/day

6+ alcoholic drinks per week

Smoke

Chemical based cleaning & personal care products

CONSIDER THIS

Try making simple changes to your life: switch to chemical free foods, skin care and cleaning products; cut right back on sugar, caffeine, and alcohol; do some form of exercise each and every day, even if it's just walking the dog; get plenty of sunshine and enough restful sleep at night; drink filtered water instead of tap; practice daily meditation, even for just ten minutes; and take time out to do simple breathing exercises and stretching when you wake, or sit for too long at your desk. Making these simple things part of your daily routine will not only reduce your risk of illness and disease in the future, but enable you to reap the rewards immediately so you can enjoy a fuller, happier life right now with the freedom to do the things you want, without restriction from health problems. So rather than simply choosing foods based on convenience, or giving into your cravings, I challenge you to start viewing your food choices as either being toxic to your health, pushing you closer towards illness and disease, or as medicine that will sustain your health for life.

The gut stuff

The Guts
of the Matter

SO. WHAT EXACTLY IS THE GUT, YOU MAY ASK?

Your gut is not just the organ your food passes through for digestion and absorption of nutrients, along with the excretion of waste. No, your gut is the core of your health, influencing everything from the function of your immune system, your mental health, your energy levels, through to your weight and metabolism. It even has a say in the diseases you may be prone to developing later in life. So as you can see, there's not much about your health that your gut doesn't influence!

The gut belongs to the digestive system, and is essentially a long hollow tube that runs from the mouth to the anus, incorporating the oesophagus, stomach and small and large intestine. It is often referred to as the gastrointestinal tract or GIT. The other major organs of the digestive system include the liver, gall bladder, pancreas, tongue and salivary glands.

The main role of the digestive system is to break down your food so that you can absorb the nutrients. These nutrients then perform a myriad of biochemical reactions, including the creation of new cells and repair of damaged tissue, required by your body to function at its best,

But, as I touched on in the introduction, it's what lives within your gut that is the real key to determining your health.

WHAT'S LIVING WITHIN YOUR GUT?

Living within your gut is a complex ecosystem of microorganisms, known as your microbiome. As I mentioned in Chapter 1, there are more bacteria living within your gut than there are cells in your entire body – around ten trillion to be precise – outnumbering our human cells by a ratio of around ten to one! These microscopic colonies of bacteria line the wall of your gut to maintain and protect it from invasion by pathogens and toxins, whilst providing nutrients and nourishment for your cells.

Up to 1000 different species of bacteria live inside your gut, varying in concentration and influence. Although scientists have known about the human microbiome for a long time, it is only since the 'Human Microbiome Project' published results in 2012 of its five year study (into how changes in the human microbiome are associated with human health & disease), that modern science has truly come to fully appreciate the powerful influence of the microbiome on our health and potential for disease.

Recent research surrounding the human microbiome also revealed that, just as we all belong to a certain blood type group, we may also belong to one of three different gut flora or 'microbiome' types. This finding could explain why some

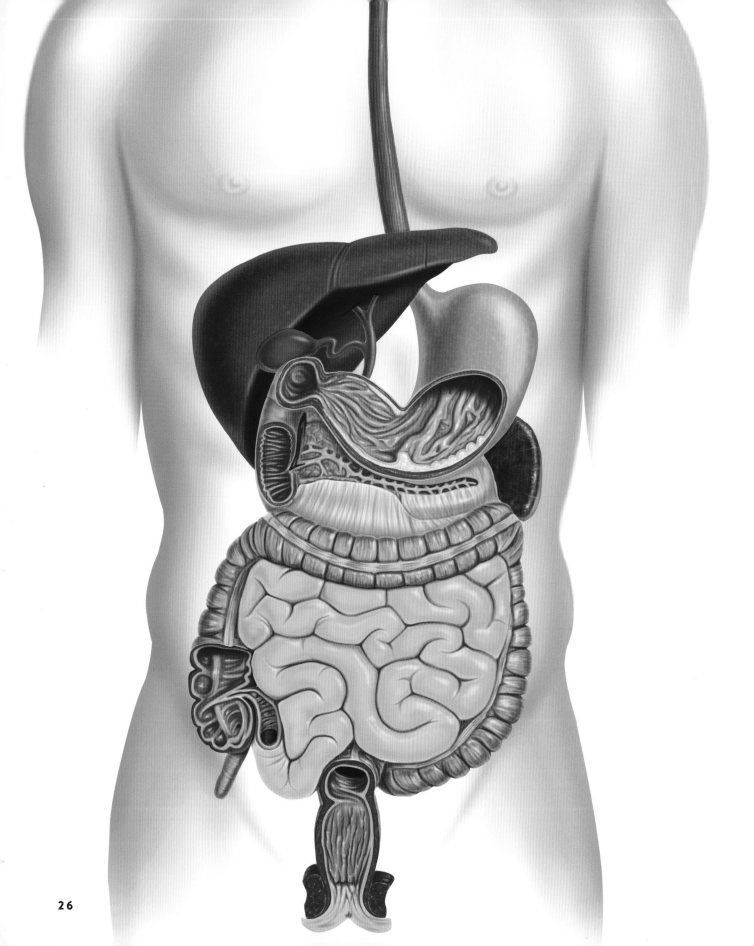

people struggle more than others to lose excess weight; why some people respond better to various diets, such as vegan or Paleo; and why some people seem able to absorb certain nutrients better than others. In time this discovery might help scientists identify which diseases we may be more prone to developing later in life, and form a basis for 'personalised medicine', with treatments and doses being determined on the basis of gut flora type.

However, not all of the bacteria living within your gut are friendly. Your gut also plays host to some not-so-friendly pathogens, specifically parasites, opportunistic or 'bad' bacteria, viruses and hostile fungi, such as Candida Albicans. You could say the world within your gut is a little like the Game of Thrones ... and as with any kingdom, the different species are all vying for power, engaged in a constant battle between 'good' and 'bad'. When the colonies of good gut flora are damaged, they become imbalanced – a condition referred to as dysbiosis – triggering a chain reaction of negative side effects. The greater the degree of imbalance or dysbiosis within your gut flora, the greater the negative impact on your health, both physical and mental. My goal in this book is to show you how to encourage the growth and survival of the good guys and eliminate the bad guys from your gut, to a point that enables your mind and body to thrive.

Believe it or not, no matter how much kale or other green goodness you may consume, when your good gut bacteria colonies are imbalanced, your body won't be able to digest and absorb all the goodness from your food. Remember what I told you in the introduction to this book – You are not just what you eat, but what your body digests and absorbs!"

Imbalances between your good and bad gut flora can also cause the tight junctions between the cells lining your gut wall to separate, causing your gut wall to become excessively permeable, or leaky like a sieve — a condition known as 'Leaky Gut' - but I'll explain more about this condition shortly.

IMMUNE SYSTEM FRONTLINE

Your gut also serves as your number one defence against all disease, with around 80 percent of your immune system located within your gut. This means a healthy gut is essential for maintaining a robust and balanced immune system. The good bacteria within your gut help to modulate your immune responses, communicating directly with your body's immune cells and enabling them to identify your enemies from your allies. Your gut flora also help to control inflammation and muster your defences against infection.

You could compare your immune system to being similar to a see-saw constantly trying to maintain equilibrium or balance. Should it tip too far in one direction for too long, your body will be exposed to either chronic low-grade inflammation, expressing as conditions ranging from allergies through to auto immune diseases or an underactive or weakened immune system, increasing the body's susceptibility to infections and diseases.

Although this is an extremely simplified explanation for one of the most complex systems in the human body, the message is that you don't want your immune system to become 'unbalanced' too far in either direction for too long, or you'll be at risk of developing chronic illness or disease..

WHAT'S LIVING IN YOUR MOUTH?

While maintaining the fragile ecosystem of your gut flora colonies is essential for maintaining a healthy immune system, there is little point in trying to eliminate pathogens from within your gut if your mouth is a breeding ground for opportunistic bacteria. There are around 500 different species of bacteria that live in your mouth, but like your gut, there are 'good' and 'bad' strains. Bad bacterial strains in your mouth can travel down your oesophagus and populate your gut, so it's essential to maintain healthy oral hygiene in your quest to maintain a healthy gut and prevent illness and disease. A common bacteria found in dental plaque - Fusobacterium nucleatum, can travel to different parts of your body causing inflammation and researchers at Harvard University have established a link between this bacteria and the initiation of colorectal tumors. If your gums regularly bleed when you brush your teeth, this is a classic tell tale sign they are overrun with pathogenic bacteria, so it's essential to get unhealthy bacteria levels in your mouth under control if you are to balance the bacteria within your gut.

Other elements of your oral health that may be impacting on your gut and overall health are amalgam fillings — those silver fillings many of us received as children. Perhaps your dentist has told you that amalgam fillings are perfectly harmless to your health, because the minute amount of mercury is encapsulated within the filling. However, the fact is, mercury is a toxic heavy metal and medical research has demonstrated that mercury is continuously released as vapor into the mouth, then it is inhaled and absorbed into body tissues, potentially affecting the function of your central nervous and immune system, liver and kidneys. I have seen patients with severe autoimmune diseases such as Lupus and MS experience a major improvement in their condition following the safe removal of their amalgam fillings.

MY CLEAN TEETH ROUTINE

I include an ancient Ayurvedic medicine practice known as 'oil pulling' as part of my dental hygiene routine. This involves swirling 1 1/2 tsp of virgin coconut oil around in my mouth for around 10– 20 minutes to eliminate pathogenic bacteria. followed by a salt water risne using 1/2 tsp Himalayan or Celtic Sea Salt and water. I also brush with natural antibacterial toothpaste that is fluoride free, and I recommend avoiding chemical based mouthwashes. Opt instead for those containing natural tea tree oil. Brushing your teeth a couple of times a week with baking soda can also work to neutralise the acid that feeds pathogenic bacteria, as well as help to naturally whiten your teeth.

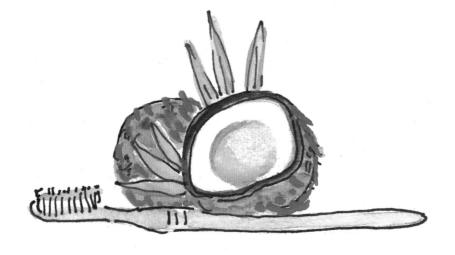

The Guts
of the Problem
Common Causes of Gut Problems

The organs within your digestive system need to work in harmony with one another in order to function at their best. Say, for example, you experience chronic constipation or diarrhoea (commonly referred to as Irritable Bowel Syndrome or IBS), this will impact on the function of all the other organs within your body, not just those within the digestive system. Over time, if left untreated, this can lead to the development of other chronic illnesses and diseases, including anxiety and depression. An article published in the Journal of Clinical Psychiatry in 2001, claims that 50 to 90 percent of people treated for IBS have psychiatric disorders, including panic disorder, generalized anxiety disorder, social phobia, post-traumatic stress disorder, and major depression. So the take home message is that the gut is typically the start and underlying root cause of most common health ailments and diseases, including autoimmune diseases and bowel cancer.

COMMON CAUSES OF GUT PROBLEMS

There are many factors that can contribute to gut and digestive problems, so in order to successfully heal your gut, it is essential to identify and address the deep underlying causes of poor gut health. Take a deep breath and grab a cup of (herbal) tea – because here follows all the whys and wherefores of a healthy and not-so-healthy gut.

A reminder: disease and illness do not stem from one single cause, nor does the origin typically lie in the organ where the problem is expressed. For instance, the underlying cause of sinus or arthritis does not begin in your sinuses or joints, but in your gut – usually many months, or even years prior. Sure, genetics can play a role, but your inherent genetic predisposition to an illness can either be expressed or repressed, depending on the balance of bacteria within your gut and the presence of

10 SIGNS YOU MAY HAVE A LEAKY GUT

1. Regular bouts of gas, bloating, diarrhoea or IBS.

2. Food allergies or food intolerances

3. Seasonal allergies or asthma

4. Regular infections - chest, ear and throat, colds or flu

5. Chronic Fatigue Syndrome or Fibromyalgia

6. Depression and anxiety

7. Acne, rosacea, or eczema.

8. Thrush

9. Diseases like Auto immune, Parkinson's and Alzheimer's, Autism and ADHD

10. Thyroid conditions

chronic inflammation - which starts long before the problem presents as a chronic condition.

Your digestive function can degenerate over time due to a combination of factors — things like exposure to antibiotics, overuse of pharmaceutical drugs, poor diet, exposure to toxins such as chemical pesticides, herbicides and fungicides sprayed on your food, chronic stress and, of course, old age.

WHAT IS A LEAKY GUT?

Think of the lining of your gut like a pair of women's pantyhose– in that it is a semi-permeable membrane – acting to enable specific substances like nutrients from your food to pass through to your bloodstream, but being tight enough to keep out unwanted microbes, allergens and toxins that can damage the delicate colonies of good bacteria within your gut.

Problems with our gut occur when the intestinal wall becomes damaged from things such as environmental toxins, antibiotics, pathogens and gluten - causing the tight junctions of your gut wall to weaken, and become excessively permeable, or 'leaky' - a little like a pair of laddered women's pantyhose. When the gut wall becomes excessively permeable, we develop a condition known as 'leaky gut syndrome'. Leaky gut increases your exposure to bad bacteria, undigested food particles and toxins which are able to leak from inside your gut wall into your blood stream. This process triggers a chronic inflammatory immune response, which can have a systemic effect on the health of other organs within the body.

Groundbreaking research in 2000 by Alessio Fasano, at the University of Maryland, discovered that a protein known as zonulin is responsible for regulating the permeability of the gut wall – a little like the bouncer at a nightclub determining who gets let in and who gets locked out. His research revealed that excess zonulin production was primarily triggered by bacteria, resulting from infection and the consumption of gluten. This research is a significant step in finding more effective treatments for diseases that are related to an exaggerated production of zonulin - including autoimmune diseases, allergies and even cancer.

GUT OFFENDERS

POOR DIET

Excessive consumption of sugar, gluten, cow's dairy, coffee, alcohol, artificial additives and processed vegetable oils can have a catastrophic effect on your digestive function, altering your gut flora colonies and triggering chronic inflammation. The various strains of bacteria living within the gut vary from person to person, depending on what they eat, as well as where they live in the world. The Japanese are thought to have some of the healthiest colonies of good gut flora in the world – largely because of their diet.

MEDICATIONS

Antacid medications, antibiotics, anti-inflammatory and steroid medications, antidepressants, pain killers and the oral contraceptive pill can all damage your gut wall and the balance of your gut flora colonies.

ANTACIDS

prescribed for reflux and heartburn are a classic example of a medication that not only fails to treat the underlying cause of the problem, but also actually exacerbates it when taken for long periods of time. If you have ever tried coming off these medications without making any changes to your diet, you will know the symptoms usually return, often worse than before.

Antacids suppress the body's production of hydrochloric acid, ordinarily produced by the stomach to assist with the digestion of protein. By repressing this mechanism, the body loses its ability to effectively digest food, resulting in a domino effect of symptoms. Rather than taking antacids to treat reflux or heartburn, I recommend treating the problem at a causative level, by following the LYG program and supplementing with a digestive enzyme. By doing so, symptoms of acid reflux and heartburn will all but disappear in the majority of cases.

ANTIBIOTICS

are a whole other kettle of fish. Society's thirst for this medication to treat every little sniffle and common cold has lead to a situation that threatens to have monumental consequences on our health. With every broad spectrum course of antibiotics you take, you are reducing vast quantities of your gut's bacterial mass. But even if you haven't been one to gobble multiple courses of antibiotics in your lifetime, you could be exposed to them through your food! Antibiotics are commonly administered to animals reared in feed lot or cages, such as beef cattle, chickens and pigs. Residual levels of these antibiotics accumulate within our system over time, causing an imbalance in our gut mircrobiome. This will not only leave you vulnerable to recurrent infection and proliferation of hostile pathogens like Candida, but the overuse of antibiotics has lead to the evolution of a new strain of super bugs that are resistant to most antibiotics. A far better approach to human infection is prevention through eating organic foods and maintaining healthy gut flora colonies to boost your immune defences. In many cases of infection, such as the common cold and flu, there are other far less destructive alternatives to antibiotics when they are not absolutely crucial for your health.

THE ORAL CONTRACEPTIVE PILL

has provided women across the world with the convenience of reliable contraception since the 1960s, and as more and more women are becoming sexually active younger and choosing to start a family later, a woman can end up on the contraceptive pill for up to twenty years. But what many women don't realise is that this convenience in a pill is decimating the good bacteria within our guts - increasing the risk of developing serious health problems. A study of 230,000 American women by Harvard gastroenterologist Dr Hamed Khalili, found women who had been on the Pill for five or more years, were three times more likely to develop Crohn's disease than their hormone-free counterparts. Dr Hamed Khalili also noted in his findings that oestrogen is known to increase the permeability of the gut wall.

Tip: If you need to take a course of antibiotics, or choose to use the oral contraceptive pill, it's essential to replenish your colonies of good gut flora by taking a probiotic for at least two to three months in the case of antibiotics, or ongoing if you are taking the Pill, as well as include naturally fermented foods in your diet each day. See page 160 for recipes.

SIGNS YOU MAY HAVE A FOOD INTOLERANCE OR SENSITIVITY

- Excess bloating, gas, frequent belching, abdominal pain, cramping or heartburn after eating

- Fatigue or lethargy after meals

- Chronic constipation or diarrhoea

- Chronic headaches or migraines

- Regular joint or muscular pain

- Catarrh, nasal congestion or mucous after meals

- Depression, anxiety or mood swings or temper tantrums in children

- Brain fog or cognitive disturbances

- Problems with sleep

Although there can be many causes behind these symptoms, if you regularly suffer from any of them there is a strong chance food intolerances are contributing. I recommend you remove all forms of gluten and cow's dairy from your diet and cut right back on your sugar intake, especially fructose, because these foods have proven to be the biggest offenders when it comes to causing food sensitivities. If you are suffering a neurological, or autoimmune disease I suggest you omit all grains and legumes from your diet, except those mentioned in the LYG recipe section.

FOOD INTOLERANCES AND ALLERGIES

The questions we need to ask ourselves are: why are so many of us suffering from allergies and food sensitivities nowadays, and why is there a dramatic rise in childhood asthma and anaphylactic reactions to certain foods, like nuts and bee stings.

I believe the answer lies in our gut, and the abnormalities that are occurring within our gut flora from our diet and exposure to excess chemicals and medications like antibiotics - creating imbalances in our immune responses. Food sensitivities and allergies are an example of an inflammatory immune response, causing us to become hypersensitive to compounds in various foods and/or pollutants and pollens in the environment.

Food sensitivities also inhibit our digestive function, and when your body can't digest food effectively, it accumulates within your stomach, which can result in acid reflux, gas, bloating, or constipation. These symptoms can be your body's way of telling you it's reacting to compounds like gluten within your food. The inflammation caused by food sensitivities and allergies can manifest over time as other conditions that stem from chronic inflammation, including high cholesterol and blood pressure, depression or arthritis.

I find many people believe they don't suffer from any food sensitivities or intolerances, because they only identify such problems with symptoms typical of a food allergy - such as hives, swelling of the tongue, or a severe gut ache or cramping - that manifests shortly after eating the offending food. But in truth only about four to six percent of children and four percent of adults, are affected by food allergies, according to the Australian Centre for Disease Control and Prevention. Food intolerances, on the other hand, can affect a much greater percentage of the population and are more difficult to pin point, because their associated symptoms can take hours, days, even weeks to fully manifest. The other difference between an allergy and a food sensitivity or intolerance lies in the way the symptoms are expressed. Food intolerances can present in the form of anything from fatigue to depression, through to gut pain, reflux, bloating or diarrhoea, even anxiety, brain fog, acne or weight gain. I've seen many of these symptoms alleviated in patients when we eliminate the foods they are sensitive to.

TRACKING YOUR FOOD INTOLERANCE

There are various pathology tests available to assess food sensitivities, however

I find these can often be inaccurate, not to mention expensive, so in my experience the most effective way to diagnose and treat food sensitivities is to listen to your gut!

By eliminating certain foods from your diet for at least four to six weeks, such as those listed in the 8 foods to avoid on page 70 you'll be able to monitor how your body responds physically, not to mention mentally. You'll also enhance your results by combining the LYG eating program with the supplements in the gut repair and detox pack (available from my website). These will help to heal your gut wall and replenish your gut flora colonies more effectively – helping to regulate your immune responses. I also recommend keeping a detailed food and symptom diary to record exactly what you're eating for a period, and track your responses, as this will help you to pinpoint any additional foods you may be sensitive to.

I also test my patients for nutrient deficiencies that can result from leaky gut syndrome, including B12 and folate, zinc, iron studies, red blood cell magnesium and iodine. Optimal vitamin D levels are also essential for healthy immune responses. I recommend finding a sympathetic health care practitioner - preferably one who practices nutritional or functional medicine, and ask for a pathology referral to assess these nutrients, as deficiencies in them can greatly impact on your body's ability to function at its best.

GUT PATHOGENS & PARASITES

If there's one pathogen that can wreak havoc on your health like no other, it's intestinal parasites. The problem with parasites is they can go undetected for years, and they can mimic the symptoms of other illnesses. I have seen many patients present with symptoms from severe IBS, through to unexplained weight gain skin rashes, and chronic fatigue, only for the turning point in their health to be traced back to a bad bout of travellers' diarrhoea, or food poisoning, years prior.

But it's not just travellers' diarrhoea that can lead to parasitic infection, parasites can be contracted simply by eating everyday foods that have become contaminated, and children and animals are great little incubators for parasites and their eggs. Parasitic infection can also be passed on simply through not washing your hands before handling food, or after going to the toilet.

But there's no need to go getting all OCD about cleanliness on me, because not all parasites are infectious or harmful to your body, and if you maintain a healthy balance of good gut flora, you will improve your immune systems defences against them. The more infectious parasites definitely need to be eliminated.

HOW TO TEST FOR PARASITIC INFECTION

Parasitic infection can be diagnosed through a stool test, using a reputable lab. Not all labs test for all species of parasites, so if you return a negative result and your symptoms persist, despite following my LYG program, you may want to visit a Clinical Nutritionist, Naturopath, or a functional medicine doctor for further testing. They can order a CDSA (comprehensive digestive stool analysis) through labs such as Great Plains Laboratories in the US, or Genova Diagnostics who have international distributors, including Nutripath labs in Australia. These testing facilities specialise in gut health-related pathology testing, using a sample of your stool, to analyze for a broad range of parasites and overgrowth of other pathogens like bad bacteria and Candida Albicans.

- Acid reflux

- Heartburn

- Abdominal pain on an
empty stomach

- Loss of appetite

- Bloating

- Burping

- Nausea

- Vomiting (vomit may be
bloody or appear like coffee
grounds)

- Black, tarry stools

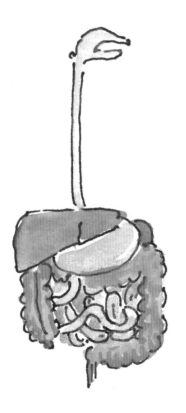

Be warned, these tests can be expensive, unless you can claim under Medicare or insurance, so alternatively you may want to try a month or two on broad spectrum anti-parasite herbs, such as those contained in my gut repair and detox pack, or those mentioned on page 62. When taken for a minimum of four weeks, these herbs will be effective in killing the eggs, as well as the live parasites, to prevent you getting re-infected.

I always recommend taking a herbal anti-parasite complex when travelling to any third world countries, as this will save you a lot of pain and problems down the track. Just be sure to replenish your good gut flora colonies with a quality probiotic for at least two months afterwards, and include some naturally fermented foods in your diet each day.

PATHOGENIC OR OPPORTUNISTIC BACTERIA

Your gut doesn't play host just to beneficial bacteria, but also to opportunistic or pathogenic bacteria – hundreds of species that we know of to date, and like other pathogens, they too can easily disrupt the balance of your good gut flora and overall gut function.

H-PYLORI

H-Pylori or Helicobacter pylori, is one such bacteria that can inhabit your gut — in fact, more than 50 percent of the world's population is believed to harbour an infection, making it the most common chronic bacterial pathogen in humans. But, amazingly, over 80 percent of individuals infected with H-Pylori display no symptoms. An overgrowth of H Pylori can be responsible for ulcers in the stomach and small intestine and a condition known as Gastro Esophageal Reflux Disease (GERD). H-pylori infection also increases your risk of developing stomach cancer by forty times, and could play a significant role in the development of Parkinson's disease. Symptoms can include bad breath, reflux, nausea, vomiting, lack of appetite, bloating and excessive belching, although many H-pylori infections can exhibit no symptoms at all. H-pylori infection can be passed on simply by kissing someone who is infected, by consuming under- cooked foods like chicken, or by ingesting excessive fructose or wheat.

HOW TO TEST FOR H-PYLORI INFECTION

Consult with your doctor who can refer you for either a stool or breath test. These are more effective at detecting active H. pylori infections than a blood test.

HOW TO TREAT H-PYLORI INFECTION

As always, prevention is the best approach. Include natural foods in your diet: fermented vegetables and/or homemade kefir, fresh extra virgin olive oil, green tea, broccoli and broccoli sprouts, unsweetened cranberry juice and turmeric to inhibit the growth of H. pylori infections. In severe cases it may be necessary to take specific antibiotics, referred to as 'triple therapy', prescribed by your doctor, but these should always be followed up with a powerful probiotic and gut repair program. An effective natural alternative to antibiotics for treating H-pylori infection may be sulforaphane, a compound contained in cruciferous vegetables, such as broccoli and broccoli sprouts, combined with oregano oil or grape seed extract.

SMALL INTESTINAL BACTERIAL OVERGROWTH (SIBO)

As its name suggests, this condition is defined by the overgrowth of bacteria within the small intestine. It is thought that SIBO has strong links with IBS, causing chronic diarrhea and malabsorption, as well as unintentional weight loss, nutritional deficiencies, and osteoporosis.

It is commonly triggered by the overuse of antibiotics and antacids, which can cause diminished gastric acid secretion, and other medications that damage your good gut flora.

SIBO tends not to be recognised by the conventional medical fraternity, meaning often people fail to get tested or properly diagnosed. Instead, many cases of chronic digestive problems such as gas, bloating, diarrhoea, and/or constipation are misdiagnosed as IBS when the underlying problem can actually be small intestine bacterial overgrowth.

SIBO can also present with non-digestive symptoms such as fatigue. It can be present in cases of chronic illness such as chronic fatigue syndrome, fibromyalgia, allergies, arthritis, autoimmune diseases, diabetes, just to name a few.

WHAT CAUSES SIBO

Excess intake of sugar or alcohol

Chronic stress

Diabetes

Hypothyroidism

Insufficient stomach acid production — a condition referred to as Hypochlorhydria, caused by long term antacid use and old age

Scar tissue in the small intestine from gastric bypass surgery; Crohn's disease or diverticulitis

Immune deficiency

Medications such as steroids, antibiotics, antacids and the contraceptive pill

Lack of dietary fibre

SIGNS YOU MAY HAVE SIBO

- Reflux / heartburn
- Abdominal cramping, pain or distension,
- Gas and bloating after meals, which is worse after eating carbs, fibre and sugar
- Diarrhoea or constipation
- Mucus in your stools
- Soft, foul-smelling stools that stick to the bowl
- Chronic illness
- Poor fat metabolism
- Fatigue
- Rosacea
- Anemia caused by vitamin B12 malabsorption
- Depression
- Nutritional deficiencies despite taking supplements
- Weight loss

HOW TO TEST FOR SIBO

I recommend getting a CDSA - comprehensive digestive stool analysis-through Genova Diagnostics in the US, or Nutripath in Australia, as this is more accurate than a hydrogen breath test.

HOW TO TREAT SIBO

If you identify with many of the symptoms associated with SIBO, start by following the LYG eating program, which eliminates high sugar/ fructose foods and assess your response after four to six weeks, before undergoing a CDSA. I also recommend combining the LYG eating program with my gut repair and detox pack, as this will work to rebalance your gut flora colonies and repair your gut.

VIRUSES

Viruses are the ultimate opportunists, striking when your immune defences are down, leaving you vulnerable to infection. Before I developed CFS and Lupus, I contracted two viral infections, EBV or Glandular fever, and CMV or Cyto Megalo virus. This double whammy was likely because my immune system was so run down from over training with my running and gym workouts, along with excess stress in my job. The problem with viruses is they can remain dormant in your body for many years and have a lingering impact on your liver function. Compromised liver function can result in the accumulation of excess toxins in your body and inadequate fat digestion, as well as hyper-sensitivity to a range of foods and environmental chemicals.

HOW TO TEST FOR VIRAL INFECTION

Consult your GP for a referral for relevant and thorough pathology tests, including EBV, CMV, HPV6, Ross River, Entero virus and Coxiella Brunetti virus.

HOW TO TREAT VIRUSES

Your best attack against a viral infection is your own immune defence, but if it has been compromised from an infection, you'll need a bit of extra help. Diet will obviously play a major role in this process, making the LYG program perfect for boosting your immune defences! I also recommend consulting with an experienced Nutritionist, Naturopath or functional medicine doctor, as they will be able to prescribe appropriate herbal complexes to help boost your immune defences to overcome the viral infection and replenish any specific nutrient deficiencies, like B vitamins and C. Rest is absolutely essential when you are suffering an

SIGNS YOU MAY HAVE A VIRAL INFECTION

- CFS or chronic fatigue
- Regular fevers
- Aching muscles and joints
- Fibromyalgia
- Autoimmune disease

acute viral infection. Don't make the mistake that I did and try to return to work, study or exercise too soon, or you will put your body at high risk of developing post viral syndrome or CFS - Chronic Fatigue Syndrome, like I did.

CANDIDA ALBICANS

Candida is a naturally occurring yeast or fungus living within your gut, unlike other pathogens that you contract externally, like parasites. Although Candida is a normal part of your gut's ecosystem, issues arise when this fungus starts to overgrow - a little like weeds in your garden taking over from the plants and flowers. It is believed that over eighty percent of us are affected by an overgrowth of this yeast, causing a wide range of, and often very debilitating symptoms, caused by the resulting inflammation and disruption to your good gut flora.

CAUSES OF CANDIDA OVERGROWTH

Candida mainly feeds off sugar, so it's little surprise that so many of us are suffering from an overgrowth, considering how much sugar is consumed as part of the modern Western diet. Many of the foods we commonly eat, like sugar, wheat and other grains, cow's dairy and processed foods, are making our system overly acidic, and Candida thrives in an overly acidic environment.

Candida overgrowth can also result from poor digestion, causing the accumulation of undigested food in the small intestine. Over time the undigested food particles begin to ferment, or rot within our gut, attracting the overgrowth of Candida.

Excess use of antibiotics, the oral contraceptive pill and antacid medications can also cause an overgrowth of Candida. It is essential to keep Candida in check to prevent it from crowding out your colonies of good bacteria and contributing to leaky gut and depleting essential nutrients and trace minerals.

HOW TO TEST FOR CANDIDA

There are several tests to assess for Candida overgrowth. I recommend the following: Anti-Candida Antibody blood test - this is your best first port of call; Comprehensive digestive stool analysis - CDSA if you want to combine testing for other pathogens and overall digestive function; Urinary organic acids test. I recommend Genova Diagnostics, or Great Plains for both Australia and the US.

SIGNS YOU MAY HAVE A CANDIDA INFECTION

- Chronic fatigue
- Bad breath
- Dandruff
- White coating on tongue
- Sugar cravings
- Joint pain
- Excess gas & bloating
- compromised immune defences
- Brain fog, depression, anxiety
- Acne / skin rashes
- Urinary tract infections
- Low libido
- Thrush
- Headaches
- Cradle cap in babies
- Jock itch
- ADHD/Austism
- Autoimmune disease

HOW TO TREAT CANDIDA

To bring Candida overgrowth under control it is important to eliminate the food sources that feed it, such as sugar, yeast and high starch carbohydrates. Otherwise your good gut flora will struggle to re-establish. But diet alone is typically not enough to effectively bring Candida under control, so I recommend combining the LYG eating program with specific herbal botanicals that target Candida. Look out for formulas that also contain herbs such as pau' d' arco, cats claw and uva ursi, or lauric acid, as these have an antifungal action. In some chronic cases of Candida, it may be necessary to take prescription antifungal medications such as Nilstat, however these should only be taken for a short period of time, or you risk eliminating friendly yeast organisms from within your gut, which are necessary for controlling Candida overgrowth. It is essential to follow up any herbal or prescription strength antifungal medication with a pre and probiotic formula, such as the one in my gut repair and detox pack, to re-establish your colonies of good gut flora.

FRUCTOSE MALABSORPTION

Fructose malabsorption is a disorder in which sufferers are unable to absorb fructose - the naturally occurring sugar in various foods, including fruits and vegetables. Fructose malabsorption results in symptoms associated with IBS, specifically bloating, flatulence, diarrhoea, reflux, nausea, vomiting, gut pain and cramping. Fructose malabsorption can cause deficiencies in certain nutrients, like tryptophan (a precursor to the production of the happy hormone, serotonin), zinc and folate.

If you find you are following the LYG Program and not experiencing total relief from IBS symptoms then you may suffer from this condition and should undergo further testing before adopting a low FODMAP's diet. See page 100 for a list of high FODMAP's foods to avoid.

HOW TO TEST FOR FRUCTOSE MALABSORPTION

Diagnosis can be made through a hydrogen/methane breath test. You can obtain this either through your doctor or visit www.hydrogenbreathtesting.com in the US or www.gastrolab.com.au in Australia.

TREATMENT FOR FRUCTOSE MALABSORPTION

If you test positive to fructose malabsorption, consult with a health practitioner qualified in counseling on a low FODMAP's (Fermentable Oligo-, Di- and Mono-saccharides, and Polyols) diet. As a reference I have included a list of the high FODMAP's foods to avoid on page 100. However, please be aware that not all of all my recipes are low FODMAP's because it would be too restrictive for those who do not suffer fructose malabsorption or severe IBS. But take heart, as the majority of my recipes can be easily adapted to be low FODMAP's if they are not already.

LIFESTYLE FACTORS

TOXICITY

In today's world we are surrounded by toxins, but thankfully our bodies come with their own inbuilt detox mechanism – primarily the liver, skin, lymphatic system, kidneys and bowel. But the problem nowadays is the excessive levels of toxins we are exposed to - far more than our body is designed to handle. This toxic overload overburdens the body's natural detox systems, leading to the excess accumulation of toxins within the body. Chemical pesticides and herbicides, smog and exhaust fumes, artificial additives and sweeteners, alcohol, caffeine, cigarettes and drugs, chemical based skin care and cleaning products are just some examples of common toxins we're regularly exposed to. Impaired liver and bowel function and poor digestion will also contribute to a buildup of toxins within the body.

DRINKING WATER WITH MEALS

Drinking too many fluids like water when you eat, can dilute essential pancreatic enzymes and hydrochloric acid levels in your stomach. Believe it or not, your stomach actually needs to be acidic when you eat to ensure you can digest your food effectively – in particular protein, the most difficult nutrient of all to digest. But too many of us have made a habit of drinking water (especially iced water), fruit juice or soft drink with our meals, and this is one of the major contributing factors to poor food digestion. Many patients report to me that they are thirsty when they eat, and this is often a sign of dehydration, and/or their meal is too high in processed salt. I recommend avoiding drinking liquids like water, 20 minutes either side of meals. If you do need to quench your thirst during a meal, stick to a few small sips of room temperature water, preferably with a few drops of bitters - as this will help to stimulate your digestion. You may have noticed that many Asian cultures will serve warm green tea after a meal, and this is because cold or iced beverages actually reduce blood flow to the gut, which depletes the production of digestive enzymes.

CHEWING TOO QUICKLY OR EATING ON THE RUN

Digestion begins in your mouth and chewing your food is an extremely important part of the digestive process, making it easier for your gut to absorb essential nutrients from food. So if you want to achieve healthy digestion and learn to eat less, then you need to start with chewing your food for longer and eating more slowly.

Too many of us are what I describe as 'unconscious eaters', meaning we are focused on everything and anything but our food at meal times, and have forgotten the art of eating slowly. Consider how people from traditional European cultures, like the French, Greek and Italians eat their food — they view meal times as an important part of their day, taking time out to enjoy a meal with friends and family, surrounded by plenty of love and laughter. Many researchers believe this may be a major contributing factor to their longevity and quality of life, because of their lower caloric intake from a diet rich in healthy fats, clean and lean proteins, plenty of fresh vegetables, and a little fresh fruit. But countries like Australia, the US and UK often approach meal times as more of a chore or an inconvenience - often opting for fast food take out, and eating on the run. Too many of us also prefer the company of Facebook or TV, rather than engaging in quality conversation at meal times. We also chew far less now than we used to because we've replaced whole, nutrient-dense foods with refined processed junk that requires little chewing. A classic example is a fast food burger that is so soft you can swallow it after just one or two chews!

If this scenario sounds familiar, then I recommend turning off your mobile phone, the TV or computer and starting to retrain yourself to chew your food more slowly by being present when you eat. Placing your knife and fork down in between each mouthful will also help you to eat more slowly and then your body will be able to extract all the nutrients and process them for maximum absorption.

OVEREATING OR EATING TOO LATE AT NIGHT

Eating too quickly will cause you to overeat, because the hormones that signal to your brain when you're satiated or full don't have enough time to kick in. Other factors such as leaving too long between meals, or skipping meals can also contribute to overeating, causing your blood sugar levels to drop too low, triggering cravings for sugar or starchy carbohydrates. It typically takes your brain twenty minutes to register that you are full, so before you load your plate with a second helping, sit back and enjoy the moment after your meal and I guarantee you will not want the second helping. Allowing three hours or more between eating and retiring to bed will also help you to lose weight and take the stress off your digestion. I've seen many folks drop several kilos simply by making dinner their smallest meal and/or eating before six pm.

EMOTIONAL STRESS

Chronic stress can have a major effect not just on your neurological health, but also on your gut health and overall digestion, because your gut is directly connected to your brain via the vagus nerve. Eating when stressed, such as eating on the run or emotional eating, can also impair your stomach's production of hydrochloric acid, which, as I've mentioned, affects the body's ability to optimally digest food and can even cause diarrhoea and reflux.

Chronic stress is a very common problem, triggering the overproduction of stress hormones - adrenalin and cortisol. Eventually this scenario can lead to your adrenal glands becoming chronically stressed or 'exhausted', resulting in compromised digestive and immune activity, and thyroid disorders. This can lead to conditions like CFS and adrenal fatigue syndrome.

BIRTHING AND FEEDING

Believe it or not, many people's gut problems start from childbirth as a result of compromised gut flora colonization. One of the most common causes of this occurs when a child is born via a caesarian birth, or is not breastfed at all, or for an insufficient period of time. When we are inside our mother's womb, our gut is actually sterile. The first implantation of good bacteria takes place during birth as we pass through our mother's vaginal canal - the bacteria adhere to our skin and we get an influx up our nose! These good bacteria continue to grow and proliferate when we are breastfed. So the health of our mother's gut flora colonies during pregnancy, how we are born, and if and for how long we are breastfed will directly determine the health of our gut flora colonies. Babies born via caesarian birth or those reared on formula can have compromised good gut flora colonies, which not only has a direct impact on optimal digestion and their immune health, both early and later in life, but also on their propensity for developing obesity.

Gastro infection at a young age or exposure to antibiotics as a baby can also have a profound effect on a child's gut and overall health, in some instances for life.

If you're a mother-to-be, it's even more essential to optimise your gut flora colonies, as this will largely determine your child's health. The period when we are breastfed is critical for shaping and determining our natural immune defences. If you are pregnant and unable to give birth naturally, or you cannot breastfeed for at least six months, I cannot stress enough the importance of building your child's microbiome through supplementing daily with the recommended fermented foods in this book and/or a baby probiotic formula. This will not only help to give their immune and digestive health the start in life needed to develop into healthy adults, but also dramatically reduce their risk of developing many chronic illnesses and diseases, both in childhood and later in life.

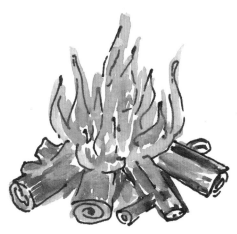

Inflammation –
The fire that burns within

If I were to give you one word to sum up the underlying cause of the majority of health problems and chronic disease states we see today, it would be 'inflammation'. Hundreds of scientific studies now reveal links between chronic inflammation within the gut and the development of the major lifestyle diseases – including obesity, heart disease, cancer, Alzheimer's, diabetes and autoimmune illnesses.

Most of us associate the word 'inflammation' with pain caused by arthritis, or a sprained ankle, or pain from a back injury, but in fact inflammation is a major driving force behind hundreds of common conditions like seasonal allergies, food intolerances, depression, high blood pressure and cholesterol and of course - the dreaded IBS.

In saying that, not all inflammation is bad, such as acute inflammation in response to an injury or infection, but it is the low grade, chronic inflammation that promotes the development of many illnesses and diseases that is highly damaging. Chronic inflammation behaves a little like a fire. At first it starts as a small smouldering camp fire. However, should conditions prevail that are conducive to that fire getting out of control, those once small flames can build into bigger and bigger flames, eventually spreading far and wide and developing into a raging bush fire, devastating everything in its path. This analogy is somewhat reflective of the inflammation that initially starts within the gut and eventually becomes systemic - spreading throughout the body, to other organs and systems.

HOW DIET AND STRESS CAN CAUSE INFLAMMATION

A diet high in acidic foods, such as sugar, gluten, alcohol, artificial additives, coffee and too much red meat are some of the major drivers of chronic inflammation within the gut. This is why it is essential to consider the powerful effects your food choices have towards combating and preventing inflammation, versus triggering it.

Chronic stress has become the twenty-first-century epidemic,

CONDITIONS CAUSED BY CHRONIC INFLAMMATION

- Obesity
- IBS
- Reflux heart burn / GERD
- Allergies and food intolerances
- Sinus and hay fever
- Asthma
- Acne
- PMS – pre menstrual syndrome
- Endometriosis and PCOS
- Type 1 & 2 diabetes
- Heart disease
- Hypertension and elevated cholesterol
- Cancer
- Depression and anxiety
- Alzheimer's and Parkinson's disease
- ADHD and Autism
- Autoimmune disease
- Osteoarthritis

wreaking havoc on the mind and body, but ironically, many of us are so stressed that we are often oblivious to the fact that we are, and the effect it is having on our lives and subsequent health - until something starts to go seriously wrong. Stress can be defined as anything that triggers an increase in your stress response hormones, cortisol and adrenalin, and it is also a major driver of inflammation.

A 2012 study from the Carnegie Mellon University. "How stress influences disease," revealed how chronic psychological stress causes the body to lose its ability to regulate inflammatory responses. These findings suggest that chronic emotional or mental stress can increase your inherent genetic predisposition to disease. Prolonged stress alters the effectiveness of your stress hormone, cortisol, to regulate inflammatory responses, so, put simply, the more stress you are exposed to, the greater the degree of inflammation within your body.

INFLAMMATION AFFECTS THE RATE OF AGING INSIDE & OUT

If you want to slow the rate you age, both on the inside and the outside, then controlling inflammation within your gut really is the secret to the fountain of youth. If you have been trying to preserve the way you look and obtain that ageless glow by slopping on expensive creams and potions and getting lasered and tasered, then I'm sorry to say, but probably the only thing you're really achieving is burning a hole in your pocket. Addressing your diet, getting plenty of restful sleep each night, reducing inflammation and your exposure to stress and maintaining your gut health - are the most effective means for slowing the aging process.

CONTROL PAIN

The same approach applies for effective pain control. The obvious remedy to ease pain is to pop a pharmaceutical anti-inflammatory or painkiller, but in fact these medications, if taken on a regular basis, can perpetuate the problem, due to the damage they cause to the lining of the gut and good bacteria colonies within. This is precisely the reason I resisted taking the anti-inflammatory steroid medications I was prescribed when I developed Lupus. As soon as I read that the associated side effects included 'gastrointestinal upset', I knew this was not the way to tackle my health problems.

No matter the cause of your pain, whether it's the dreaded monthly period cramps, headaches, arthritic or back ache caused by physical injury, you need to tackle it on a biochemical level through diet and maintaining your gut health, because these have a direct influence on the way physical pain and inflammation not only manifest, but express down the track.

CONTROLLING INFLAMMATION FOR DISEASE PREVENTION

Controlling chronic inflammation won't just slow the rate you age on the outside, but also on the inside, by preventing disease. Say you suffer from hypertension or elevated cholesterol, or even if you have a genetic predisposition to these conditions, then controlling inflammation within your gut is the key to treating the underlying cause of these conditions. Taking a statin or antihypertensive medication is not targeting the problem at the source and may only provide symptom relief at best.

AUTOIMMUNE DISEASES

Autoimmune diseases are increasing at an alarming rate, along with neurological conditions such as depression, anxiety, ADHD, Autism, Alzheimer's and Parkinson's. The common dominator with all of these conditions is again - inflammation that starts within the gut. Maintaining a healthy pH within your body by eating more alkaline foods, such as those I recommend on the LYG program, will have a powerful influence in preventing all illness and diseases.

The gut-brain connection

I'm sure you've heard the term 'gut instinct', an expression used to describe that feeling you get in your 'gut' when you have a sense of knowing about something or someone? Well far from being your imagination, there's actually something in these instincts, because your gut also functions as your 'second brain'. Your brain and gut are directly connected through the vagus nerve, which runs between your brain stem and your abdomen. The trillions of bacteria living within your gut not only influence how your gut and immune system function, but they have a direct impact on the way your brain functions as well.

The 'brain' embedded in the wall of your gut is referred to as your enteric nervous system (ENS), and works independently of, and in conjunction with, the brain in your head. Your gut and your brain are actually created out of the same type of tissue, so it's hardly surprising that their function is so intertwined.

To put it simply, the 'gut-brain connection' translates to 'happy gut, happy brain'! According to the Black Dog Institute, (an organization specialising in research and treatment of mood disorders) one in five Australians are affected by mental illness each year, as are 50 percent of us at some point in our life. Most alarming of all, depression is now the leading cause of disability worldwide.

But it's not only conditions like depression and anxiety that are on the rise, we've also seen a dramatic worldwide increase in childhood neurodevelopmental disorders such as ADHD and autism, as well as neurodegenerative diseases like dementia and Alzheimer's increasing at an alarming rate. According to leading American Neurologist, Dr David Perlmutter, Alzheimer's is now the third leading cause of death in the US, affecting some 5.4 million Americans, and this statistic is expected to double in the next 15 years.

So as you can see, illnesses of the brain are an increasing problem. The question is why? Obviously there are many factors that can contribute to neurological disorders, but consider for a second that over 90 percent of your serotonin receptors reside in your gut, specifically your bowel, and the trillions of bacteria within your gut are actually responsible for manufacturing neurochemicals like serotonin and dopamine. This goes a long way to explaining why your gut flora has the ability to significantly influence the way your brain and mind function. Serotonin is your happy hormone and it influences everything from your mood and behaviour, to your sleep and appetite. A deficiency in serotonin can contribute to depression, anxiety, mood swings, sugar cravings and sleep disturbances.

So if the majority of your serotonin receptors reside in your gut and your gut bacteria produce these 'happy' hormones, then maintaining a healthy balance of good bacteria, along with the integrity of your gut wall, should be a 'no brainer' - if you want to optimize your neurological health.

In addition, external stressors can also influence your gut and digestive function. Have you ever been so stressed that you've experienced diarrhoea, or had butterflies in your tummy caused by nerves before giving a speech or presentation?

So the take-home message is that if your gut health is suffering, and inflammation is running rampant, then your brain function will also be compromised — whether it's your mood or motivation, or ability to learn and concentrate, the hormones in your brain can go haywire when your gut is not healthy. In this instance your brain function can make it difficult to focus and process information in a clear and concise manner. I experienced this for a period as a child and was consequently diagnosed with ADD (Attention Deficit Disorder), but it turned out the cause of my 'unfocused behavior' was inflammation within my brain, caused by the effect multiple food intolerances were having on my gut health. Luckily for me, my mother had the insight to remove the offending foods from my diet and give me plenty of probiotics in order to heal my gut. This was effective in switching off the systemic inflammation and the impact it was having on my cognitive behavior.

SOME STORIES TO LEARN FROM

Our food choices, and the state of our gut function, have the power to cause absolute devastation to our health and our lives. Through my practice, I have been fortunate enough to witness some incredible stories of recovery – simply through replenishing underlying nutrient deficiencies, restoring optimal gut function and following the LYG eating program. Many of these success stories include significant improvement in debilitating neurological conditions, including ADHD, MS, Parkinson's, depression and anxiety.

One such example was a patient who came to me with advanced Parkinson's. Her neurologist had all but given up on ways to assist her further, after she had begun to react to the pharmaceutical medications prescribed to treat her Parkinson's. This woman, who was in her sixties, was often reliant on a walking frame to get around. Her tremors had become progressively worse and she was no longer able to do many of the things she enjoyed including cross-stitch, which required fine motor skills. When 'Mary' consulted me, I naturally enquired about her diet, which turned out to consist of 7-11 cups of black coffee a day, virtually no water, and white bread and cheese sandwiches, capped off with a few mints. But it wasn't just her diet that nearly saw me fall off my chair, but the fact that when I asked if she had 'normal' bowel movements, she replied 'Yes.' I decided to rephrase the question and asked, 'Mary, how often do you have a bowel motion?' to which she replied, 'Every 10 days to 2 weeks.' I was shocked, not just because her doctor had failed to ask this most basic of questions, but because she thought this was 'normal' bowel function! 'Sweet Jesus Mary,' I said, 'your body is literally poisoning itself from all the toxic waste you are storing up inside!' It was little wonder that she was unable to tolerate the medications prescribed for the Parkinson's, let alone the fact that she had developed Parkinson's. Now this may sound like an extreme case, but once we were able to get Mary's bowel moving every day through healing her gut and overhauling her diet, she no longer had to rely on her walking frame and her tremors reduced to the point that she was able to return to cross-stitch — largely because she started to poo every day and we healed her gut!

People with chronic gastrointestinal problems also have a higher risk of developing mood imbalances and psychological disorders, including anxiety and depression. Although there are many factors that can contribute to mental illness, based on my clinical experience and research, I am convinced of the major role gut health plays in the expression of neurological disorders.

WHAT CAUSES INFLAMMATION IN THE BRAIN?

As you've just read in the case of Mary, diet and digestive function played a significant role in her condition, which had roots stemming from chronic inflammation within the gut. You'll recall I explained how your gut wall can become 'leaky', a condition known as leaky gut, well, the same can occur with your brain! Just as your gut is protected by the mucous membrane that surrounds it, the brain also has a protective barrier or layer, known as the blood brain barrier. This acts like a filter - retaining the nutrients that need to be absorbed for use by

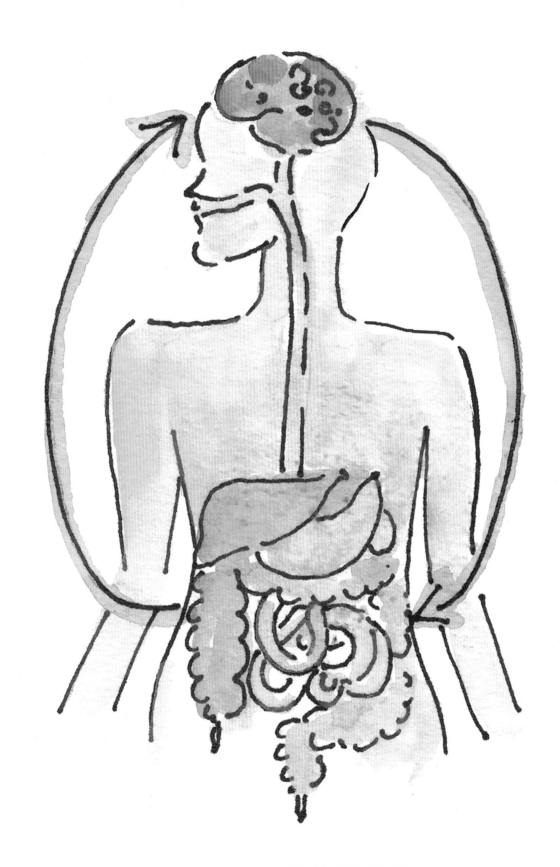

THE GUT-BRAIN CONNECTION

UNDERLYING CAUSES OF CHRONIC BRAIN INFLAMMATION

- Chronic stress

- Food intolerances / Gluten sensitivity

- Chronic insomnia or sleep deprivation

- Blood sugar imbalances

- Excess exposure to chemicals

- Autoimmune conditions

- Hormonal imbalances

- Elevated homocysteine levels

- History of head or neck injuries

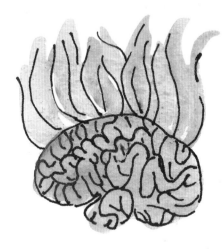

the brain, whilst protecting it from neuro toxins and other substances that can damage it. The protein involved in leaky gut, zonulin, can also open up the blood-brain barrier, causing a 'leaky brain'. The resulting inflammation between the gut and the brain is a complex feedback loop that can drive the development of a myriad of neurological conditions. This can range from simple brain fog and poor concentration, through to serious neurological disease states such as Alzheimer's and Dementia. Inflammation within the brain can also impact on its ability to communicate with your endocrine (hormonal) system, affecting the function of your thyroid and adrenal glands. The presence of opportunistic bacteria within the gut can also cause neurological and cognitive problems.

As with the gut, certain foods and chemicals can cause inflammation within the brain. Certain foods including gluten, sugar, and artificial additives, can have a neurotoxic affect on the brain, and damage the blood brain barrier. Gluten is one of the major offenders when it comes to causing inflammation in your brain. According to a 2012 study published in Psychiatric Quarterly, as many as 57 percent of people with neurological dysfunction of unknown origin, test positive to gluten antibodies and 22 percent of Coeliacs develop neurological or psychiatric disorders. Research has also revealed a connection between the incidence of autoimmune disease occurring in many cases of Coeliac disease and gluten sensitivity disorders.

One of the main reasons we have experienced such a rapid increase in the incidence of neurological conditions and mental illness since the Second World War, is because of the changes to our diet and gut flora. The modern Western diet is now largely based on the foods I recommend you avoid — sugar, gluten, cow's dairy, artificial additives, soy, corn, yeast, caffeine and alcohol. Considering these foods can have a negative impact on your gut function, it should come as no surprise to hear they can also have a negative effect on your brain function and neurological health.

Don't believe me? Well let's look at another case study from a patient I treated. 'Fred', as I'll refer to him, presented to me suffering severe panic attacks that at times led to convulsions. He also experienced constant depression and anxiety to the point that he sometimes could not walk into a crowded restaurant or drive in heavy traffic for fear of suffering a panic attack. Fred had consulted countless doctors and psychiatrists for his condition, yet the only treatments offered were prescription drugs

– five different medications at the time he came to see me, including anti-depressants, anti-anxiety meds, anti-psychotics, Nexium, and the amphetamine Adderall, which includes side effects of dizziness and nervousness (remember, this was a man that suffered severe anxiety and panic attacks!), weight loss, increased heart rate, low blood pressure and decreased libido. Basically Fred was on a daily chemical cocktail of uppers and downers that left him feeling unmotivated, fatigued, sleepless, irritable, and of course anxious. Fred was far from functional and struggled to go to work more than a few days a week and spent much of his day sleeping whilst lying awake much of the night. But perhaps the most alarming thing about Fred's case was the fact that none of his doctors had asked him about his digestive function or diet, and had instead continued to medicate him with more and more drugs when he failed to respond. In the end, many of Fred's symptoms became a product of his medication.

Fred was also constantly bloated and constipated, averaging two to three bowel movements a week, eating no more than two meals a day, thanks to the appetite-suppressant effects of the Adderall. Fred also enjoyed a healthy appetite for beer, drinking up to 24 cans a day and smoking up to a packet of cigarettes, whilst consuming a diet based mainly on processed foods laden with sugar, refined salt, soy and gluten. It was evident Fred wasn't just a functioning alcoholic, but also a gluten and sugar addict, and, in my view, he was a textbook case for subclinical or 'silent' Coeliac disease. But doctors had dismissed gluten as being an issue for him, thanks to a previous negative pathology result for coeliac disease.

Chronic inflammation caused by a severe gluten intolerance can decrease blood flow to the frontal lobe, or executive centre of the brain - the part responsible for our emotions, including empathy and compassion, focus and comprehension, sequencing, and even short term memory. Fred's neurological symptoms of severe anxiety and depression were clearly a product of what I refer to as an 'inflamed brain', triggered by inflammation from within the gut, which in his case was caused by multiple food intolerances – namely gluten - and severe dysbiosis.

When I first saw Fred I observed his teeth, as well as his tongue, fingernails and complexion. I noticed that Fred's teeth had no enamel, his nails were weak and brittle with white flecks, and his tongue had a thick white-to-yellow coating at the back, with red pinprick dots at the front and dental indentations or scalloping, along the sides. What did all

SIGNS YOU MAY HAVE AN INFLAMED BRAIN

- Depression
- Anxiety
- Brain fog
- Poor concentration
- Poor memory
- Mood swings
- Learning difficulties
- Cravings for sugar, caffeine, alcohol, or nicotine

NEUROLOGICAL CONDITIONS DIRECTLY RELATED TO INFLAMMATION IN THE BRAIN

- ADHD
- Autism
- Anxiety
- Alzheimer's
- Ataxia
- Bipolar
- Dementia
- Depression
- Multiple Sclerosis
- Schizophrenia
- Parkinson's

this tell me about Fred's health you ask? Well for one, Fred's guts were excessively 'damp' (a term used in TCM Traditional Chinese Medicine) and inflamed, thanks to the undigested food that was busily rotting or fermenting inside his gut, attracting an overgrowth of Candida and opportunistic bacteria - SIBO. He was also deficient in nutrients such as B vitamins and zinc, and wasn't digesting or absorbing his food properly - all of which was later confirmed with a CDSA. Despite Fred's poor appetite, he had managed to gain twenty kilos, largely due to the effect the pharmaceutical drugs were having on his thyroid and metabolic rate, in conjunction with the undiagnosed Coeliac disease that had severely damaged his gut lining and microbiome.

Fred's gut and brain were entwined in a state of total chaos, driven by the effects of his diet, alcohol and nicotine addiction, sleep deprivation, and capped off by the effects of the prescription medications. So I set about slowly unraveling the maze of biochemical chaos he had been enduring over the years by overhauling his diet using the LYG program, replenishing the major nutrient deficiencies, and most importantly, repairing his gut!

After six months of treatment, Fred was able to be weaned off all prescription medications, he started sleeping soundly for eight hours a night, regained his energy and lost over 15kg/33lb, and most importantly, he was able to move his bowels easily, twice a day, and return to full time work.

Like so many sufferers of depression and anxiety, Fred was told by his doctors that his condition was irreversible and a likely consequence of his 'inherent genetic profile', and there was nothing he could do beyond take prescription medications for the rest of his life. So if Fred's case is not an example of the devastating effect chronic gut problems and food intolerances can have on neurological function, then his recovery must be nothing short of a miracle.

I am not claiming that the sole cause of all psychological and neurological conditions originate solely from gut imbalances and poor diet, because certain conditions like Bipolar, Alzheimer's and Post Traumatic Stress Disorder have significant genetic and environmental links, and it may be necessary for sufferers to take certain pharmaceutical medications, combined with psychological therapy. But what I am saying is that the severity of these conditions can be significantly expressed through imbalances in your gut flora, a diet high in inflammatory foods and excess exposure to chemicals. So in the case of any neurological condition or illness, no matter how mild or severe, I would always advise incorporating dietary and nutritional therapy, including healing your gut, whilst minimising your exposure to chemicals in your environment.

Setting aside more extreme cases like Mary, and Fred, if you have children in your life then I'm sure you have witnessed the effects sugar can have on their behaviour – turning a calm, happy child into a raging, tantrum-throwing beast! In my view, no matter how mild or severe, we can no longer address neurological problems and diseases through pharmaceutical medicine alone, and as with any illness or disease, it is essential to combine other therapies with a dietary and nutritional approach in order to truly heal the brain.

FOODS THAT NOURISH YOUR BRAIN HEALTH

The microbes found in fermented foods and quality probiotic supplements, (such as Lactobacillus and Bifidobacteria species) may have a powerful and positive influence on your brain health. By including these in your diet every day, you will replenish and maintain your good gut flora colonies, and this will help to improve your brain function.

Just how happy
is your gut?

If you regularly experience any of the symptoms below then chances are your gut is not functioning as well as it should be. Whatever the reason – and it could be because of food intolerances, an imbalance in your good gut flora, medications, excess toxicity, stress, or poor digestion – if you answer yes to more than three of the questions below then you've got one unhappy gut! So go through the checklist below and get a gauge on just how happy your gut is.

Answer Yes or No to the following questions. If you feel it's a 'maybe' then it's more than likely a yes than a no..

1. Fatigue or lethargy	YES	NO
2. Cravings for sugar and starchy carbs	YES	NO
3. Gas, bloating, abdominal pain or discomfort/stomach aches	YES	NO
4. Diarrhoea or constipation	YES	NO
5. Sleep disturbances such as insomnia or broken sleep	YES	NO
6. Mood swings or irritability	YES	NO
7. Problems with concentration, memory and comprehension	YES	NO
8. Lack of motivation	YES	NO
9. Depression or anxiety	YES	NO
10. Frequent hunger or lack of satiety despite regular meals	YES	NO
11. Skin complaints, acne, rashes, rosacea eczema or psoriasis	YES	NO
12. Acid reflux/heart burn (GERD)	YES	NO
13. Joint pain	YES	NO
14. Headaches or migraines	YES	NO
15. Difficulty losing weight, despite regular exercise	YES	NO
16. Dandruff or thrush	YES	NO
17. Period pain	YES	NO

What does your poo say about you?

There's an old saying in life, and it goes something like this ... 'If you don't sh#@ you die' and as crude as that may sound, there's a lot of truth in it. The bowel is part of the gut, and it's where the majority of our gut flora reside. It's from the bowel that we eliminate the bulk of our body's waste material – aka poo – and absorb vital nutrients and water to feed our cells. We might not like to admit it, but we all need to do it!

If you're like most people the talk of poo may be a somewhat embarrassing or unsavoury topic of conversation, but the sooner you become familiar with your number twos, the sooner you will learn a lot about you! Well, at least about the inside of you, in particular your digestive health. Quite simply, understanding what your poo is saying about you will give you the power to know what you need to do to improve it, should everything not be moving along as it should.

People's bowel habits are another one of those things that I have paid very careful attention to during my years in private practice, and believe me, most folks do not move their bowels as often as they should, nor does the poo come out looking as it should. The problem with not moving your bowel as often as nature intended is that you become a walking nutrient-deficient, dehydrated, toxic waste dump ... because quite literally you are not 'emptying the garbage' as often as required.

Your poo is mainly comprised of food debris and bacteria. The bacteria in your poo helps to synthesise various vitamins, process waste products and food particles, and protect you against harmful bacteria. The way that your poo comes out, and the frequency, tells us a lot about your gut and overall health. So here is the A- Z of poo, to help you learn exactly what yours says about you!

THE A-Z OF POO

BLOOD IN POO OR BRIGHT RED POO

Blood in your poo can appear in the form of dark or fresh red blood, depending on which part of your digestive tract it has come from. Blood from the upper part of the digestive tract, such as the stomach, will look dark by the time it is eliminated in your poo. Blood that is fresh-looking and bright or dark red, is more likely to have come from the large intestine or rectum, perhaps caused by a tear or hemorrhoid, or because you have been straining too hard from constipation.

CAUSES OF BLOOD IN THE STOOL INCLUDE:

- Hemorrhoids
- Anal fissures
- Diverticulitis
- Colon cancer
- Ulcerative colitis and Crohn's disease.

Another word of warning: I've had many patients become alarmed by their stools being red – panicking that they had bowel cancer – but on further questioning it turns out they have eaten a meal containing beetroot, so be sure to consider this before you jump to conclusions! But if you do start to experience blood in your stool, fresh or dark in colour, be sure to consult your doctor immediately for further investigation.

CONSTIPATION

I've come across plenty of doctors who consider having a bowel movement every second day as perfectly healthy and 'normal', but in my opinion, that's a little like only taking out the garbage every other day, even though it needs taking out daily because its full. For optimal health and digestion, you should be moving your bowel at least one or two times a day, ideally three, including on or around waking.

Constipation or sluggish bowel movements can be caused by a number of factors, ranging from parasitic infection, dehydration and insufficient fibre intake, through to an underactive thyroid, poor digestion and, of course, an imbalance in your gut flora colonies. Constipation also creates a haven for pathogens to exist, thanks to the accumulation of poo within your bowel, which ends up polluting the environment in which your good bacteria live. So until you get your bowel moving at least once or twice a day, your other body systems and organs won't function optimally. A word of caution: I see a lot of people relying on laxatives to get their bowel moving, but these do nothing to address the underlying cause of the problem and can become psychologically and physically addictive. Laxatives can damage your excretion reflex, making you dependent on them for normal evacuation, as well as depleting the body of essential nutrients like potassium.

DARK OR BLACK POO

Really dark, or black poo with a thick consistency can be caused by bleeding in the upper digestive tract, or poor elimination, causing your poo to sit in the intestines for too long.

Duodenal, peptic or gastric ulcers, gastritis, oesophageal varices, and even alcoholism can also cause dark, tar-like poo.

Certain supplements and medications can also change the colour of your poo, including:
- Iron tablets
- Aspirin and NSAIDS (which can cause bleeding in the stomach)
- Bismuth subsalicylate
- Activated charcoal
- Dark foods like black licorice

If you experience dark black tar- like poo for a prolonged period of time, you should consult your doctor for further investigation.

DIARRHOEA (OR LOOSE POO)

This is commonly your body's way of telling you there is inflammation within your gut. Inflammation can be caused by a variety of factors, but most often it comes down to food intolerances, and or an imbalance in your gut flora colonies, or even an infection from an opportunistic bacteria, virus or parasite. Emotional stress can also cause loose or explosive bowel movements – a sure sign your gut is not happy Jan! Loose poo can also be linked

to chronic fatigue and weak digestion, brought on by stress and poor diet..
Typical foods that can contribute include:
- Gluten
- Fried or greasy foods
- Cow's dairy
- Coffee
- Raw fruits and vegetables – avoid these until your poo solidifies
- Cold drinks

FLOATING POO
Soft, floating stools that are difficult to flush can be a sign of undigested fat in your stool. Poor fat digestion can again be caused by insufficient bile production from poor liver and gall bladder function.

FOOD IN YOUR POO
This is a sign of poor digestion either from eating too quickly, or from a deficiency in pancreatic enzyme and hydrochloric acid production. There are some foods, like corn, that are normal to see in your poo because the body can't digest the outer hull.

GREEN POO
Green poo is an indication of the amount of bile in your stool. Bile is a yellow-green fluid produced by your liver to aid fat digestion. As bile pigments travel through your gastrointestinal tract, they are chemically altered by enzymes, causing the pigments to change in colour from green to brown. If your food travels through the large intestine too quickly, due to perhaps diarrhoea, the bile doesn't have time to break down completely. Green poo can also be an outcome of what you eat, for example certain green vegetables or spirulina.

MUCUS IN POO
Whitish mucus in your poo can be an indication of inflammation of your gut wall, caused by food intolerances or allergies, or bacterial overgrowth. It can also be present with constipation or diarrhoea.
Conditions commonly associated with mucus in the stool include:
- Ulcerative colitis
- Celiac disease
- Crohn's disease
- Ulcerative colitis
- Diverticulitis

PENCIL THIN POO
This can be caused by a physical obstruction in your bowel, such as rectal polyps, prostate enlargement, colon or prostate cancer. If you regularly experience pencil thin stools, consult your doctor for further investigation.

RABBIT PELLET POO

If your poo resembles something more like a rabbit would do - dry, small pellets - this can be an indication of stress, dehydration, poor circulation, a deficiency in dietary fibre, excess red meat intake, food intolerances, or excess sugar and alcohol intake causing a buildup of heat in the body.

SINKING POO

This can indicate a lack of fibre in your diet due to insufficient fruits and vegetables, or dehydration – drink more water!

SMELLY POO

Believe it or not, your poo shouldn't necessarily always smell, or not too badly anyway! A nasty smell coming from your poo typically indicates the degree of toxicity within your gut from undigested food, or even an infection from a pathogen, or poor fat digestion.

STICKY POO

Poo that sticks to the toilet bowl is generally an indication of poor fat digestion and/or excess toxins due to a lack of water and possibly fibre.

YELLOW OR PALE POO

Yellow poo is typically caused by an alteration in the amount of bile pigment and/or the amount and composition of the pancreatic enzymes that are being released into the colon. If your poo is persistently yellow, this might be related to liver or pancreatic problems and you should consult your doctor for further investigation.

Yellow stools can also indicate that the transit time of your food – the time it took to pass through your digestive tract – is too quick. Yellow-to-pale stools can also occur in sufferers of GERD. Antacids prescribed for symptoms of GERD can also turn your stools pale. Acute onset of yellow stools can also be a sign of a bacterial infection in your intestines.

SO WHAT DOES A HEALTHY POO LOOK LIKE?

'The perfect poo' as I like to refer to it, is medium brown in colour, is easily passed with no straining or discomfort, has the consistency of toothpaste, and is approximately four to eight inches long. Okay, so I don't expect you to get out the tape measure here, but your morning poo should typically be your largest and you should experience a sensation of 'complete emptying of the bowel' – you know, that feeling like there's nothing left inside your bowel you feel you want to get rid of. Your poo should also slide directly into the toilet bowl, as opposed to getting stuck on the sides, and there should be minimal stench or odor.

So now that we have had this rather gross, but fascinating conversation, you will be well equipped to understand what your poo says about you! No matter what the current colour, shape, or frequency of your stools, following the LYG program and combining it with the supplements in the gut repair and detox pack, will help to get your bowels on track as nature intended!

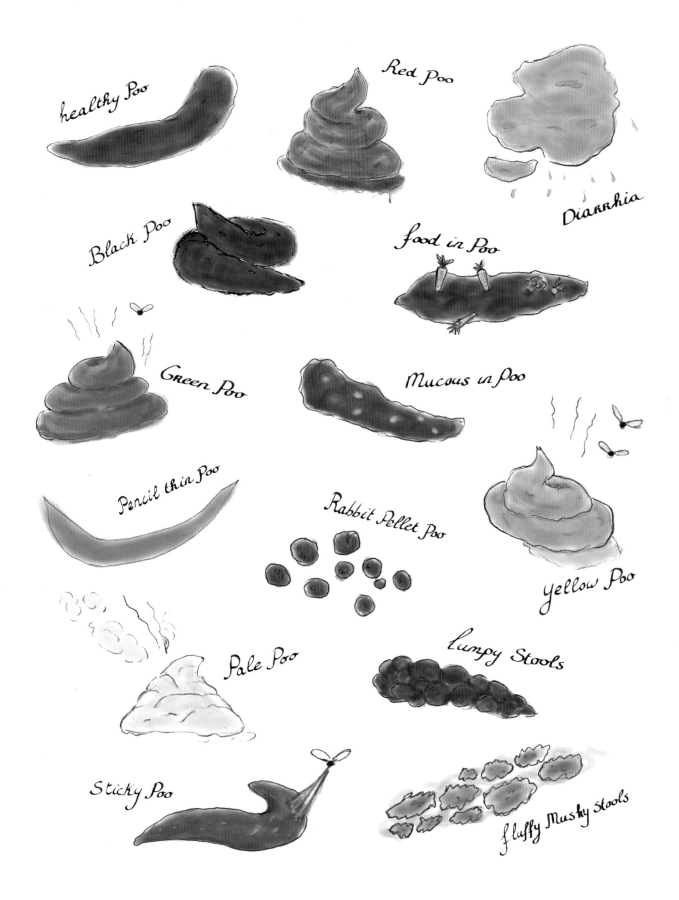

healthy Poo

Red Poo

Diarrhia

Black Poo

food in Poo

Green Poo

Mucous in Poo

Pencil thin Poo

Rabbit Pellet Poo

Yellow Poo

Pale Poo

Lumpy Stools

Sticky Poo

fluffy Mushy Stools

WHAT ELSE IS YOUR BODY SAYING?

You may not realise it, but your body is constantly talking to you. Perhaps not in a language you're used to speaking or hearing, but in the way you function emotionally and physically day-to-day, along with the appearance of everything from your skin, to your hair, nails and even your tongue!

These physical signs and symptoms were traditionally used by doctors to diagnose health before pathology tests, scans and x-rays came along, but with the advent of modern medicine many of these very useful functional diagnostic tools have been forgotten. When was the last time your doctor asked to inspect your tongue, or took a close look at your nails, or palpated your tummy during a general check up?

A healthy body will feel and look good most days, and you should generally feel physically energised, vibrant, happy and calm in your mind. Sure, external factors or people may come along which may upset you, triggering negative emotions – that's perfectly normal – but if you expose yourself to an unhappy or unhealthy environment for too long, then don't expect your body to function at its best.

So, aside from your poo, here are some body parts that can tell a story about you:

NAILS

These should be strong, clear, and free from ridging, pitting or pin prick dots, flaking or peeling. White flecks in your nails are a classic sign of zinc deficiency and dry, brittle nails that frequently crack have been linked to thyroid problems, poor protein digestion and a lack of essential fatty acids. Redness in the skin directly around the nail can be an indication of Candida overgrowth. Yellow nails can be an indication of fungal infection in the nail and pale or white nail beds can indicate liver problems, including hepatitis.

EYES

The whites of your eyes should be clear and a bright white, although they will naturally yellow with age, like your teeth. Puffy eyes, caused by fluid build up below the eyes, can either be due to illness, allergies or simply excessive salt consumption which can result in the body retaining more fluid than usual.

Discolouration of the skin under your eyes can be an indication your health is out of balance. Dark, bluish circles are typically indicative of problems or disorders with the kidneys, and adrenal and gonad hormones. A yellowish tone in the eye area can be related to an over-functioning liver and gallbladder often caused by excess dairy consumption.

Discolouration of the skin under the eyes should fade over time if you are following the LYG's eating program, although a degree of discolouration is natural with age.

TONGUE

A healthy tongue should be smooth and a light pinky-red in colour, with a light film covering it. Different parts of your tongue reflect the health of different organs within your body:

The right side relates to the health of your gall bladder and the left to that of your liver. Dental indentations or scalloping along the sides of your tongue can be an indication of nutrient deficiencies, usually caused by leaky gut or malabsorption.

The middle correlates to your stomach and spleen.

The back correlates to your kidneys, intestines, bladder and uterus.

The very tip of your tongue is representative of your heart and, just behind it, the lungs.

If you notice your tongue is covered in a thick, furry, yellow or white coating this is usually an indication of excess heat and/or dampness in your gut, typically the result of the fermentation of undigested food and an overgrowth of Candida, caused by – you guessed it – an imbalance in your good gut flora. So the best way to address this is to follow my eating plan and consider combining it with my gut repair and detox pack to improve digestion and balance your gut flora.

There are plenty of other signs and symptoms your body will express when your health is imbalanced in some way – too many to list in this book, but use these as your main indicators, and practice being more connected with your body. Also, be sure to consult your doctor or health care practitioner if you are experiencing any ongoing symptoms – it's your body's way of trying to communicate with you!

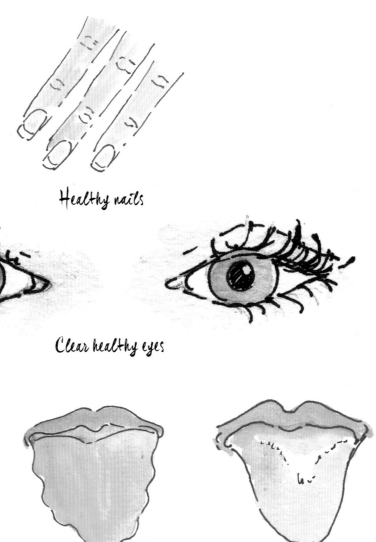

Healthy nails

Clear healthy eyes

Healthy tongue   Scalloping tongue   White coated tongue

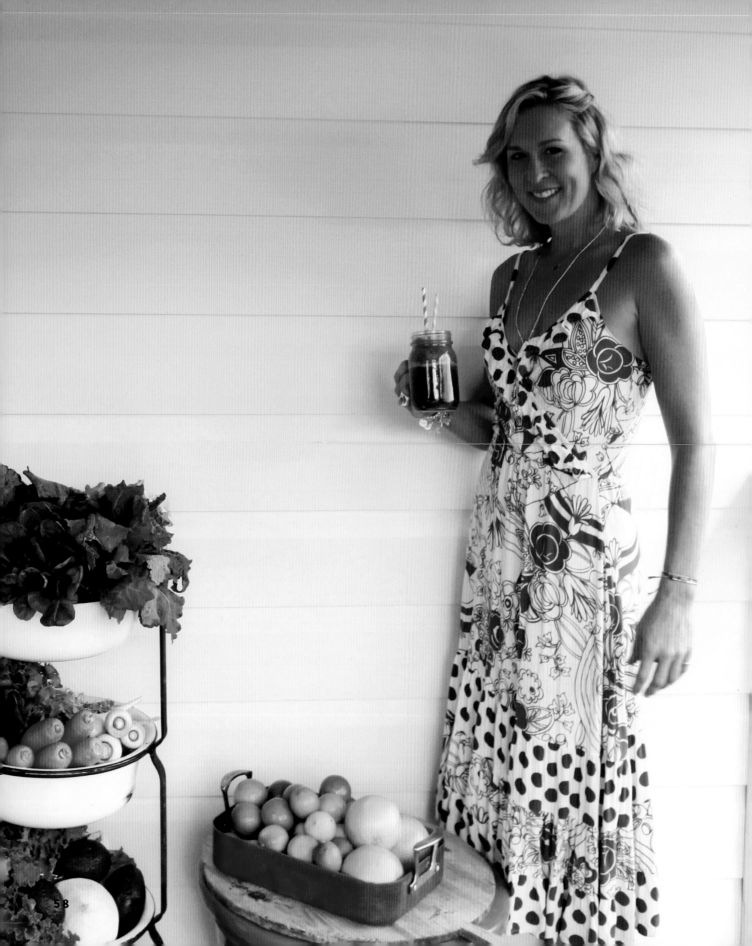

Get with the program!

Welcome to the LYG program, which sits at the heart of this book and my health philosophy as a Clinical Nutritionist.

There is so much conflicting and confusing information about what we should and shouldn't be eating, and I know many people throw their hands up in frustration, so I designed this program with one purpose in mind — to help you change your health as you know it today, and in the future, simply by eliminating certain foods and replacing them with heaps of delicious, healthy alternatives, along with a system to help you heal your gut and overall digestive function. The best part is, healing your gut will have a flow on effect to maximizing the health of all your other body systems so you can function at your best each and every day.

Remember, this program isn't just another 'diet' where you have to starve yourself of calories and enjoyment to achieve a shift in your health. Oh no, this is all about eating for enjoyment as much as it is to be healthy – after all, eating is one of life's greatest pleasures. But if the cost of that pleasure is leaving you feeling tired, or gassy and bloated afterwards, gaining weight, or getting sick later in life, then surely there has to be a better alternative? So that's exactly what I have designed the LYG program to do – to provide you with food choices that not only taste delicious, but are also healthy for you – now that's what I call having your (gluten-free) cake and eating it too!

In fact, if you're like many folks out there, you may not even realise you have a problem with your gut until you experience life without your specific health problem/s, but that's ok, stick with me for the next 28 days and hopefully beyond, because I promise you'll experience a shift in your health that will have a profound effect on your day-to-day life.

HOW THE PROGRAM WORKS

You've heard the saying 'you are what you eat'? And whilst this is true, it's only half of the story because in my view 'you are what you eat and what you digest and absorb!' There is little point in getting your diet right if your digestive system isn't functioning optimally. This would be a little like switching your car fuel to premium unleaded to enhance its performance, without cleaning out the fuel lines that process that fuel to all the different parts the engine - the car still wouldn't perform at its best. So in order to get the maximum benefit from the LYG program, it's best to combine eating the right foods with repairing your gut and detoxing your digestive system. Remember, without an optimally functioning digestive system, even good food has the potential to cause problems with your health.

I'VE SPLIT THE LYG PROGRAM INTO TWO EASY STAGES:

Stage I – 'Strip Back & Alkalise' - week 1-2
Stage II – 'Maintenance Phase' - week 3-4 & beyond

I also recommend combining stage I & II with the '4SGR' gut repair & detox nutrients and herbs – detailed on page 62 for maximum results.

Stage I

'STRIP BACK & ALKALISE' – WK 1- 2
THE 28 DAY LYG EATING PROGRAM

We're going to kick off the program by giving your body an initial spring clean. I refer to this stage as the "Strip Back and Alkalise" because it works to flush any accumulated toxins from your liver, bowel lymphatics and kidneys, as well as alkalise your body systemically – which is highly effective for reducing chronic inflammation. After all, every good renovation begins with a spring-clean!

When the body's pH is more alkaline, every cell will function better and that translates to the prevention of chronic illness and you feeling and looking great every day!

Many of us eat too much animal protein, especially from red and white meat, and this places excess stress on the digestive system. The aim of this stage is to give your digestive system a well-earned break from sources of difficult to digest animal proteins, in addition to eliminating the 'eight essential foods to avoid.' If you suffer from particularly bad IBS, I also recommend you eliminate any high FODMAPS vegetables during this period (see list on page 100.

I've included lots of homemade soups and fresh vegetable juices and smoothies in the Strip Back and Alkalise stage, because being liquid, they are not only easy to digest - to optimize nutrient absorption - but they're also highly alkalising and will work to stimulate your natural detoxification processes.

I recommend following this stage for the initial two weeks of the program, or longer if you feel your body needs it. If eliminating all animal protein does not suit you right now, for whatever reason – perhaps you are pregnant or breastfeeding, or you have a demanding job, or exercise regime that requires more energy from animal protein – that's totally ok, feel free to incorporate non-farmed, low mercury varieties of fresh fish and organic eggs (as long as you don't have an intolerance to them) and a little slow cooked meat one to two times per week. You can come back to the Strip Back and Alkalise stage anytime it suits you, or even repeat it when you feel your body needs a quick detox, or you want to regain that healthy glow from eating more alkaline foods.

Stage II

'MAINTENANCE STAGE' – WK 3-4 & BEYOND
THE 28 DAY LYG EATING PROGRAM

I refer to this as the 'maintenance phase' of the program, because it is designed to help you form healthy eating habits for life. Whilst you'll continue to eliminate the 'eight essential foods to avoid' throughout Stage II, you can reintroduce animal proteins from 100 percent grass-fed beef and lamb, along with organic chicken and free range pork, if desired.

Beyond week 4 on the LYG program, you can loosen the reigns a little, by applying the LYG eating principles at least 80 percent of the time. That way you'll continue to feel your best for life and continue to heal your gut, which can take up to six to nine months and, in some cases of chronic illness, even longer.

How to heal your gut

In order to heal your gut we need to do two things – eliminate the foods from your diet that cause inflammation and leaky gut, in combination with repairing the function of your gut. I've identified eight specific foods that are essential to avoid throughout the LYG program because they are highly inflammatory and damaging to your gut. These are the foods most responsible for contributing to common health problems, including weight gain, fatigue, bad skin, pain and an unhappy brain, especially when consumed in excess.

The purpose of eliminating these eight specific foods on the LYG program is to help your gut to heal, and restore balance to your overall digestive system, by shifting the biochemistry of your body from an overly acidic state to a more alkaline state. This will work to minimize inflammation, restore your energy, reboot your metabolism, banish the bloat and excess gas, and give you that youthful glow... all while helping you to feel happier and clearer in your head.

I don't want you to be concerned about what you can't eat during the LYG program, because I've included a handy list of healthy alternatives under the 'swap it don't drop' section on page 102 as well as over 100 delicious recipes to provide plenty of inspiration and guidance. Also included are two delicious sample meal planners, along with a healthy pantry shopping list to guide you on exactly what to eat.

In conjunction with removing the gut offending foods from your diet to reduce inflammation within your body, it's essential to heal your gut as well. By this I mean the elimination of any pathogens you may have developed, such as an overgrowth of Candida, SIBO or parasites, as well as repairing your gut wall and replenishing the colonies of good bacteria within your gut. These steps are critical to fully optimise your gut health - enabling you to feel totally revitalised and energised.

The process of repairing your gut requires a specific approach that I have called the **'4SGR' program – which stands for '4 Step Gut Repair'.**

THERE ARE 4 SPECIFIC STEPS TO THE 4SGR PROGRAM.
REMOVE, RESTORE, REPLENISH, REPAIR.

Let's start with a little analogy so you can understand the reason we need to go through each of the four steps in the order I recommend. Say you wanted to build a house, you wouldn't start by painting the walls, laying the carpet and hanging the curtains would you? No, you'd start by laying the foundations, then installing the plumbing and electrics, so the house is functional and inhabitable. This is exactly the same approach we take to rebuilding your gut: first we need to get the 'plumbing', your digestive system, and the 'electrics', your nervous system, sorted!

Step 1.
REMOVE
(OFFENDING FOODS, PATHOGENS AND TOXINS)

We're going to begin the gut repair journey at the bottom… quite literally! The first issue I tackle when it comes to a patient's health, aside from removing all the toxic inflammatory foods from their diet, is their bowel function. Until this is functioning well, producing nice solid, healthy coloured stools, that are easy to pass, you won't be removing the waste and toxins from your body at the rate you need to, making it impossible to heal the rest of your body. So how do we get your bowel functioning effectively? Obviously we start with feeding your body the right fuel, and we do this by following the LYG eating program. And to help give things a little 'push' in the right direction, I recommend including herbs such as slippery elm and aloe vera. We also need to remove any pathogens like parasites, bad bacteria, viruses and excess Candida from your gut, as their presence will negatively affect your health. Until you 'weed the garden', so to speak, you cannot expect any plants to thrive and survive! Luckily nature can provide once again, this time by way of specific nutrients and natural compounds. These can be found in herbs such as garlic, Chinese wormwood, oregano and black walnut and the friendly yeast saccharomyces boulardii - which collectively work to remove unwanted pathogens and bring Candida overgrowth under control.

The formulas contained in my gut repair and detox packs, (available from my website sallyjoseph.com), will support the elimination of pathogens and aid elimination and detoxification of your liver and bowel.

Step 2.
RESTORE
(DIGESTION)

The second step in the 4SGR program is to restore optimal function to your digestive system. This includes improving the production of hydrochloric acid (HCL) and pancreatic enzymes. As I've mentioned, one of the most common causes of poor gut health is insufficient production of HCL and pancreatic enzymes which help to break down your food, enabling the nutrients to be absorbed and utilised by the body. This is why I typically prescribe digestive enzymes to my patients, as well as recommend foods that encourage better digestion, such as apple cider vinegar and bitter greens like rocket (arugula) and adding bitters to water before a meal.

Step 3.
REPLENISH
(GOOD GUT FLORA)

This step involves replenishing your good gut flora colonies through the use of probiotic cultures, but this cannot be done effectively before completing Steps 1 and 2, because it's difficult for probiotic cultures to survive and thrive if they're introduced into a hostile environment. When choosing a probiotic formula, it's important to look for one that has a broad variety of good bacteria strains, preferably with a minimum count of 45 billion CFUs - colony-forming units - per day. I recommend taking a probiotic in capsule form vs powder, to ensure more bacteria survive your stomach acid and reach your lower intestine.

Combining a quality probiotic with a prebiotic, is more effective for establishing your good gut flora colonies, because prebiotics act like food, or fertilizer for the good bacteria in your gut to grow. Prebiotics like inulin, are a type of indigestible starchy carbohydrate. In large concentrations, inulin occurs naturally in chicory root (which is where it's extracted from) and in lower quantities in Jerusalem artichokes, onion, garlic, asparagus and banana.

Just as you would top up your lawn with fertiliser to keep it healthy and lush, I recommend topping up your gut flora colonies with a quality probiotic formula for a minimum of two to three months, or longer - depending on your pre-existing health condition. Once you have established healthy gut flora colonies, you could reduce your frequency to two to three times per week, in combination with including quality fermented foods in your daily diet.

The same recommendation applies after taking a course of antibiotics, because of the damage these cause to your good gut flora colonies. If you are taking the oral contraceptive pill, or suffer from a chronic illness, autoimmune condition, or neurological disease, then I recommend taking a probiotic supplement ongoing, as a powerful defence against chronic inflammation, and to help regulate your immune responses.

Step 4.

REPAIR
(YOUR GUT WALL)

The repair of your gut wall is one of the most crucial steps in the 4SGR program, even though each stage is dependent on the other to be fully effective. The 'Repair' stage of the 4SGR program pulls the whole gut repair program together; otherwise it's like trying to fill a bucket up with water that has holes in the bottom.

There are specific nutrients and herbs that aid the gut repair process, including high quality collagen protein, L-glutamine, slippery elm, turmeric, aloe vera and zinc, Licorice root.

HOW WILL YOU KNOW WHEN YOUR GUT HAS REPAIRED?

The duration of the gut repair process will depend largely on how closely you follow the LYG eating program and for how long; whether you combine it with the '4SGR' program; your pre-existing health condition; and successful elimination of any pathogens.

It typically takes around 2 – 3 months to see a significant improvement in the integrity of your gut wall, but in some chronic cases it can take up to 12 months to see a full improvement. If you return to regularly eating foods that cause damage to your gut, like gluten and sugar, this could jeopardise your efforts to repair your gut wall.

When your gut begins to effectively heal, you should not experience regular bloating, gas or abdominal upset, your bowel should be eliminating waste easily, at least twice daily, and your stools should be well formed with minimal odour. You should also find it easy to reach and or maintain a healthy weight without dieting, and any cravings for foods like sugar, caffeine and alcohol should be reduced to just here and there, rather than every day. Your mood and general cognitive function should also improve.

You should feel more balanced and you should wake each day feeling energised after a deep, restful sleep. Your skin and complexion should be clear and your hair free of dandruff and excess oil. Your body odour should be sweeter and your tongue should lose any heavy mucousy coating.

WHAT SHOULD I DO IF I AM STILL EXPERIENCING ONGOING GUT SYMPTOMS?

If you have been closely implementing all of my recommendations on the LYG program, in combination with the '4SGR' supplement program and you are still experiencing ongoing gut problems, I recommend consulting a qualified health practitioner, (preferably experienced in functional medicine, or gut health), for further testing and assessment of your individual case.

If you have not already done a CDSA – Comprehensive Digestive Stool Analysis, that includes parasitology testing, this is a good place to start. But remember, you need to wait at least two weeks after taking any anti-microbial herbs before testing. From there your practitioner can decide if you require any additional tests to help assess and treat your individual needs. Remember, each person's health is unique and one case will vary from another, but getting your gut health in order is the first place to start when addressing ANY health issue.

NOTE

Although the gut repair process takes time, you should notice progressive improvements, starting as early as week one! But remember that restoring your health is like removing the layers of an onion and then replacing them with new healthy layers one-by-one, and this takes time – in some cases up to 12 months, so be mindful about being patient and consistent, and your dedication will pay off with incredible results! I'm walking proof of that myself, as are thousands of my patients who have followed the LYG program.

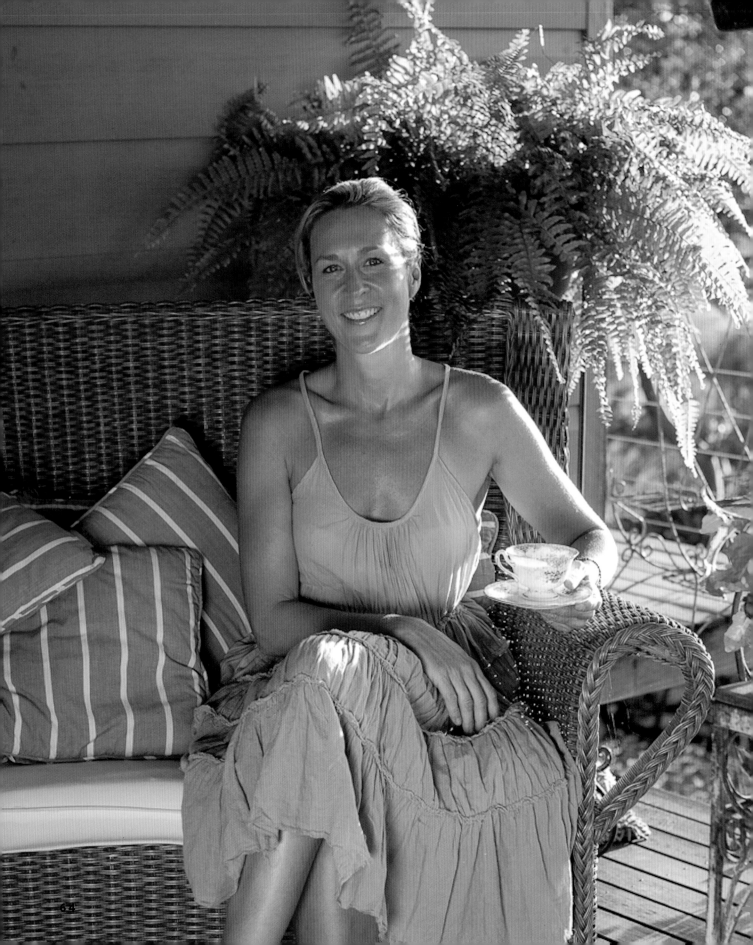

A friendly little pep talk before you begin

Okay, so we are about to jump into the program, but before you panic and cry, 'But what am I am going to eat?' whoa back tiger, because the program will only seem daunting for a short while, until you get the hang of it and it becomes second nature. Like any change in life, I admit it will be challenging initially, especially if you have been consuming the standard Western diet, or, as it's known in the US, the SAD (Standard American Diet) diet – a rather appropriate abbreviation, wouldn't you say? The SAD diet is standard fare in most Western countries nowadays and it generally contains processed, packaged foods – out of a box, bottle, or wrapper – with an ingredients list as long of your arm, most of which is made up of sugar, artificial additives, gluten, soy, corn and processed vegetable oils.

But there is a whole world of food out there just waiting to be discovered. And, before you ask, no, it doesn't all taste like cardboard and bird seed! You see, I'm not just a Nutritionist but also a foodie who is as big on flavour as I am on nutrition and convenience, so I am not going to ask you to eat anything that doesn't taste delicious and doesn't help to make life simple and easy when it comes to preparing your food.

Of course you don't need to suffer from a chronic illness or disease to benefit from the program. In fact you may be a really health conscious peep, consuming what you believe to be a healthy diet – eating low fat dairy, wholegrain bread and pasta with fresh fruit juice, and snacking on dried fruit and low salt this and that. If that sounds like you, well, hopefully you'll learn a few things from this book about what really classifies as healthy food choices (hint: those things aren't included!).

WHAT WILL THE LYG PROGRAM DO FOR YOU?

The LYG program will not only help you to lose that spare tyre around your middle (if that happens to be your issue), but it will teach you the secrets to achieving your full health potential, no matter if you are suffering from a chronic illness, such as an autoimmune disease, or battling anxiety and depression, or you simply want to enjoy the best of health in your old(er) age. You'll learn about how your gut influences the function of every cell, organ and system in your body, in particular your brain and immune system, and the links it has to regulating healthy blood sugar and insulin levels, balancing your hormones naturally and, perhaps most importantly of all, controlling the number one threat to your health – inflammation.

The fact is, there is no single way of eating that suits everyone in the world, and you may need to tweak a few things on this program to suit your individual needs, especially if you have a specific food intolerance, or suffer IBS and react to certain vegetables that I have not recommended you eliminate entirely from your diet. However I have marked any high FODMAPS recipes as best as possible with a 'Gut Alert' tag if this happens to be your health issue and removed the major dietary offenders when it comes to causing inflammation, fatigue, weight gain, illness and disease, so you should feel a heck of a lot healthier than if you were to keep eating these bad boys!

By the way, this program doesn't mean you can't enjoy a pizza or a glass of wine with friends every now and again, or indulge in a coffee and a piece of chocolate cake. (In fact, I have even included a chocolate cake recipe as part of my 'Nothing Naughty Treats', just to keep you smiling.) What I am hoping though, is that by sticking to the program for the next 28 days at least 90 percent of the time, and hopefully at least 80 percent of the time beyond, you will actually lose your physical and mental desire to eat unhealthy foods. After the initial 28 days, if you do feel like a bit of a blowout here and there, go for it, just don't do it too often. I've no doubt your body will tell you, more loudly and clearly than I can, just how bad those foods are for you, because you are likely to feel as 'rough as guts', as they say!

GO AT YOUR OWN PACE

The best advice I can give you when you approach the list of '8 Foods To Avoid', is to ask yourself, 'What am I prepared to do to look and feel as good as I can?' Then consider if you want to tackle this journey head on, with everything you've got, or bit by bit in stages. The choice is yours and there's no right or wrong way to do it – just as long as you do it! The only difference will be the rate you achieve your health goals. If jumping straight in the deep end just isn't your style, then no problem, start by eliminating the most challenging foods first (also the most detrimental to your health) – that'll be sugar, gluten and artificial additives. Then you can tackle the rest in the order and at the pace you feel comfortable with. As you successfully eliminate one food type, progress onto the next and then the next, until eventually you have removed all of the '8 Foods To Avoid'. Remember that by leaving any of them in your diet, you may not experience the full effects of the program. LYG is all about making the transition to a healthy way of eating for life, so work at a pace that works for you.

TASTE THE DIFFERENCE

Another thing to bear in mind, is that as your gut flora begin to tip back into balance and your body starts to detox and become more alkaline, your palette will improve and you will lose your cravings for sugar, caffeine or salt. Your food will taste better. Your digestive system will start to work how nature intended and the hunger signals from your brain will begin to normalize, preventing you from overeating. Or, if your problem has been that you don't have much of an appetite (maybe because you have been relying a bit too heavily on coffee or nicotine), then your appetite for healthy, nutrient-dense foods will return. You may even find that you will be eating more food, whilst losing fat at the same time! Sounds too good to be true? Try it and see.

ASK YOURSELF: WHAT IF?

I've had many of my patients tell me they don't want to be 'inconvenienced', or a burden on family and friends by having to make changes to their diet, or they worry they will never be able to enjoy eating out because, 'There's nothing I can eat.' A question for those of you reading this because you are searching for answers to unrelenting health problems – if you are concerned you might be inconvenienced by having to eliminate certain foods, consider this, 'How much is your health inconveniencing you right now?' Maybe you can't lose weight and as a result don't dare don a pair of shorts and a singlet top, thanks to those wobbly thighs and bingo wings. Would changing your diet be such an inconvenience if you could fit into the clothes you want to wear? Or what about having more energy to do the things you want to do each day? Maybe your health is impacting on your relationship with your kids, spouse, work colleagues, or even yourself? What would you give to have harmony and joy in your life again? Or maybe you're suffering with fatigue and depression? Perhaps you have experienced a heart attack, or been diagnosed with a chronic illness? Would changing your diet seem so difficult and inconvenient if it meant being able to overcome all of these troubles and live the life you desire? That's what's really at stake here. After all, who wants to eat food that makes you fat, tired and bloated, or even sick? So rather than worry about what you won't be eating on the program, lets adopt a glass-half-full attitude and focus on all the delicious, healthy foods that you will be enjoying over the next 28 days, which will help you to feel alive and vibrant every day.

Oh, and for those of you afraid of getting into the kitchen, I'll admit you may be cooking more than you're used to, especially if you have been in the habit of eating takeout most of the time, but I'm not going to ask you to spend hours in the kitchen, nor send you on a wild goose chase in search of exotic ingredients. Nope, I will only recommend practical, healthy and readily available foods that taste great and are quick and easy to prepare.

So now that we've had this little pep talk, and you have considered your personal 'what if' I hope you're feeling supercharged and geared up to begin your new life, just as I did all those years ago. I too had to overcome certain mental blocks, and I am so glad I did because my life changed for the better as a result and yours can too, if you truly want it. Even if you're still feeling a little nervous, that's ok, just focus on taking one day at a time, one change at a time, and before you know it, new habits will form and big changes will be just around the corner.

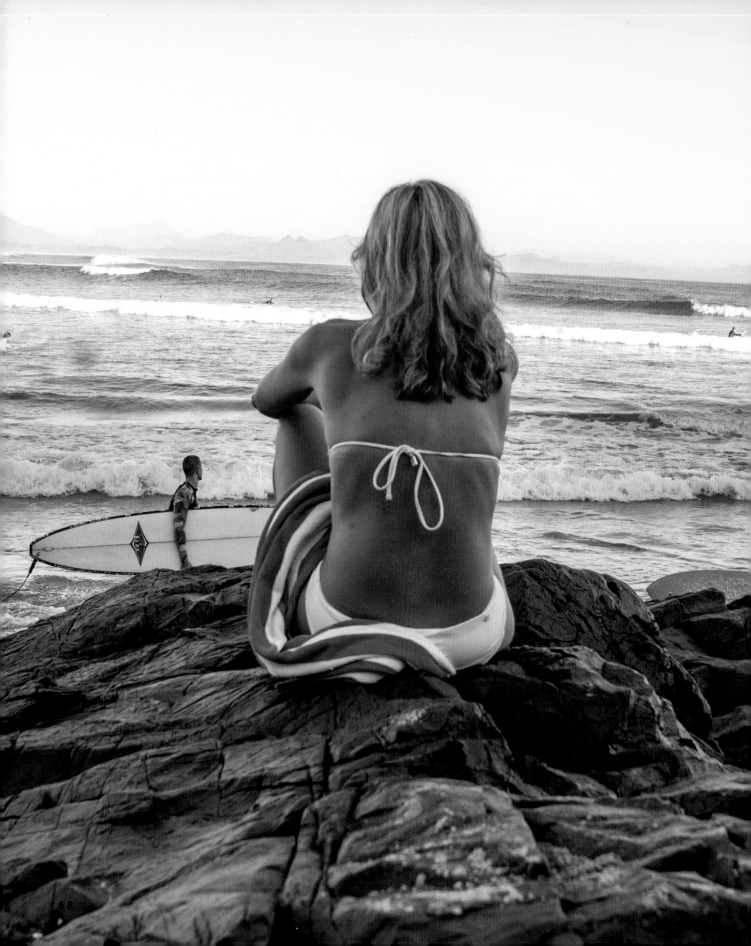

FOR THOSE SUFFERING FROM A CHRONIC ILLNESS...

A special word to those of you reading this book because you're looking for answers to a chronic illness like I was: I want you to be prepared to work a little harder and to be a lot more patient, as it may take longer for your body to heal. I usually say a good gauge is around three to six months for every year you have been unwell, depending on your condition. It may take less, it may take longer, but your road to recovery will also depend largely on YOU and how well you address the contributing factors on a whole. Keep in mind that you will get out what you put in, and what you put in might well be influenced by your attitude towards yourself. Look out for that voice in your head that is trying to do it's best to sabotage your efforts to get healthy. Getting your mind in shape is just as important as getting your body in shape. But luckily for you, your brain is connected to your gut, so by fixing your gut you will start to notice big changes in how your brain functions, including your general mood and cognitive function.

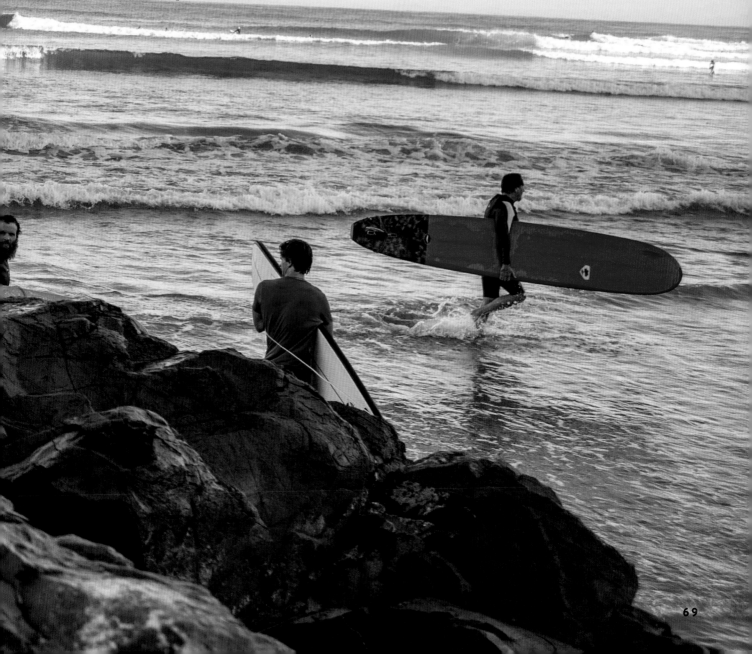

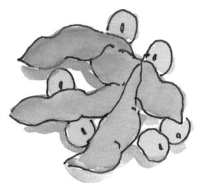
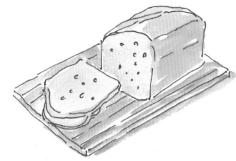
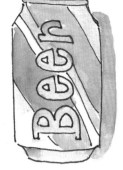

The 8 Foods to
Avoid on The
28 Day LYG
Eating Program

Okay, so now that we've had that little pep talk and I've prepped you for what's ahead on the LYG program, lets get this show on the road! Following are the '8 essential foods to avoid' for the next 28 days, at least ninety percent of the time if you want to experience the full effect, so read on and you'll discover why!

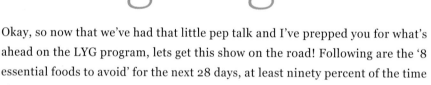

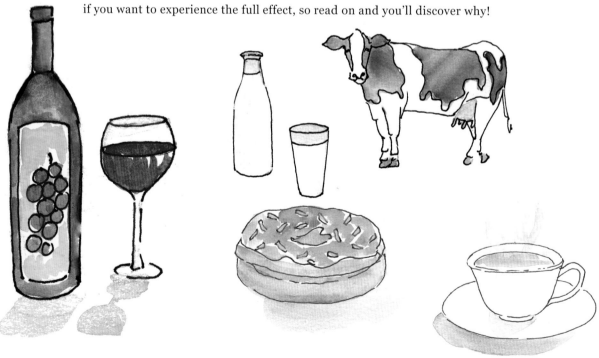

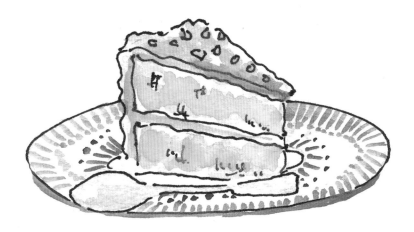

Sugar

Unless you've been sleeping under a rock lately, you've probably caught all the bad press surrounding sugar. Sugar is one the most addictive substances we can consume, with some medical experts arguing you may as well be shooting up heroin as far as its addictiveness goes – and I have to say, I totally agree!

HOW DID WE BECOME SO ADDICTED?

The main reason so many of us have become sugar gobbling gremlins boils down to the amount and type of sugar we're now consuming. Latest statistics reveal America is the largest consumer of sugar in the world, averaging 126 grams per day - equivalent to around three 375 ml cans of Coca Cola, more than twice the daily intake recommended by the World Health Organisation, for someone of normal weight. Australia falls fifth on the list of sugar-addicted nations, averaging 95.6 grams per day, or 24 teaspoons! These statistics make sugar responsible for creating the biggest health crisis in human history. So if we didn't used to have an issue with our dietary consumption of sugar, how did it become such a big problem today? There are three main reasons:

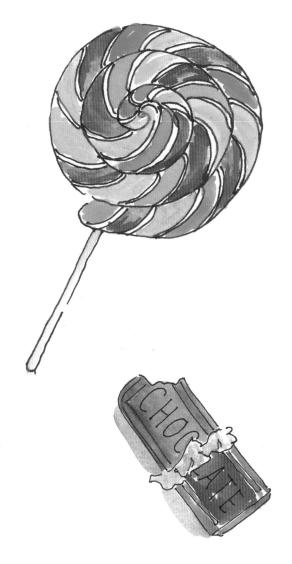

- **AVAILABILITY** – sugar has been part of our diet since caveman days, but back then we ate it sparingly because it was not always readily available. We also consumed only natural, unprocessed forms of sugar, like raw honey and fruit. But with the evolution of processed foods, Western nations slowly but surely abandoned their traditional wholefood diet in favour of processed 'convenience' foods, and sugar became the predominant ingredient. Americans consume as much as 70 percent of their diet from processed food, so it's little wonder they rank as the biggest consumer of sugar in the world !

•   **WE REPLACED DIETARY FAT WITH SUGAR** – in 1958, scientist Ancel Keys performed a study known as the 'Seven Countries Study' in pursuit of how dietary fat influenced rates of cardiovascular disease. Professor Key's study revealed that the countries where fat consumption was the highest had the most heart disease, and hence the theory that dietary fat caused heart disease was born. The problem with his research was that he cherry picked his data to support his theory, by leaving out countries where people eat a lot of fat, but have little heart disease, such as Holland and Norway, as well as countries where fat consumption is low, but the rate of heart disease is high, such as Chile. Unfortunately for us, Professor Key's research has since shaped the dietary guidelines of Western countries - recommending we eat less fat and avoid dietary cholesterol. But with the advent of a low fat diet, came low fat processed foods, and when food manufacturers removed the fat from their products to make them 'healthier', the products lost their flavour! Their solution to improve the palatability? Add sugar! This was the beginning of the end for skinny waistlines!

•   **WE SWITCHED TO PROCESSED SUGAR** – as agriculture and technology evolved, we became exposed to processed or refined forms of sugar, such as corn syrup and high fructose corn syrup. Refined forms of sugar derived from fructose impact our hormones in a totally different way to unrefined forms, specifically our appetite and mood regulating hormones, leptin and ghrelin, causing us to lose our 'off switch' when it comes to sugar consumption, impacting our health on a whole new level. Although excess consumption of sugar in any form, (unrefined or refined), can lead to obesity and

disease, not all forms of sugar are created equal as far as the way the body metabolises them, and this is what determines the impact sugar has on your appetite, and overall health - including your waist line! Sugar can be split into two predominant types: glucose and fructose.

GLUCOSE

Sugar in the form of 100% pure glucose is the body's number one and preferred source of fuel over any other nutrient, required for energy by every cell and every bacteria, in every living thing on earth. Without it, life would not exist! When you consume foods containing glucose, an insulin response is triggered from the pancreas to transport the glucose from the blood to your cells for energy. The remaining glucose will either be stored in your muscle cells or liver as glycogen for later use, or as fat. Excess glucose intake will also stimulate the production of excess insulin, and chronically high levels of insulin, are directly linked to heart disease and diabetes, as well as cancer.   But unlike fructose, glucose suppresses your hunger hormone ghrelin and stimulates leptin – the appetite-suppressing hormone. This means you are less likely to overeat foods containing pure glucose, such as rice malt syrup or glucose powder, than those containing fructose, or a combination of both such as honey, maple syrup or table sugar, even fruit, because glucose accelerates fructose absorption.

FRUCTOSE

is the sugar found naturally in many fruits and vegetables, but it is the processed form of fructose added to many processed foods and beverages like soft drinks or sodas and fruit-flavoured drinks in the form of high fructose corn syrup (HFCS), that is the most fattening and dangerous form of fructose. Unlike glucose, fructose does not trigger an insulin response; instead 100 percent of the fructose you consume is metabolized in the liver. Because it is not the preferred energy source for your muscles or brain, it is far more rapidly converted to fat, compared to glucose.

Not only is fructose converted to fat more readily, but unlike glucose, fructose does not stimulate the production of leptin, the key hormone for telling your body when it is full. So in short, the more fructose you consume in your diet, the less likely you are to feel full and the more likely you are to keep on eating, which is why fructose in particular is so highly addictive. Overconsumption of sugars like fructose also increases the growth of pathogenic bacteria and yeasts like Candida Albicans, promoting gut dysbiosis (an imbalance in gut flora colonies). When your colonies of gut flora are out of balance you will crave more sugar - and so the vicious cycle begins - as the more sugar you eat the more you'll fuel the growth of these bad bacteria and yeast.

The overconsumption of fructose also causes your body to deposit fat around your abdomen and organs. It's this type of as visceral fat that specifically increases your risk of developing a condition known as insulin resistance - where your body loses the ability to burn fat. Insulin resistance significantly increases your risk for developing a string of lifestyle diseases, including diabetes, heart disease and cancer.

HOW MUCH SUGAR DO YOU REALLY NEED?

In reality your body can meet its daily energy requirements from sugar by eating a couple of pieces of whole fresh fruit and plenty of vegetables, which have the added benefit of containing vital nutrients, fibre and enzymes. Keep in mind that eating too much fruit, particularly high fructose varieties such as dried fruits, grapes, mangoes and bananas can still be fattening and upset the balance of your gut flora.

HOW MUCH SUGAR ARE YOU REALLY EATING?

Many of us are oblivious to how much sugar we are consuming each day, thanks to the hidden forms contained in packaged foods. When I ask my patients how much sugar they think they're eating in a day, the common response is, 'Not much, aside from a teaspoon or two in my morning coffee and maybe the odd sweet or chocolate,' and that's the problem right there: we lack the understanding of which foods contain sugar and how much we're really consuming.

HIGH SUGAR ALERT!

Here are a few examples of not-so-obvious sources of high sugar foods that may cause you to reassess your sugar intake: flavored yoghurts, fruit juice, potato chips, processed mayonnaise, bottled salad dressings and BBQ sauce, breakfast cereal, muesli bars, low fat dairy products, muffins and pastries, bananas, dried fruit and semi dried tomatoes, spreads, chutney, marmalade, jams and Thai food. If you regularly eat anything on this list, you're eating lots of sugar!

SUGARS TO LET INTO YOUR LIFE (IN MODERATION)

Remember one of the main aims of the LYG program is to reduce your desire and taste for the sweet stuff and the best way to do this is to avoid sugar, but these healthier, fructose free sugar alternatives are ok in moderation.

STEVIA - a natural sweetener derived from a South American plant. It contains no calories but is infinitely sweeter than sugar. If you've never tried it, be sure to use very sparingly, as it is 200 times sweeter than sugar gram for gram and has a nasty bitter aftertaste if you're too heavy handed. Personally, I prefer using the drops over the powder.

RICE MALT SYRUP – made from cooked rice it gets a big tick being fructose free - but it does contain a blend of glucose and maltose, so it will still impact on your insulin and blood sugar levels. The key is not to overdo it and remember it is STILL a form of sugar!

GLUCOSE POWDER – pure glucose, or 'dextrose' as it's sometimes known, contains no fructose, making it a safer alternative to fructose-based sweeteners, but be sure to use sparingly as this is not an invitation to overindulge, as excess consumption will still end up on your hips and spike your insulin levels.

SUGAR ALCOHOLS – GLYCEROL, SORBITOL, MALTITOL, MANNITOL, ISOMALT, ERYTHIRTOL AND XYLITOL.

–common sugar alternatives derived from plants like fruits and vegetables. They are promoted as low calorie sweeteners because they are not completely absorbed by the small intestine, but a percentage is still metabolized as if it were fructose. The problem with sugar alcohols is they can often irritate your gut, causing bloating, diarrhoea, and flatulence, because of the fermentation of sugar alcohols by your gut bacteria. Tolerance for sugar alcohols often improves after a month or two. If you are going to use sugar alcohols, my preferred choices are erythirtol and xylitol, but be sure to stick to occasional consumption only in say, baking. If you are prone to IBS or suffer fructose malabsorption, I recommend you avoid these sugar alternatives altogether to be on the safe side.

LABELLING TRICKS

Manufacturers use a lot of sneaky tricks to make their products appear 'low sugar' or 'sugar free'. Familiarise yourself with the tricks below so you can avoid being mislead!

NO ADDED SUGAR - this doesn't mean 'no sugar', but rather that the manufacturer has been kind enough not to add any more sugar than what's already naturally occurring in the product, such as in bottled fruit juices. Many products advertising 'no added sugar' are commonly still too high in naturally occurring sugar.

LOW SUGAR - says who and compared to what? Use this simple guideline to gauge if a food really is low in sugar: A food should contain no more than 6 grams of sugar per 100 grams or mls.

SUGAR FREE - sure sounds good, but double-check this does not mean it contains artificial sweeteners instead! If it does, give it a big swerve. Alternatively the product may contain sugar alcohols, but be sure to stick to erythirtol and xylitol in this case and only consume occasionally.

LOW FAT OR 99% FAT FREE - this typically translates to HIGH sugar! This is a clever labeling technique food manufacturers use to seduce you into thinking their product is healthy, so be sure to read your labels to check it's not loaded with sugar!

GLUTEN FREE - doesn't mean sugar free. Many gluten free products are laden with sugar or other nasty's such as soy, artificial additives and vegetable oils, so always be sure to check for these.

CONTAINS NATURAL SUGAR - the natural sugar in question is usually sugar cane, honey, maple syrup or some other forms of unrefined sugar. These are 'natural', yes, but they still contain fructose and glucose, which has the potential to inflame your gut and expand your waistline if consumed in excess, so go easy and avoid any natural sugars containing fructose for at least four to eight weeks to help break your addiction!

By eliminating fructose from your diet your taste buds will be restored to normal and your tolerance for the sweet stuff will dramatically decrease. Not only will you desire less sugar, but, if you do eat something really high in sugar, it will quickly taste sickeningly sweet and very unpleasant, not to mention leave you with a sugar hangover.

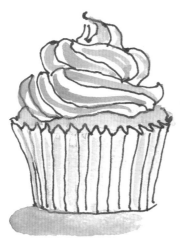

MY NIFTY TIPS AND TRICKS TO KICK YOUR SUGAR CRAVINGS

As you make the transition from sugar, gluten and coffee and alcohol, you will notice your body will experience what some refer to as a healing crisis, or what I like to refer to as a biochemical adjustment. Believe it or not, the food you have been feeding your body has been determining, to a large degree, how you think, how you sleep how you feel and what you crave. This is because food affects the biochemistry of our body. I have a saying…. "Eat crap, feel like crap." It really is THAT simple!

Here are my top tips to bust the sugar cravings!

• **EAT FAT** – because unlike high sugar foods, fat is filling and will satisfy your hunger whereas eating sugar will keep you crying out for more! Include foods rich in healthy fats such as avocado, coconut oil, plain coconut or sheep's yoghurt, goat or sheep's cheese, to help to switch off your hunger hormones.

• **RAW COCOA NIBS** – are 100 percent unprocessed chocolate, without the cream and sugar of course. To the sweet tooth they will taste bitter at first, however this will improve as your palette changes and becomes sensitive to sweetness again. Alternatively try 85 percent dark chocolate.

• **TOP UP YOUR NUTRIENTS** - L-Glutamine, magnesium, chromium and B vitamins are essential for supporting healthy nervous system function and regulating healthy blood sugar and insulin production.

• **LOAD UP ON GREEN LEAFY VEGETABLES AT MEAL TIMES** - these are rich in fibre to help keep you feeling fuller for longer.

• **CLEAN YOUR TEETH AFTER A MEAL** - I know it may sound silly, but I tend to find this really works.

• **TRY A GLASS OF WARM WATER WITH LEMON AND APPLE CIDER VINEGAR** – this will help to alkalise your system and neutralise sugar cravings.

• **EAT PROTEIN** – include a serving of healthy protein with every meal or snack. Consider snacks such as raw nuts, hummus with celery sticks or my recipe for Bellissimo Balls.

• **EAT A SPOONFUL OF FERMENTED VEGETABLES** – often sugar cravings are a sign our gut flora colonies are out of balance, so by feeding your microbiome foods like this, you'll be helping to restore the balance of good bacteria, starving the growth of excess Candida and bad bacteria.

• **DRINK HERBAL TEA** -in particular licorice tea. This is a great tonic for your adrenals and has a natural sweetness to it that can satisfy sugar cravings.

• **ADD CINNAMON TO YOUR FOOD** - this helps to regulate blood sugar levels and stops sugar cravings. Sprinkle some over your food or in a smoothie, soups or in chai tea.

• **DISTRACT YOURSELF** -go for a walk, phone a friend, or grab some sunshine. Exercise does wonders for regulating your insulin and feel good hormones like serotonin and endorphins.

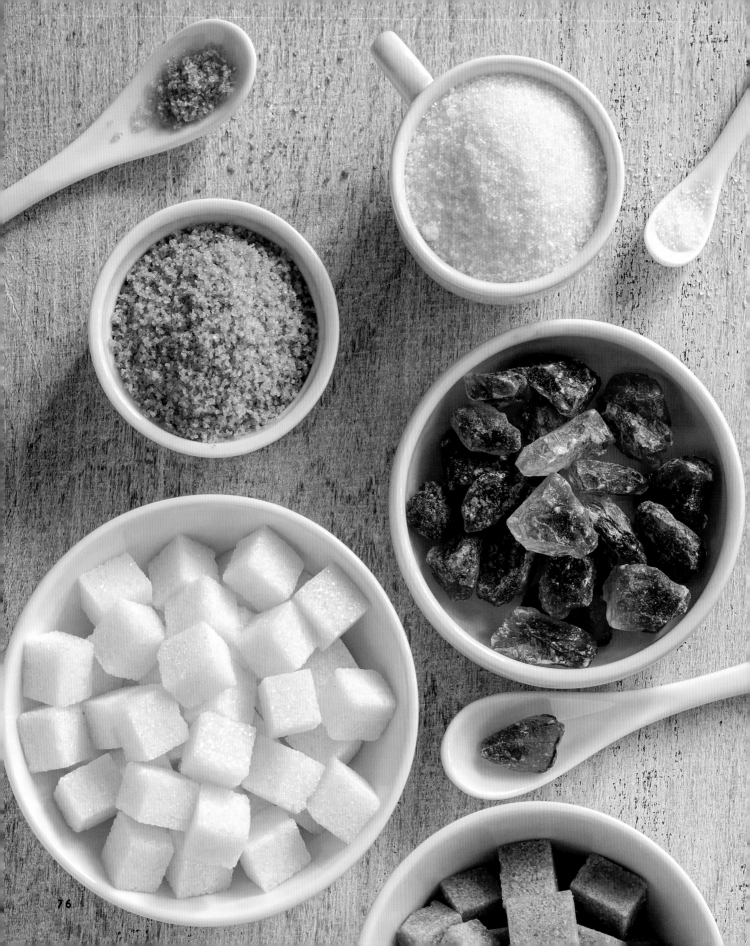

Fructose Offenders

If fructose is the big offender, it makes sense to know where to find it and in what quantities. Here is your handy guide to fructose offenders.

FRUIT JUICE
Contains naturally occurring fructose, which converts very rapidly to fat, because the fibre has been removed during juicing. Fructose content depends on the variety of fruit..

SUCROSE
That's common sugar to you and me. Contrary to popular belief, brown sugar isn't better for you, it's just a little less refined than white.

50% fructose

HONEY
Despite being a natural sugar, honey is not fructose free, so avoid it at least initially, to break your sugar habit and cravings.

40% fructose

GOLDEN SYRUP
Made during the process of refining sugar cane juice into sugar..

40% fructose

PALM SUGAR
Made from boiling the sap of coconut sago, and arenga pinnata palms, a common ingredient in Asian food.

40 - 50% fructose

FRUCTOSE
If you see this sweetener in the ingredients list of any packaged food, that's a signal to bin it!

RAPADURA
The pure juice extracted from sugar cane (using a press), which is then evaporated and ground to produce a grainy sugar.

50% fructose

MAPLE SYRUP
Made from the sap of maple trees.

40% fructose

MOLASSES
A by-product of the refining of sugar cane, grapes or sugar beets into sugar.

40% fructose

COCONUT SUGAR
A natural sugar made from the sap of the coconut plant.

48% fructose

HIGH FRUCTOSE CORN SYRUP
A cheap industrialised food product, extracted from corn stalks. This is the most fattening of all sugars.

55% fructose

AGAVE
This popular form of sugar used in many raw dessert recipes is one of the highest sources of fructose.

70 - 90% fructose

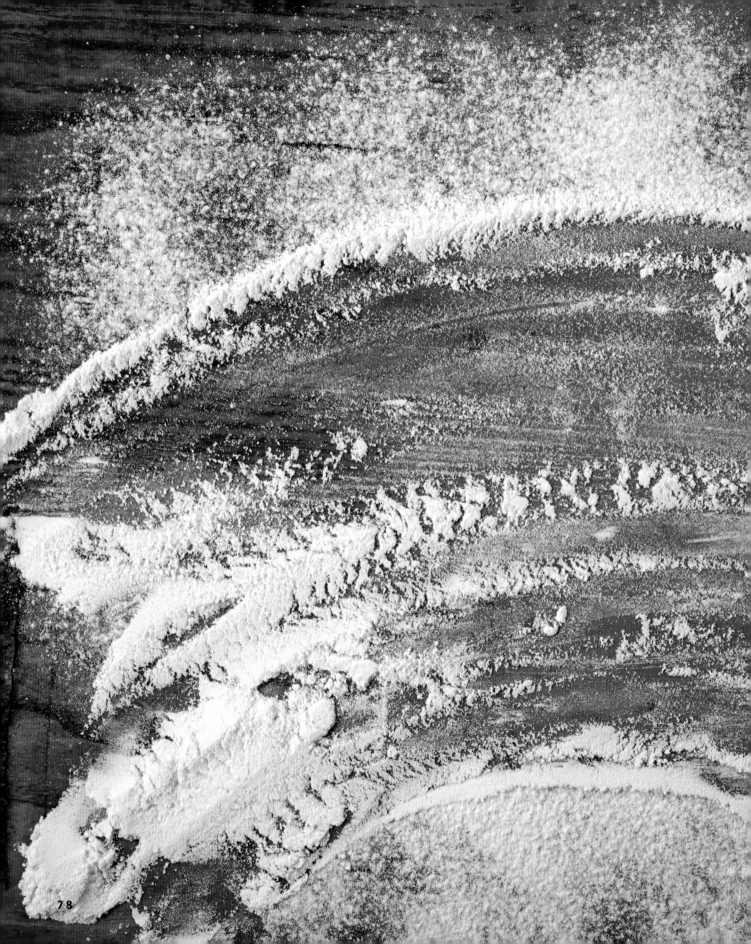

Gluten

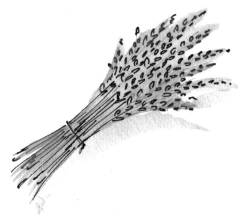

Step aside, sugar. It's time to make way for your partner-in-crime, gluten. If there are two foods I recommend eliminating from your diet most of all, it's these two. Sugar and gluten are the most pro-inflammatory and gut-damaging foods you can eat. Like sugar, gluten can be highly addictive, thanks to the morphine-like compounds present in grains known as 'exorphins'. These exorphins make it very difficult to moderate your intake, because of the impact they have on the neurology of your brain.

Gluten is also one of the most common offenders when it comes to food sensitivities, however the symptoms of gluten sensitivity will vary from person to person and they don't necessarily have to express as gut-related, or display immediately after consumption. With my history of autoimmune disease, I am very sensitive to gluten, so I avoid it 90 – 100 percent of the time, even though I am not Coeliac. For me, any exposure will typically express as lethargy, brain fog, dark rings and puffiness under my eyes and fluid retention, even weight gain, well before I experience any gut-related symptoms like bloating, flatulence or loose bowels. Regluar gluten consumption would also trigger an increase in my thyroid antibody levels.

Another major downside to gluten is the effect it can have on your mood and cognitive function. Many people are susceptible to feeling irritable, depressed or anxious and gluten can be one of the major culprits behind these symptoms. If you are prone to experiencing any sort of neurological symptoms like these, I recommend you look straight to your diet, because even the smallest amount of gluten exposure can be enough to express neurologically, if you're especially sensitive.

Throughout my years in clinical practice, not one of my patients reported feeling worse, or experienced no improvement in their health after eliminating gluten from their diet. The majority lost significant amounts of weight, overcame IBS, allergy symptoms, headaches, even chronic illnesses, and normalized their blood pressure and cholesterol in the process.

WHAT IS GLUTEN?

So what is gluten and why is it having such a profoundly negative effect on our gut and overall health? Put simply, gluten is a naturally occurring protein (made up of the peptides gliadin and glutenin) found in grains such as wheat (including durum and semolina), rye, spelt, kamut and barley. Although oats don't naturally contain gluten, they are typically contaminated with gluten, thanks to being grown on the same land as gluten-containing grains and processed in the same facilities.

WHY IS GLUTEN A PROBLEM TODAY?

You might be wondering why wheat and other gluten-containing grains have become a problem for so many today, considering they have been a staple part of the human diet for centuries?

In a nutshell, the wheat we consume today is very different from the wheat our ancestors ate. In the interests of producing softer, fluffier bread, and a higher yield, wheat now contains much higher levels of gluten, as well as phytates which can block the absorption of essential minerals. Also, new crossbreeding techniques, developed to make wheat more disease-and-pest-resistant, are exposing us to higher levels of gluten and chemical pesticides.

Think about a typical day in the modern Western diet ... the average Joe might begin their day with a bowl of high sugar, wheat-based cereal, maybe a slice or two of toast, followed by a mid-morning biscuit or muffin to help bridge the gap until lunch time, which typically involves a sandwich or bread roll, followed by another afternoon snack, of, say, potato crisps flavoured with artificial ingredients containing gluten, or even another biscuit or two, topped off with a pasta or pizza for dinner, or a stir fry made with bottled sauces (laden with hidden forms of gluten) and perhaps a couple of beers to wash it all down. If this scenario sounds even a little bit like you, you're consuming a plethora of gluten, which could be triggering an inflammatory immune response, or 'fire' within your gut. If you've been packing on the pounds or struggling to lose weight, feeling tired, bloated or gassy, or even a bit cranky and foggy in the head, gluten could very well be the reason why!

AM I SENSITIVE TO GLUTEN?

I often get asked, 'Do you need to be a diagnosed Coeliac to avoid gluten?' The short and answer is, 'No!' A common assumption people make with gluten sensitivity is that if they don't test positive to Coeliac antibodies then they don't have a problem with gluten in their diet. It is estimated that 30 to 40 percent of the population experience some degree of gluten sensitivity and are unaware, making gluten intolerance far more common than Coeliac disease, which has also risen more than fourfold in the past 50 years.

So no, you don't need to be a Coeliac to suffer the physiological and neurological effects of gluten. After seeing so many negative pathology results for gluten sensitivity or Coeliac disease in clients with gut problems, I eventually gave up testing and now mainly rely on the elimination method for evidence, because I find physiological symptoms more reliable than blood tests in this instance.

To establish if you have a gluten sensitivity, and the degree of your intolerance, you need to avoid all foods containing gluten for at least 28 days, preferably six weeks, because this is the period it will take your body to eliminate all traces of gluten from your system and for the effects to subside. I also recommend you avoid corn during this period as it can 'cross react' with gluten, mimicking the same symptoms of gluten sensitivity. After four to six weeks, you can try reintroducing gluten to test your tolerance, but steer clear of the other 'foods to avoid' so that you can accurately assess your degree of sensitivity. It is often not until you reintroduce gluten after a period of abstinence that you will experience the acute effects it is having on your health.

Don't fall into the trap of thinking you can get away with eating small amounts of gluten here and there, as there are no halfway measures when it comes to treating a gluten sensitivity or Coeliac disease. A serving of gluten, just once a month, can be enough to trigger an inflammatory immune response that can last for weeks in very sensitive individuals. As I say to my patients, 'Remember it only takes one match to light a fire!'

HOW DOES GLUTEN IMPACT ON YOUR HEALTH?

Gluten can cause 'leaky gut syndrome', as discussed in greater detail on page 30 of this book. Increased gluten consumption can also trigger an imbalance in your microbiome or gut flora, triggering inflammation within your gut, which can then express in the form of many common health conditions. A 2002 paper by Farrell Kelly in The New England Journal of Medicine stated 55 diseases are known to be potentially linked to gluten consumption. These ranged from heart disease and cancer, autoimmune disease, IBS and neurological disorders, just to name a few. Aside from wreaking havoc on your gut, gluten also has a powerful inflammatory effect on your brain. In particularly sensitive individuals, it can significantly contribute to, or exacerbate, many neurological conditions, as detailed on pages 43 - 49.

Tips to remember when going gluten-free

KNOW WHAT YOU ARE EATING

It's essential to read food labels and check the fine print for hidden sources of gluten, and when you're dining out, don't be afraid to ask which dishes are gluten free, as increasingly restaurants and cafes are catering to this request. But the simplest and healthiest way to avoid hidden sources of gluten is to cut out all packaged, processed or fast foods from your diet, and just stick to eating whole, fresh foods – like the ones included in all my recipes.

GLUTEN FREE DOESN'T ALWAYS MEAN HEALTHY!

Many food manufacturers, restaurants and cafes are jumping on the bandwagon, promoting their products as 'healthy' because they are gluten free, but often this is just a disguise for mounds of sugar, artificial additives, even processed vegetable oils, so be vigilant and read the ingredients list and check the nutrition table for sugar content, or check with the waiter for the information you need.

LOOK OUT FOR HIDDEN SOURCES OF GLUTEN

It's not just the obvious sources of gluten that you need to be on the look out for, as there are many hidden sources too, and you may be eating it, or even rubbing it onto your skin or hair, without realizing. You will typically find these hidden sources of gluten lurking inside many processed, packaged foods in the form of stabilizing agents and bottled sauces, such as salad dressings, mayonnaise and soy sauce, just to name a few.

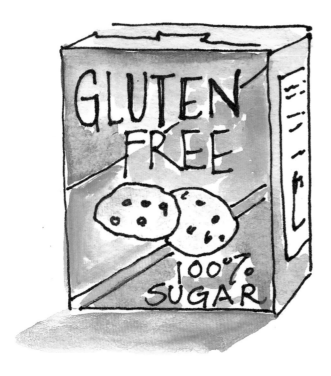

Believe it or not, gluten has made its way into medications, beauty and personal care products, such as moisturizers, shampoos and conditioners and body wash! Because the skin is the largest organ, whatever you rub or spray onto it, will make its way into your bloodstream, triggering the same inflammatory immune response over time as when you ingest it orally. It's a challenge identifying these hidden sources, because they are often disguised under unrecognizable names or forms.

DIGUISES FOR GLUTEN FOUND IN PROCESSED FOODS

- Artificial colours and flavours (typically displayed as a number)
- Baking powder (unless it specifies gluten-free)
- Caramel colour/flavoring
- Citric acid (can be fermented from wheat, corn, molasses or beets)
- Dextrin
- Diglycerides (look out for this one on food labels)
- Emulsifiers
- Enzymes
- Food starch (including corn starch and seitan – another one to keep an eye out for)
- Glucose syrup
- Glycerides
- Hydrolyzed/textured vegetable protein
- Malt extract/barley malt
- Maltodextrin
- MSG
- Modified food starch
- Stabilizers
- Starch /wheat starch

OTHER HIDDEN SOURCES OF GLUTEN YOU MAY NEVER GUESS

- Personal care products – some brands of makeup, shampoo and conditioner, moisturizers, sunscreen and baby powder
- Medications and nutritional supplements - unless stated, many of these contain gluten based fillers like dextrin, derived from corn or wheat
- Sauces and condiments – some brands of mayonnaise, ketchup, salad dressings and gravy
- Stamps and envelopes – gluten is contained in the sticky adhesive
- Many luncheon meats and imitation crab meat - such as in California rolls
- Licorice and solid candy
- Kids' playdoh

WHAT SHOULD I DO IF EXPOSED TO GLUTEN

If you are knowingly or unknowingly exposed to gluten you can speed up its elimination from your system, and reduce the associated inflammatory symptoms, by taking a digestive enzyme and loading up on probiotic foods and/or a quality probiotic.

GUT RECOVERY AND GRAIN CONSUMPTION

If you have major gut problems, suffer a chronic illness, are trying to lose weight or are having difficulty falling pregnant, I recommend avoiding all grains even gluten-free varieties like rice during the gut healing process, as these can hinder your ability to lose weight and repair your gut wall. If you have been avoiding legumes and lentils throughout the gut repair stage, feel free to test your tolerance, by reintroducing them back into your diet separately and in small quantities.

A WORD ON REINTRODUCING GLUTEN

If you want to test your tolerance to gluten after completely avoiding it for four to six weeks, I recommend avoiding commercial brands of bread, because these typically contain artificial additives and are not organic. Instead opt for breads made from sprouted grains such as kamut or spelt or a quality organic sourdough, baked using the traditional method, using probiotic cultures.

Soy

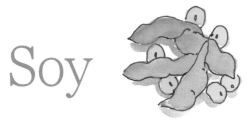

Soy is another hot topic of debate. Although small amounts of fermented soy has traditionally been part of a healthy Asian diet for centuries, the issue with soy today stems from the farming and production methods. These have altered the biochemical composition of soy, along with many other foods, with negative consequences for our health.

THE PROBLEMS WITH SOY

The case for soy as a supposed 'health food', is not looking pretty as Dr. Kaayla Daniel, author of The Whole Soy Story points out, thousands of studies link soy to malnutrition, digestive distress, immune-system breakdown, thyroid dysfunction, cognitive decline, reproductive disorders and infertility, even cancer and heart disease.

One of the reasons soy is so widely included in processed foods nowadays is because it is a very cheap and profitable grain to grow, making it very attractive to commercial food manufacturers. But to add insult to injury, the majority of soy bean crops are genetically modified – 91 percent of soy grown in the United States is GM soy - and the US being one of the biggest exporters of soy around the world, means much of the soy contained in processed foods is genetically modified. GM soy contains high levels of glyphosate from the toxic herbicide Roundup. I have explained the issues with consuming GM foods in more detail on page 118.

But the problems with soy don't stop there. Soy contains high levels of isoflavones - natural plant compounds known as phytoestrogens that resemble human estrogen and can disrupt endocrine function, cause infertility, and increase the risk of breast cancer.

SOY CAN BE BROKEN INTO TWO TYPES – FERMENTED AND UNFERMENTED

Whilst I am not a fan of unfermented soy, organic fermented sources of soy, like miso, tempeh and natto in small quantities does not wreak havoc on your body to the extent unfermented soy products do.

Unfermented soy products on the other hand are high in phytic acid which inhibits the absorption of certain minerals into the body, including magnesium, copper, zinc and iron, resulting in deficiencies.

Fermented soy products are better for your health than unfermented varieties, because they are lower in phytic acid and other "anti-nutrients" making them easier to digest. The molecular structure of the naturally occurring plant oestrogens has not has not been altered in fermented soy products the way they have in non-fermented soy.

However, beware, because soy in either form - fermented or unfermented - contains goitrogens, substances that block the production of thyroid hormones through inhibiting the uptake of iodine, thereby interfering with your thyroid function. This is a problem particularly for people suffering from an underactive thyroid (hypothyroidism), as iodine is crucial for healthy thyroid function. Iodine deficiency is becoming more and more prevalent, and could be one of the reasons behind the increase in hypothyroid conditions. If you suffer from hypothyroidism I recommend avoiding all soy products.

If you choose to consume some fermented soy products, such as tamari (wheat-free soy sauce), tempeh, or miso soup, ensure they are non-genetically modified and organic and consume in moderation.

HOW TO AVOID SOY

Like gluten and sugar, you could be consuming soy without even realizing, because it is such a common ingredient in so many processed foods. Lecithin (additive 322), for example, is used as an emulsifier in chocolate, ice cream, margarine, baked goods, potato chips, and mayonnaise. So the simplest way to ensure soy is not sneaking into your diet is to steer clear of all processed, packaged foods and get back to eating fresh wholefoods and preparing more home cooked meals.

FERMENTED FORMS OF SOY:

- Natto
- Miso
- Tempeh
- Soy sauce

NON-FERMENTED FORMS OF SOY SOY:

- Whole dry soybeans
- Soy flour
- Soy bean oil
- Soy milk
- TVP (texturized vegetable protein) or soy protein isolate, which also contains a large amount of MSG
- Soy infant formula
- Edamame
- Tofu

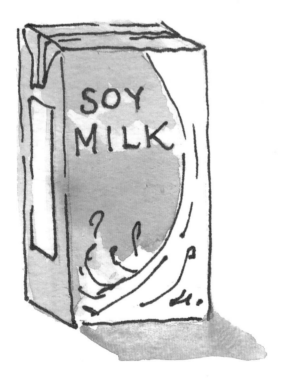

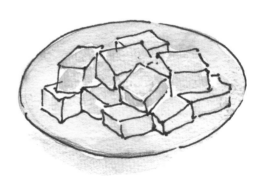

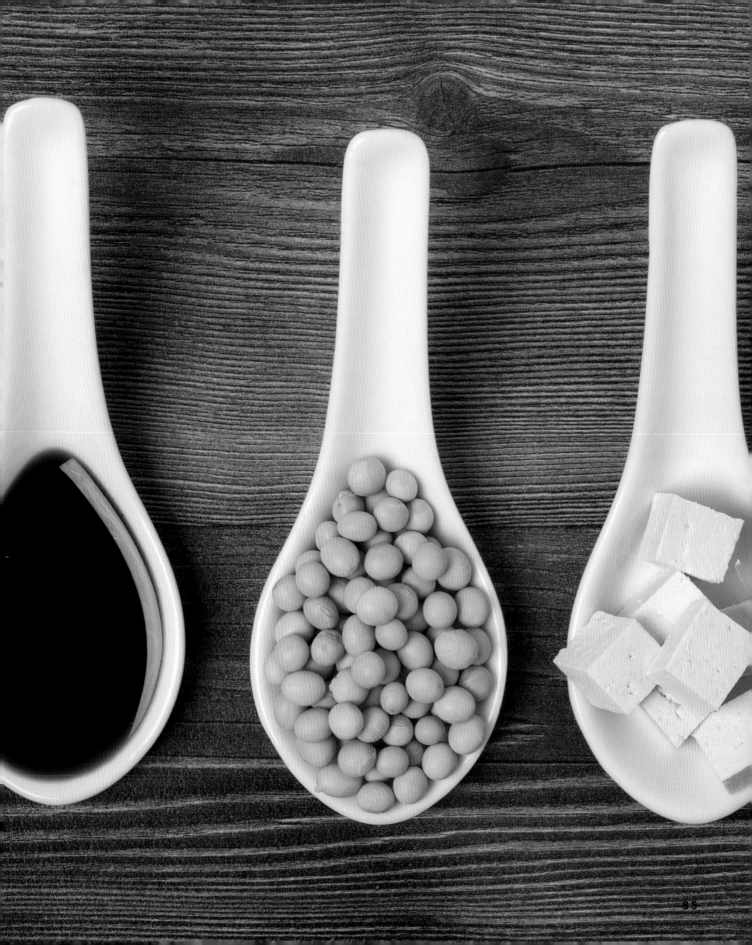

Artificial Additives and Sweeteners

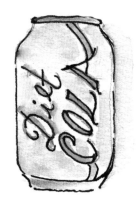

Artificial additives and sweeteners add nothing sweet to your diet, let me tell you! They are a noxious blend of chemicals and general all round nastiness that will do weird stuff to your palette, upset your body's biochemistry and have the potential to seriously damage your health. The good news is that there is real food, glorious fresh food, out there that you can eat instead of a bunch of chemicals!

If you want to improve your health by eliminating toxins and artificial additives from your body, then the answer is simple: eat clean, wholefoods that are prepared from fresh ingredients, rather than food-like products made in a factory by a bunch of scientists.

So steel yourselves and read on for the facts on artificial additives and sweeteners, which I hope will send you running to your pantry for a purge on any packaged foods!

ARTIFICIAL ADDITIVES

Artificial additives are made from chemicals for the purpose of preserving a foods' shelf life, enhance its flavour, texture or colour, or to artificially sweeten it.

WHAT'S UP WITH ARTIFICIAL ADDITIVES?

Lots of things! For a start, they contain chemicals with links to a long list of health conditions, including learning and behavioural disorders (hyperactivity) in children. This link was confirmed in a 2005 study by researchers at Liverpool University in the UK which identified the harmful effects of artificial additives including aspartame, msg, and artificial colours on the nervous system. Artificial additives can also trigger allergies and headaches, negatively impact on liver function and cause weight gain.

HOW TO AVOID ARTIFICIAL ADDITIVES

If you eat processed or packaged foods, then it's almost guaranteed that you are consuming artificial additives in the form of preservatives, flavours, colours and, of course, the dreaded artificial sweeteners.

One of the best tips I can offer for eliminating artificial additives and processed foods from your diet is to 'shop the perimeter' of your supermarket, because nearly all processed, packaged foods are located in the middle aisles, designed to lure you deeper into the processed food vortex, whilst fresh wholefoods are usually located around the edges of the store.

A good rule of thumb for identifying artificial additives in the ingredients list of packaged food is to look out for names and numbers that essentially sound as if they are from outer space! But if in doubt, pick up a copy of a little book called The Chemical Maze by Bill Statham, for details on every artificial additive and sweetener and start familiarizing yourself with the world of artificial ingredients.

HERE IS A LIST OF THE MOST COMMON, TOXIC AND ALLERGENIC ARTIFICIAL ADDITIVES:

- MSG (E62) monosodium glutamate. Commonly found in many packaged and Chinese foods.

- Sodium Nitrate (250) and nitrite (251). Found in processed and cured meats like bacon, ham, hot dogs, sausages and salami. Look for brands that state 'nitrate free' or 'naturally smoked'.

- Note: Nitrates have been classified as 'probably carcinogenic to humans' by the International Agency for Research of Cancer (IARC). Eek!

- Sulfites (221, 220, 222, 223, 228). These anti-fungal preservatives are found in wine and beer, soft drinks, dried fruit, fruit juice, cordial, wine, potato products and vinegar.

- Food colourings (including E122, E124, E102, E110, E129, E124)

- Preservatives. Look out for Sodium Benzoate (211), used as a preservative and bacteria-destroying agent in diet soft drinks, and (320), added to many commercial brands of breakfast cereal, potato chips, chewing gum and vegetable oils for colour and flavour.

- Potassium bromate (KBrO3). A rising agent used in some brands of bread.

- Trans fat – is made by adding hydrogen to vegetable oil and although these have been banned in Australia, the US will not have banned ALL trans fats from foods until 2018. Although Americans consume 80 percent fewer trans fats than they did a decade ago, there are still some food manufacturers using them. Trans fats are listed as partially hydrogenated oils under the ingredients list. Trans fats are generally found in french fries, battered or fried foods, pastry crust of pies, some brands of ice cream, pancake and waffle mixes, cake mixes and frostings, margarine and shortening, non dairy creamers, crackers, microwave popcorn, canned chilli.

ARTIFICIAL SWEETENERS

Hands up if you have been drinking diet soft drinks or food products sweetened with artificial sweeteners in the belief they're not fattening, or will help you to lose weight? Well I'm sorry to rain on your party, but that's certainly not the case.

WHAT'S UP WITH ARTIFICIAL SWEETENERS

More like, 'What's NOT up with artificial sweeteners!' First off, countless studies have found the consumption of artificial sweeteners can negatively impact on your liver and brain function, increase the risk of obesity, insulin resistance, diabetes, high blood pressure and heart disease, even cancer. Like sugar, artificial sweeteners are highly addictive and will only feed sugar cravings rather than curb them. In fact, artificial sweeteners can make you gain the same or more weight than regular sugar because of the effects of non-caloric sweeteners, like aspartame, saccharin or sucralose on the physiology of your brain, inducing hormonal responses that lower metabolizm rate and increase appetite. This finding was detailed in a study published in 2013 in which rats fed artificially-sweetened yoghurt gained more weight and greater body fat than rats that ate sugar-sweetened yoghurt, even though they consumed fewer calories overall.

But the effect of artificial sweeteners doesn't stop at your brain, hips and thighs. A report published in The American Journal of Industrial Medicine in April 2014, concluded that there was, 'enough evidence to support the potential carcinogenic effects of aspartame to warrant an international re-evaluation of aspartame's safety as an urgent matter of public health.'

So I think the evidence pretty well speaks for itself in the case against artificial sweeteners — making them a definite 'no go zone'.

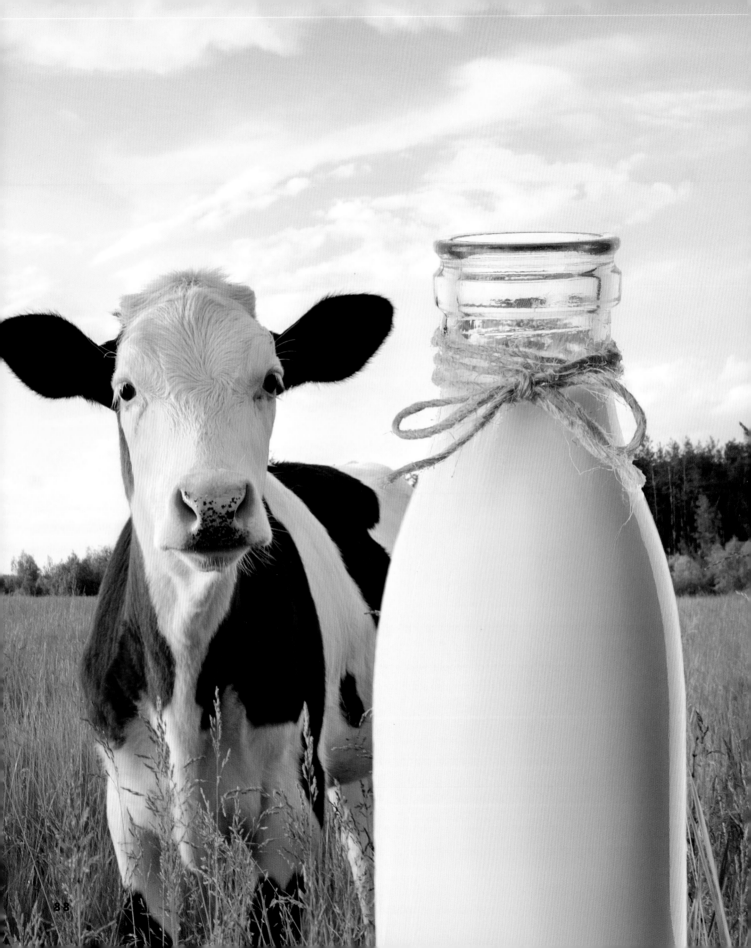

Cow's Dairy

The debate over whether humans should consume cow's dairy is up there with soy. My advice is to allow your body to do the talking, as it will never lie, or sway you because of a vested interest!

THE PROBLEM WITH COW JUICE

The truth is, we are the only mammal to drink the milk of another, and cow's dairy is a common cause of irritation to the gut for many. An intolerance to cow's dairy can be expressed in the form of a wide range of ailments, including stomach cramps, diarrhea, catarrh, sinus congestion, eczema, acne, sleep and behavioral changes in children, even asthma.

A 20 year study reported in the New Zealand Journal Of Medicine in 2003, stated that consumption of conventional cow's milk containing the A1 beta-casein protein, was significantly and positively correlated with type 1 diabetes in 20 affluent countries. Five international cohort studies found significant associations between cow's dairy consumption and the incidence of prostate cancer. One particular study involving nearly 4000 men found those who consumed five or more servings of cow's dairy per week, were more likely to suffer from prostate cancer than those who ate one serving or less. So what is it about cow's dairy that doesn't agree with human health?

IMMUNOLOGICAL 'CROSS REACTIVITY'

It is estimated that at least 50% of people who are sensitive to gluten, commonly find they are also sensitive to cow's dairy, due to a 'cross reactivity' process known as molecular mimicry. Proteins found in cow's milk, (namely casein) have similarities to the gluten protein present in grains like wheat, so when you consume a 'cross-reactive' food like cow's dairy, it can irritate and inflame the immune system as if gluten was being ingested.

LACTOSE

Lactose is the naturally occurring sugar in cow's dairy and is a common cause of digestive complaints for many who lack the enzyme to digest it. But as you'll see below, there are reasons beyond lactose intolerance to avoid cow's dairy.

ANTIBIOTICS, HORMONES, PASTEURISATION AND HOMOGENISATION

Just as wheat and many of the grains we eat today have been altered, compared to the form our ancestors ate, the way we now consume cow's dairy is also vastly different from the milk we drank when it came straight from Betty, the backyard cow. Today cow's milk is a mass-produced commodity, and a powerful, multibillion-dollar industry. With mass production comes intensive farming methods that not only alter a food's nutritional value, but also come with a lot of unwanted extras. These include residual levels of antibiotics, and in the case of US dairy cattle, growth hormones like rBST, recombinant bovine somatotropin, and genetically modified feed such as corn. It is worth noting that Australia forbids the use of the rBST hormone in dairy cattle. Although some research argues the residual levels of antibiotics and hormones in cow's dairy are too low to impact human health long-term, there have been no well-controlled population studies to explore the possibility of risks from hormones in food-producing animals, largely because they are too difficult and expensive to conduct.

Mass production of cow's milk also saw the introduction of pasteurization and homogenization, intended to produce bacteria-free, smooth pouring milk, with a longer shelf life. The heating process of pasteurisation also kills off any friendly bacteria cultures and delicate enzymes, altering the structure of the milk proteins and compromising its nutritional value.

Homogenization also increases the portion of casein and whey proteins, which may account for the increased allergenicity of modern processed milk. So what was once a gut friendly food is now little more than the cause of many health problems, rather than a source of valuable nutrition in my professional view.

THE 'DAIRY FOR CALCIUM' MYTH

The main nutritional argument for consuming cow's dairy is for maintaining strong bones, but the reality is you can easily meet your dietary calcium needs through plenty of other foods, including nuts and seeds and green leafy vegetables without the consumption of cow's dairy. A 2005 review published in Pediatrics showed that milk consumption does not improve bone integrity in children, and the Harvard Nurses' Health Study, which followed more than 72,000 women for 18 years, showed no protective effect of increased milk consumption on fracture risk. The real key to maintaining healthy bones is in fact Vitamin D, but the problem is few foods naturally contain vitamin D. Vitamin D deficiency is now a worldwide epidemic, being blamed as responsible for everything from increased rates of cancer to depression. Vitamin D deficiency also leaches calcium from muscles and bones, increasing the risk of bone weakness, fractures, and osteoporosis.

It's essential to obtain vitamin D from safe sun exposure - five to fifteen minutes of sun each day, without sunscreen, depending on your skin tone. Without sufficient vitamin D levels, only 10-15 percent of dietary calcium is absorbed, so considering many of us don't get our healthy dose of daily sun exposure, I recommend supplementing with a combination of Vitamin D and K2 in liquid or capsule form for maximum cellular absorption, especially in winter.

RAW MILK

Many health experts are now arguing for a return to raw milk, which is milk in its natural unprocessed state, because it's such a rich source of nutrition, complete with naturally occurring immunoglobulins, enzymes and live friendly bacteria cultures. Raw milk was banned, and pasteurization introduced with the mass production of milk, because of the increased incidence of bacterial infection, and this is when milk stopped being the complete food it once was.

You may find your gut can tolerate the consumption of raw milk products, without triggering any inflammation or digestive related problems, but I recommend avoiding even raw milk in the first 28 days of the LYG program, and be sure to test your tolerance by introducing it slowly and in isolation of the other foods I recommend you avoid. Many people who can't tolerate conventional pasteurized milk due to lactose intolerance find they can tolerate a little raw cow's milk because it contains a natural enzyme lactase, which digests the milk sugar lactose

A1 VERSUS A2 MILK

Setting aside the argument over raw vs pasteurized and homogenized cow's dairy, there's another contender in the great dairy debate - 'A2' cow's milk. You see, not only did we change the way milk was produced, but we also changed the species of cow we got it from. Milk from Jersey and Guernsey cows, goat, sheep, buffalo, and Asian cowsis naturally richer in the A2 beta-casein protein, but in the 1970s the dairy industry switched to using Holstein and Friesian cows, because they are bigger and better milk producers. But these cows produce milk predominantly high in the A1 beta-casein protein.

The difference between conventional 'A1' milk and 'A2' milk, lies in the chemical structure of the beta-casein proteins, which determines how they impact on our health. The A1 beta-casein protein found predominantly in conventional milk contains a peptide known as BCM-7. The significance of this peptide is that whilst it's not significantly absorbed into the bloodstream of people with healthy GI tracts, BCM7 has been shown to significantly affect people with compromised gut function, including autistic children, and people with other neurological conditions, auto immune conditions, or anyone with a leaky gut, because it has proinflammatory opiate - like properties. Opioids in the gut may affect bowel motility and the absorption processes, making the A1 beta-casein protein, gluten's partner-in-crime. Its similar structure and effect on gut health in sensitive individuals may result in diarrhoea, constipation, gas and bloating, headaches and migraines ,and skin conditions like dermatitis and eczema.

But it seems the inflammatory effects of the A1 beta-casein protein may go beyond our gut. Multiple studies are revealing populations which consume milk containing high levels of the β-casein A2 variant, found in goats and sheep milk, have a lower incidence of cardiovascular disease and Type 1 diabetes compared to those countries that consume milk containing the A1 beta-casein protein.

So until the jury is out on the safety of long term consumption of conventional milk containing the A1 protein, if you choose to consume cow's milk, my tip is to go for a brand of full fat, A2 milk (commercial producers of A2 milk are yet to release an organic, non-homogenised variety), or, if you can access it legally, organic raw milk - preferably from cows that predominantly carry the A2 protein. But again, I recommend waiting at least 28 days before re-introducing either of these forms of cow's dairy back into your diet to allow sufficient time for any food intolerance symptoms to settle

WHAT ABOUT BUTTER?

Despite what Fabio says, there's nothing wrong with including a little pure, organic butter in your diet, because it's so low in casein compared to milk. Alternatively, substitute butter with fresh olive oil or use avocado as a spread instead. But, whatever you do, don't go buying spreadable butter blends, as these contain dreaded vegetable oils like canola and soy. Instead, simply make your own by blending a little extra virgin olive or macadamia oil with your butter.

The best fats to cook with are virgin coconut or macadamia nut oil, or ghee. Because extra virgin olive oil has a lower smoke point, it's best to use it fresh over salads and steamed vegetables, or add to homemade mayonnaise, sauces and dips. If you do cook with olive oil,use it on low to moderate heat to avoid

oxidizing it, and like all oils, store it away from direct sunlight in a glass, airtight bottle, and use within three to four weeks for maximum freshness.

WHY LOW FAT DAIRY IS NOT LOW-FATTENING

If you think you're doing your hips and heart health a favour eating low fat or skim dairy products, think again, because by removing the fat you're left with the naturally occurring sugar – lactose - and with less or no fat left, low fat and skim dairy products can actually be more fattening. They are far less filling, so you're likely to eat more than you would a serve of full fat dairy. If you choose to eat any form of dairy, be sure to steer clear of low fat varieties and always go for full fat, organic varieties and never choose fruit flavoured yoghurts, as these are laden with sugar.

WHAT ABOUT SHEEP & GOAT'S DAIRY?

I find many people who cannot tolerate cow's dairy have no reaction to dairy from goats or sheep, or even buffalo. Milk from sheep or goats is much easier to digest than cow's milk, because they produce milk predominantly higher in the A2 beta casein protein. Goat and sheep's milk also does not contain the BCM7 peptide. The casein in goat's milk is also more similar to human milk, which is also classified as A2 milk and may explain why it's better tolerated, especially in young children who react to cow's milk.

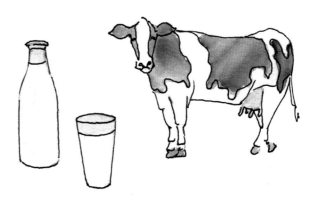

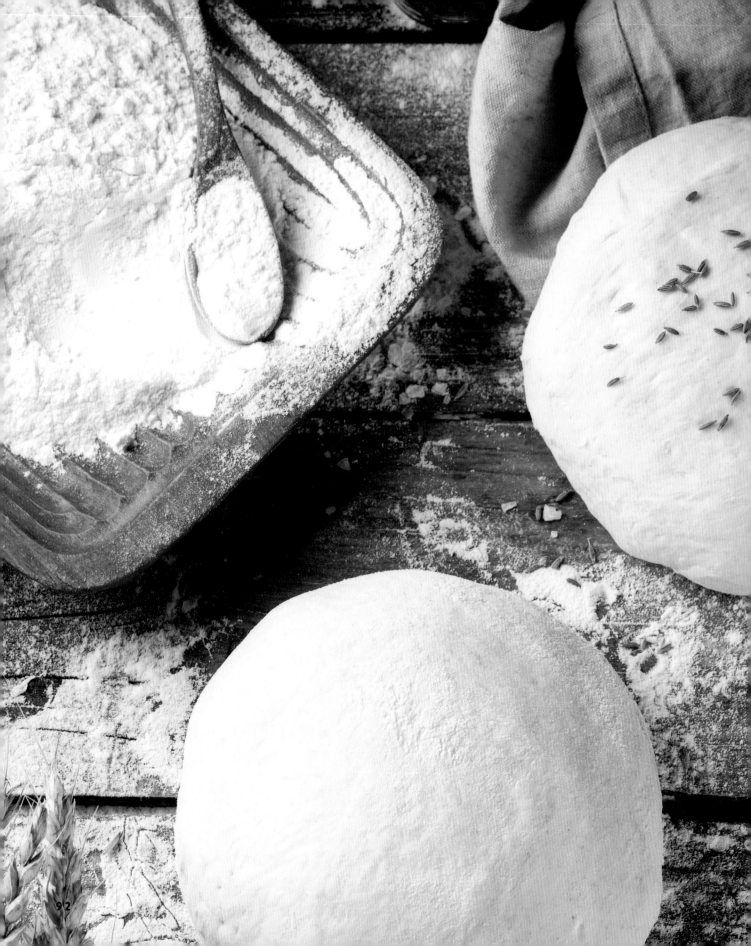

Yeast

Yeasts are a form of fungi, but not all sources of yeast are bad for us, or feed Candida Albicans. There are also beneficial yeasts contained in probiotic foods, which can help to knock out some bacterial infections and control Candida by feeding your good gut flora colonies. The reason I want you to avoid the food sources of 'bad yeast' below is to help restore the balance of your gut flora by eliminating excess Candida. Many food sources of bad yeast also contain gluten, sugar and artificial additives.

BENEFICIAL SOURCES OF YEAST...

- Naturally-fermented foods such as cultured vegetables
- Kefir
- Yoghurt (sugar-free, non-cow's dairy)
- Probiotic supplements
- Saccharomyces Boulardii – a 'friendly' yeast found in supplement form that acts as a natural prebiotic and helps reduce the growth of Candida

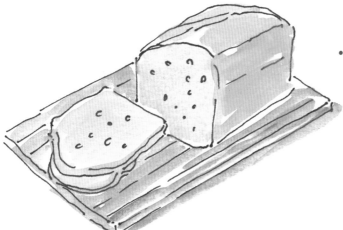

SOURCES OF YEAST TO AVOID ...

- Bread, including sourdough (Baker's yeast)
- Vegemite, beer, distilled spirits, cider (Brewer's yeast)
- Soy sauce, miso, tamari and tempeh
- Nutritional yeast (also known as yeast flakes)
- Salad dressings, seasonings on potato and corn chips, stocks and bouillon cubes (yeast extracts)
- MSG
- Balsamic, red or white wine vinegar, or vinegar added to pickles, mayonnaise, chutneys
- Certain fermented or ripe foods - these can harbor a form of naturally occurring yeast such as on (very) ripe fruit and vegetables, dried fruit, barely malt, peanuts, buttermilk, cow's dairy products, ripe cheeses, or any food that has been opened and stored for a long period, for example jams may develop yeast on the surface.
- Kombucha tea can contain wild airborne yeast, which can harbour Candida Albicans (despite also containing beneficial yeast) so I recommend avoiding this initially if you have a chronic problem with Candida overgrowth.

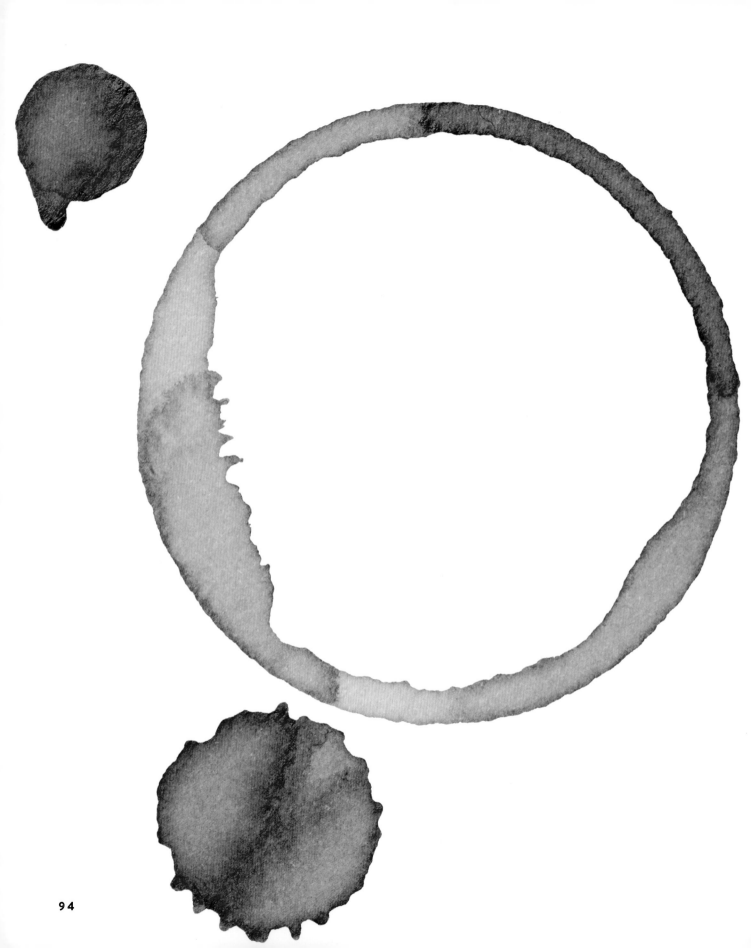

Alcohol

To put it bluntly, alcohol is a toxin, which is why it is metabolized differently by the body compared to food, bypassing normal digestion where it goes straight to the liver. The liver prioritises the elimination of alcohol over food, so while there is alcohol in your system, your liver will not effectively process and digest your food. So if you are trying to lose weight or even just maintain your ideal weight, drinking alcohol is one of your worst enemies, being a trigger for inflammation and causing impairment of your liver and brain function.

Additionally, one of the primary functions of the liver is to process toxins for elimination from your body, but if you overstress it with toxins like alcohol, your liver's natural detoxification mechanism becomes compromised. This will lead to a buildup of toxins in your body – a sure fire way to accelerate aging and disease, reduce your libido and to gain weight!

Alcohol is made by fermenting sugar and fruits, such as grapes to make wine, apples to make cider and grains to make beer and spirits, or potatoes in the case of some vodkas. The fermentation and distillation process converts the sugar to alcohol, also removing any gluten from spirits, but not from beer! Whilst wine and straight spirits contain very low amounts of sugar, this does not mean they contain no calories, so they can still be fattening. Wine and beer in particular can feed the growth of Candida within your gut. Cocktails and pre-mixed alcoholic drinks

on the other hand, are generally loaded with sugar, thanks to the added sugar syrup, fruit juice or sodas like coca cola with rum, tonic with gin, or ginger ale mixed with scotch. A 375 ml can of gin and tonic, for example, contains around five teaspoons of sugar whereas a rum and coca cola can contain up to 10 teaspoons of sugar!

Alcoholic beverages like wine and beer also contain artificial preservatives, which many people have an intolerance or allergy to. Symptoms associated with preservatives in alcohol include headaches, sinus, hay fever, skin rashes, acne and behavioural changes. So if you really want to get your gut health and liver function shipshape, then I recommend kicking the bottle for at least 28 days, and you will look and feel so much better!

If and when you do consume alcohol again, I recommend sticking to organic wines and sugarless mixers with gluten-free spirits like vodka mixed with soda water and fresh lime or lemon. If you insist on returning to beer, try a gluten-free beer, or at the very least, stick with a brand that is preservative free.

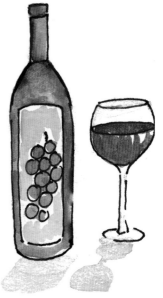

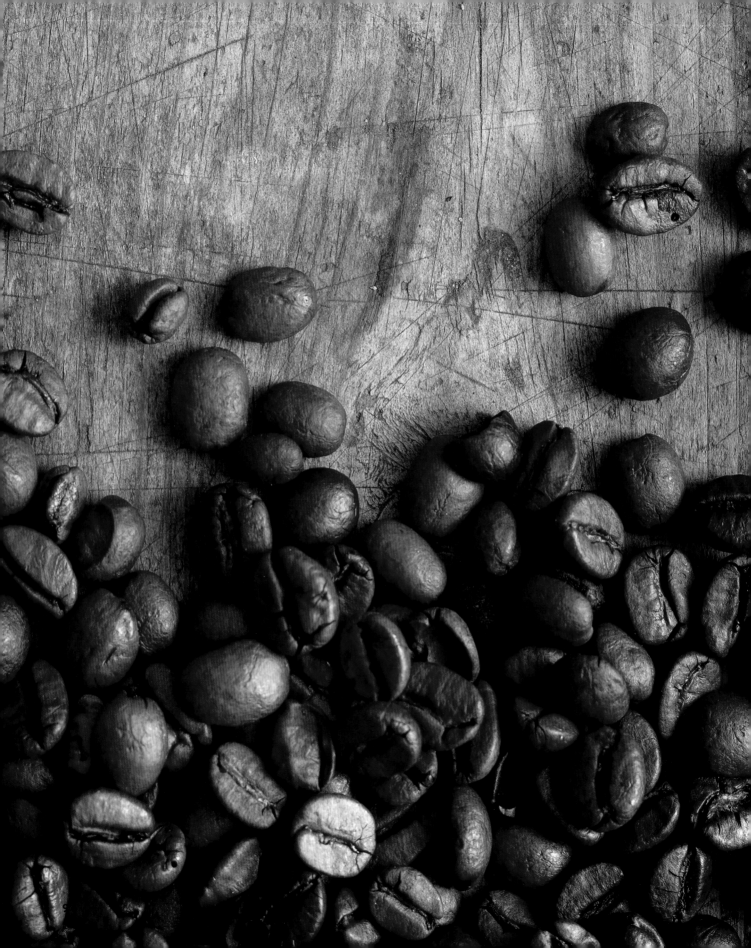

Caffeine

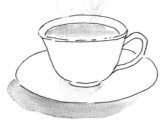

Now I know, coffee tastes delicious. I love it too! But the problem is that your liver, gut and adrenals may not be loving this daily ritual in quite the same way as your taste buds. Caffeine is actually a drug and, although it may be a socially acceptable one, because of its addictiveness our body requires more and more over time, in order to experience the energy boost so many of us crave. So let's use the next 28 days to give your body a break from the stimulating effects of caffeine.

If you've been turning to coffee for your morning pick-me-up because you're lacking the natural energy to get going in the morning, or you typically experience an energy slump in the afternoon, this can be an indication of a deficiency in essential nutrients, in particular B vitamins and minerals like iron and magnesium. These nutrients are required by your body for the production of natural energy, and drinking coffee or caffeinated soft drinks is not the answer to this problem, and will only make it worse!

Caffeine can also put a strain on your adrenal glands by stimulating the production of the stress hormones adrenalin and cortisol. Over time excess cortisol production begins to take its toll on your body, a little bit like the effect of driving a car in first gear at high speed all day – you wouldn't drive your car this way, knowing the wear and tear it would have on the engine, so why do it to your precious body? It's not like you can just trade it in if it falls apart!

Furthermore, caffeine is treated as a toxin by the liver and is metabolized differently by each individual, so for some people caffeine can contribute to insomnia, irritability and even anxiety. Compounds in coffee can also interfere with the metabolism of certain medications and normal detoxification processes in the liver, and another little known fact is that coffee crops are some of the most heavily sprayed with chemical pesticides in the world!

Habitual coffee consumption can decrease your sensitivity to insulin, making it difficult for your cells to respond appropriately to blood sugar. Elevated blood sugar levels are linked to an increased risk of Type 2 diabetes and cardiovascular disease.

Coffee is also highly acidic and can upset your gut, causing loose bowels or diarrhoea, indigestion and heartburn.

So whilst there is no denying that coffee in fact carries some proven health benefits, your body is not designed to consume it the way many of us do – in excess! Nor is its purpose to get you out of bed in the morning.

The other thing to consider about coffee consumption is the milk and sugar you might be adding. If your daily coffee ritual involves chugging down a couple of large lattes with an added sugar or two, then you're only adding fuel to the fire. And your poor old adrenals and gut will not be feeling as happy as you from your caffeine high.

So my suggestion is to give the caffeine a break for a while, in order to focus on getting your gut health and adrenals sorted, and this will help to leave you feeling brand spanking new again! If you're worried about the side effects of going cold turkey with caffeine, try cutting back gradually over a week to ten days, (depending on your level of consumption), to soften the blow from any potential headaches and fatigue. I also recommend you switch to a piccolo or espresso size - that way you'll also be cutting back on the milk and you may as well just ditch the added sugar straight up! Remember to drink plenty of water to help your liver process the caffeine more effectively for elimination.

Healthy Coffee Alternatives

Don't freak out about losing your morning ritual or your excuse for a break from the office, because there are plenty of healthy coffee alternatives you can try. Use the next 28 days to explore the world of amazing herbal teas and I know you'll find one you like!

HERE ARE A FEW OF MY FAVOURITES:

CHAI TEA - this soothing blend of aromatic spices mixed with black tea is a delicious option if you're craving a warm creamy beverage. I make mine with frothed sugar-free almond or coconut milk and sprinkle with fresh cinnamon on top see page 315.

DANDELION TEA – personally I think this is the closest flavour to coffee and it's great for supporting your liver function! It tastes delicious mixed with unsweetened almond or coconut milk, and I love adding raw cacao powder for a mocha-type flavour. Check out my Dande Mocha recipe on page 319.

FRESH LEMONGRASS, GINGER AND MINT TEA - the perfect anti inflammatory combination, I think you may develop a daily habit for this combo. I brew up a pot using fresh ingredients for the ultimate flavour, and drink warm or iced ,depending on the weather. See recipe on page 313.

BLACK AND GREEN TEA - like coffee, black and green tea also contain caffeine. However, unlike coffee, they contain an amino acid called 'L-Theanine' which has a calming effect on the nervous system. I actually prescribe L-Theanine in supplement form when treating patients with anxiety and nervous tension. It is because of the calming effects of L-Theanine that we don't experience the stimulation or shakes that can occur with drinking coffee or other sources of caffeine.

GOLDEN MYLK - made from fresh turmeric and black pepper, it not only tastes delicious, but this beverage also acts as a natural anti-inflammatory and helps your liver to eliminate toxins from your body. See recipe on page 316.

DECAF COFFEE – Switching to decaf coffee from caffeinated is not always a healthy alterative, due to the process used to extract the caffeine. A lot of decaf coffee brands have undergone a decaffeinating process known as 'Direct Process' which uses the chemical methyl chloride to remove the caffeine. The National Cancer Institute of America lists methyl chloride as a possible carcinogen. If you really want to drink decaf coffee, go for an organic brand that has undergone the Swiss water process, as it only uses water, but be sure to avoid adding cow's dairy and sugar.

Other 'Not So Nice Foods' To Lose

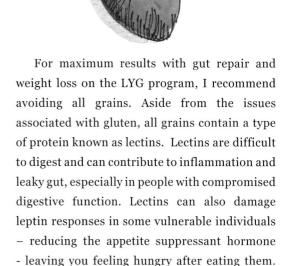

In the case of suffering a chronic illness, or inflammatory condition like IBS or arthritis, or if you're struggling to lose weight on the LYG program, you may find it necessary to avoid these additional foods, especially in the initial stages of the gut repair process.

NIGHTSHADES

These are a group of vegetables that include:

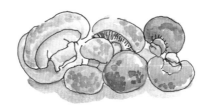

- Tomatoes
- Eggplant
- Mushroom
- White Potato
- Capsicum

The purpose of avoiding the nightshade group of vegetables relates to cases of severe Candida overgrowth and other inflammatory conditions. Nightshade vegetables can feed the growth of the Candida fungus and irritate the gut, because they contain a compound known as solanin. Some people find the nightshade group of vegetables can exacerbate arthritis, as well as other chronic inflammatory based illnesses like autoimmunity and autism. If you fit into any of these categories, experiment with eliminating these vegetables along with the 8 essential foods to avoid, and note if your symptoms improve.

GRAINS

These include:

- Wheat
- Rye
- Kamut
- Spelt
- Oats
- Rice
- Corn
- Millet

For maximum results with gut repair and weight loss on the LYG program, I recommend avoiding all grains. Aside from the issues associated with gluten, all grains contain a type of protein known as lectins. Lectins are difficult to digest and can contribute to inflammation and leaky gut, especially in people with compromised digestive function. Lectins can also damage leptin responses in some vulnerable individuals – reducing the appetite suppressant hormone - leaving you feeling hungry after eating them. Grains are also high in starch which can contribute to excess weight gain.

Acceptable grains on the LYG program include buckwheat, amaranth and quinoa, because they are technically not grains, but what's referred to as pseudo grains. You may need to avoid these pseudo grains initially, especially in cases of neurological disorders, insulin resistance and Type 2 diabetes. When you do try introducing them, I recommend soaking them in water overnight with a splash of apple cider vinegar before cooking them, or you can try sprouting or fermenting them, to make them more 'gut friendly'.

High FODMAPS

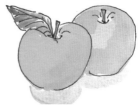

In addition to the '8 foods I recommend you avoid' on the LYG program, it may necessary for some people with bad IBS or Fructose Malabsroption syndrome to also avoid foods high in FODMAPS - Fermentable Oligosaccharides, Disaccharides, Monosaccharides And Polyols. FODMAPS are short-chain carbohydrates that are incompletely absorbed in the gastrointestinal tract and can be easily fermented by gut bacteria, causing excess gas, bloating, diarrhoea and abdominal cramping. I have not ensured all my recipes on the LYG program are low FODMAPS, because it is only necessary for those suffering pretty acute IBS and or Fructose Malabsorption Syndrome to eliminate these high FODMAPS foods from their diet. You can easily adjust any of my recipes to be low FODMAPS. For a full list of low, medium and high FODMAPS foods; additional low FODMAPS recipes and information on following a low FODMAPS diet, I recommend downloading the Monash University Low FODMAPS app. Below is a list of all the high FODMAPS foods.

VEGETABLES & LEGUMES

Asparagus

Beans – broad, kidney, lima, soya

Broccoli and broccolini

Cabbage - savoy

Cauliflower

Cassava

Chicory root

Choko

Corn - sweet

Garlic

Leek bulb

Mushrooms

Onions

Snow Peas

Sweet potato

Taro

Scallions/spring onions/shallots - bottoms only

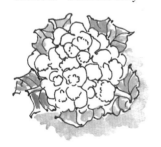

FRUITS

Apples

Apricot

Avocado

Blackberries

Boysenberry

Cherries

Custard apple

Dates

Fresh coconut water

Fresh figs

Grapefruit

Guava

Lychee

Mango

Nectarine

Papaya

Peaches

Pears

Plums

Pomegranate

Raisins

Sultanas

Tamarillo

Watermelon

NUTS & SEEDS

Almonds

Cashews

Pistachio

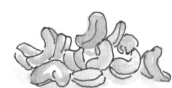

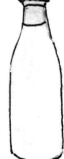

DAIRY

Cow's milk

Goat Milk

Sheep's milk

Soy milk

Butter milk

Cream

Custard

Greek yoghurt

Ice cream

Sour cream

Yoghurt

Cream cheese

Cottage cheese

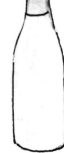

High FODMAPS

 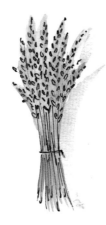 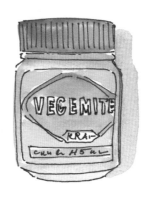 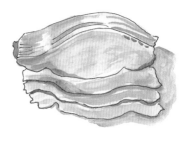

SWEETENERS

Agave

Honey

High Fructose Corn Syrup

Inulin

Isomalt

Malitol

Mannitol

Sorbitol

Xylitol

GRAINS

Barley

Bran

Couscous

Gnocchi

Granola

Muesli

Muffins

Rye

Semolina

Spelt

Wheat

CONDIMENTS

Hummus

Jam

Relish

Tzatziki dip

MEAT SUBSTITUTES

Sausages and chorizo

Processed meat – ham, salami, bacon

Swap it don't drop it

Just because you have to eliminate certain foods, it doesn't mean you can't replace them with a far healthier and delicious alternative! See my quick reference guide below:

Swap regular wheat bread for grain free Paleo bread (page 142.) or gluten free bread made from sprouted grains

Swap rice for cauliflower rice (page 216)

Swap potato chips for baked sweet potato chips (page 180) or kale chips (page 179)

Swap white mashed potato for cauliflower mash, (page 216) pumpkin or sweet potato

Swap pasta for zucchini or summer squash noodles (page 241), or simple quinoa (page 254)

Swap breakfast cereal and toasted muesli for grain free granola (page 149)

Swap oat porridge for quinoa porridge (page150) or chia seed pudding (page 167)

Swap soft drinks / sodas and fruit juice for green vegetable juice (page 163), mineral water with fresh lemon and mint or cucumber

Swap sugar for rice malt syrup, dextrose, stevia or xylitol

Swap cow's milk for unsweetened nut (page 148), coconut milk (page 139) or goat's milk

Swap cow's cheese and yoghurt for sheep, goat or coconut yoghurt, or kefir

Swap ice cream for coconut ice cream (page 309)

Swap coffee for dandelion coffee (page 319), herbal or chai tea (page 315)

Swap fruit juice for fresh whole fruit

Swap dried fruit for goji berries

Swap vegetable oils for coconut, olive, or macadamia oil

Swap margarine for ghee or cultured butter

Swap deep fried chicken for baked organic chicken (page 235)

Swap processed meats – salami, ham and bacon for grass fed roast beef, organic roast turkey or free range, nitrate free bacon

Swap peanut butter for almond butter (page 175)

Swap refined salt for Himalayan or sea salt

Swap wheat flour for coconut and almond flour

GUT HEALING FOODS

Many natural whole foods can help to heal your gut, maintain a healthy balance in your good gut flora colonies, boost immunity and combat inflammation — this is what is referred to as using 'food as medicine'. Below are my favourite gut healing foods. I encourage you to incorporate some of these into your diet every day.

Bone Broth – see page 189

Fermented Vegetables – see page 288

Grass Fed bovine collagen powder

Turmeric – see page 316

Garlic – see page 329

Kefir – see page 329

Apple Cider Vinegar – see page 75

Green Vegetable Juice – see page 163

Lemon – see page 75

Peppermint Oil – see page 313

Building A Healthy Pantry

You've probably got some of these items in your pantry already. But you can use this list to top up any missing items to build on your healthy pantry. For those of you starting from scratch, here is a handy shopping list to help you get started.

When shopping, be sure to read your labels on the back and check your nutritional panel for grams of sugar- remember its best to avoid any products containing more than six grams per 100 grams or mls. And if you are wondering about which foods to buy organic – and what's not so important – then check out my recommendations for this on page 115.

Keep your pantry stocked with these goodies and you'll have all the basics on hand to cook up most of the yummy recipes in this book.

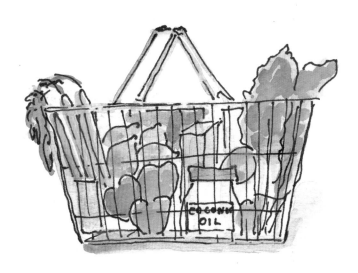

FATS AND OILS

Virgin coconut oil (avoid odourless)

Extra virgin olive oil (avoid 'light')

Macadamia oil

Sesame oil

Organic pure butter

Ghee

FLOURS

Almond flour

Coconut flour

White rice flour

CONDIMENTS

Nut butter – almond/cashew/ABC* spread

Whole egg mayonnaise

*Almond, brazil nut and cashew butter

Apple Cider Vinegar for salad dressings and as a digestive aid

SUPERFOODS

Raw cacao powder

Raw cacao nibs

Goji berries

Maca root powder

Spirulina

TEAS

Green tea

Peppermint tea

Ginger and lemongrass tea

Licorice tea

Rooibos

Your favourite herbal tea

HERBS & SPICES

Cinnamon

Nutmeg

Ginger

Cumin

Caraway seeds

Cayenne pepper

Cardamom pods

Dried Rosemary

Turmeric

All spice

Black peppercorns

Celtic sea or Himalayan salt

Mixed herbs

NUTS & SEEDS

Make sure you these raw and unsalted

Almonds

Cashews

Brazil

Walnuts

Macadamia

Pepitas

Sesame seeds

Sunflower seeds

Chia seeds

Quinoa

Dried coconut (shredded and/or desiccated coconut flakes)

COW'S DAIRY ALTERNATIVES

Sheep's yoghurt (plain)

Coconut yoghurt (plain)

Nut milks (tetra pack)

eg: cashew, almond or coconut - must be unsweetened and carrageenan free

Goat's cheese

Sheep's cheese

Haloumi Cheese (made from sheep's milk if possible)

Eggs

DRY GOODS

Stock – organic liquid, yeast free

Baking powder – gluten free

Olives (in brine or oil)

Canned Goods

Coconut milk

Coconut cream

Brown lentils

Navy beans

Chickpeas - if tolerated

Adzuki beans - if tolerated

Capers

Tuna

Salmon

Anchovies

Sardines

FRESH FOOD ESSENTIALS

Avocados

Salad vegetables: lettuce, rocket, baby spinach, celery, cucumber, sprouts – alfalfa and mung beans, beetroots, radish, fennel

Leafy green vegetables: broccoli, beans, spinach, kale, bok choy, snow peas

Sweet potato, pumpkin

Lemons, grapefruit, limes

Young fresh coconuts

Fresh turmeric and ginger

FREEZER ESSENTIALS

Frozen berries

Frozen berries - organic

Frozen Peas

Organic Free-range chicken thighs and/or breasts

Fish fillets (fresh, not crumbed or battered) avoid farmed varieties

Lean red meat (lamb, beef, kangaroo) must be 100% grass fed, hormone and antibiotic free.

NATURAL SWEETENERS

Rice malt syrup

Stevia

Xylitol

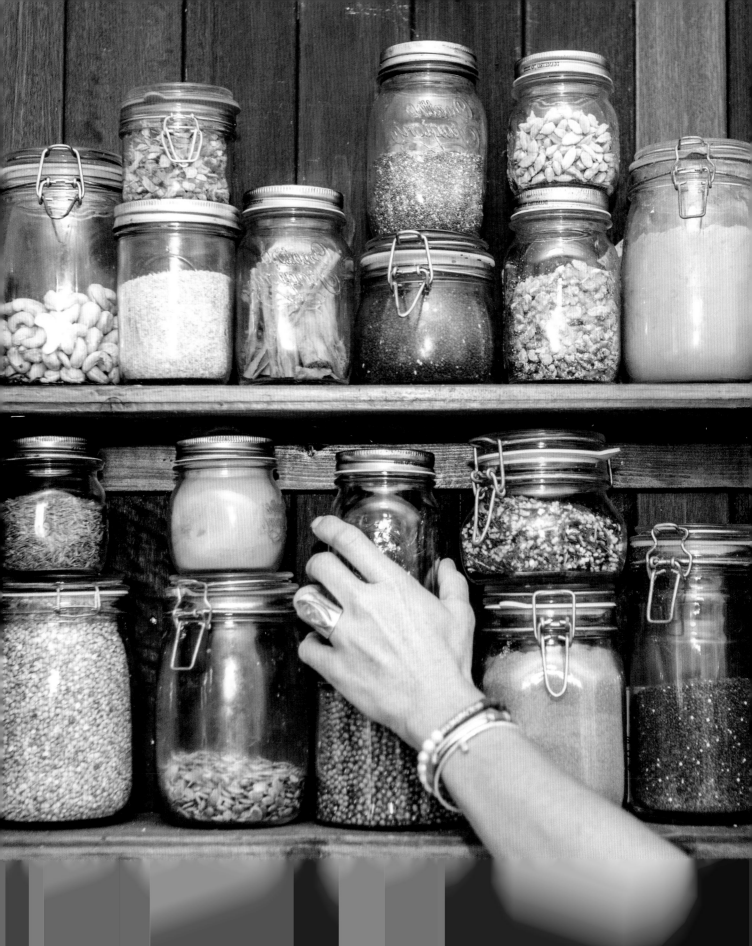

Stage I
Strip Back and
Alkalise Cleanse

WHAT TO EXPECT

Because your body will detox more intensely during this stage, it is not uncommon to experience various side effects. These will vary from each individual, depending on how acidic and inflamed your system is to begin with.

- Light-headedness
- Headaches
- Fatigue
- Changes to your bowel movements
- Nausea
- Skin breakouts
- Aching joints
- Feeling emotional or easily irritated

It's important to take it easy and get plenty of rest as needed during the two week Strip Back and Alkalise stage, because your body will be hard at work offloading the accumulated toxins you decided were a good idea to guzzle, gobble or inhale over the years. If you experience an intense headache or fatigue, I recommend trying a teaspoon of aluminum free bicarbonate of soda in water. This works to naturally alkalise your system and may ease any pain caused by inflammation as you detox, in place of taking pharmaceutical painkillers.

Limit any exercise to simple stretches, light yoga or gentle walks – no more than 45 minutes and consider doing meditation or breathing exercises.

You can decide whether you want to include fish during Stage I, or to stick to vegetarian meals only. Just be sure to only consume wild fish varieties, as opposed to farmed, and limit shellfish or crustaceans to occasional consumption to minimise your exposure to heavy metals, like mercury.

You can, of course, choose to follow Stage I for longer, depending on your desired health goals and existing level of health. If you have a chronic health condition, suffer from particularly bad IBS, chronic constipation or diarrhoea, or you have been consuming a lot of red or white meat, then you may benefit from continuing Stage I for another one to two weeks, or until you feel a significant improvement in your digestion, before progressing onto Stage II. You can consume unlimited herbal teas during the program, except I recommend limiting green tea to one cup per day during 'the detox period, if it is tolerated, due to the caffeine content. Feel free to rearrange any of the recipes from the Stage I meal planner to suit your personal tastes and lifestyle, and remember you can include any other meat free recipes from the book during this period. You can, of course, repeat any of the evening meals for lunch the next day, just as long as you don't get bored, as variety is the spice of life! Be sure to experiment with new recipes that are aligned with the philosophies of the LYG program, and most of all, have fun!

BEFORE YOU START...

I recommend measuring your urinary and salivary pH using litmus paper test strips, (available online or from health food stores or pharmacies), first thing in the morning, before eating or drinking anything. You can continue to do this throughout the LYG program to assess the shift in your body's pH level. As your body starts to become more alkaline, you should see your pH reading shift towards the optimal range of between 7.30 – 7.45. You won't necessarily reach your optimal pH level by the end of the LYG program, as this may take longer to attain, depending how acidic your system is to begin with.

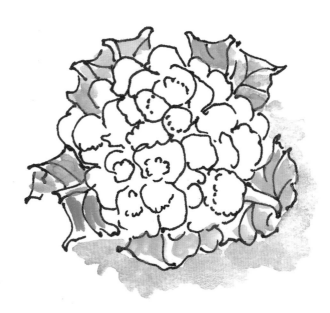

Weeks 1-2 meal planner
(DETOX PERIOD)

MEALS	SUNDAY	MONDAY	TUESDAY
ON WAKING LEMON JUICE, APPLE CIDER VINEGAR & WARM WATER GREEN GODDESS VEGETABLE JUICE PG. 163 METABOLISM BOOSTER PG. 317			
BREAKFAST GREEN GODDESS POWER SMOOTHIE PG. 153 BERRY DELICIOUS SMOOTHIE PG. 144 CHOC COCONUT SMOOTHIE PG. 157 GRAIN-FREE BIRCHER MUESLI PG. 134 CHIA SEED BREAKFAST PUDDING PG.167 GRAIN FREE GRANOLA PG. 149 GRAIN FREE PANCAKES PG. 160			
LUNCH ZUCCHINI NOODLES WITH PESTO PG.241 CAULIFLOWER SOUP PG.198 SALLY'S SUPER FOOD SALAD WITH QUINOA PG.273 ZUCCHINI AND PEA FRITTERS PG.258 ZUCCHINI AND COCONUT CREAM SOUP PG.196 SPINACH AND FENNEL SOUP PG.186 SALMON & KALE FRITTATA PG.214			
DINNER CAULIFLOWER SOUP PG.198 PAN FRIED WHITING FILLETS PG.267 ZUCCHINI NOODLES WITH PESTO PG.241 CAULIFLOWER RICE VEGETABLE STIR FRY PG.264 FISH CAKES WITH GREEN GODDESS DRESSING PG.224 PUMPKIN AND ADZUKI BEAN CASSEROLE PG.230 PRAWN ZUCCHINI LINGUINE PG.228			
SNACKS ½ AVOCADO, WITH FRESH LEMON JUICE, SALT & PEPPER ALMOND HUMMUS WITH CELERY STICKS PG.134 MIXED NUTS AND SEEDS PG. 172 WITH FRESH GINGER LEMONGRASS TEA PG. 313 2 TABLESPOONS OF FERMENTED VEGETABLES PG. 288 1 CUP OF BONE BROTH PG. 189 ROAST BRUSSEL SPROUTS S PG. 267 BEETROOT AND MINT DIP WITH CELERY STICKS PG.169			

Weeks 1-2 meal planner
(DETOX PERIOD)

WEDNESDAY	THURSDAY	FRIDAY	SATURDAY

Stage II weeks 3-4 Maintenance Stage

WHAT TO EXPECT

After you kick start the program with the 2 week Strip Back & Alkalise cleanse, you can start to reintroduce some animal protein from red and white meat, and fish and eggs – if you have been avoiding them. Your body will continue to detox as you will continue to avoid these foods:

- Gluten
- Cow's Dairy
- Sugar
- Soy
- Artificial additives
- Yeast
- Corn
- Alcohol
- Coffee

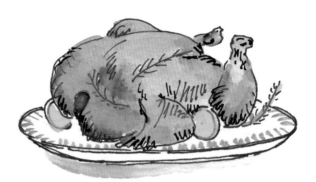

I recommend you use the weeks three to four sample meal planner to guide you on the types of meals and snacks I recommend consuming during this stage and beyond.

Congratulations on making it half way through the 28-day LYG program. Hopefully you are over the worst of any detox symptoms and you are noticing some real improvements in your digestion, energy, sleep and complexion. There's still a way to go with healing your gut, but depending on the size of the job, and how hard your liver has been working, the scales may be looking a little lighter by now. If you're yet to see any significant weight loss, be patient, as your body is still likely to be hard at work, processing unwanted waste and toxins, and your metabolism will start to kick in as your hormones catch up. Stay calm and trust that your body knows exactly what to do to heal now that you're creating a healthy environment to enable it to do so.

HANDY TIPS FOR WEEKS 3 AND 4

When you reintroduce animal protein from red and white meat, it's best to consume them slow-cooked where possible, as this will tenderise the meat, making it easier to digest. If you experience any excess bloating or gas, or a change in your bowel movements, try taking a digestive enzyme and/or a probiotic, and if symptoms persist, it may be that you may have an intolerance to eggs — so try avoiding them for a couple of weeks before re-introducing them.

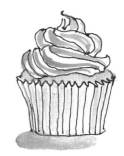

SUGAR CRAVINGS GETTING TO YOU?

Refer back to my 'tips for beating sugar cravings' on page 75 and ensure that you are including enough healthy fats to satisfy your hunger and regulate your blood sugar and insulin levels.

You can try experimenting with a little sweetness over the next couple of weeks by introducing some of my Nothing Naughty Treats, such as the Bellissimo Balls, Nothing Naughty Rocky Road, Choc Coconutty Clusters, Beetroot and Chocolate Brownies, or Coconut Chocolate Mousse, as these are super low in sugar and fructose free, so they shouldn't put you at risk of feeding those sugar demons. After week 4, feel free to celebrate your success on the program with one of my more decadent Nothing Naughty Treats like the Gluten-free Apple Grumble, Flourless Orange Cake or Chocolate Cake.

If you have been incorporating any gut repair supplements from my website, consider starting the probiotic now, but only if you have finished taking any anti-microbial herbs, as these will counteract the probiotic.

Remember, feel free to swap around any of the meals and snacks from the week three and four meal plans to suit your personal tastes and lifestyle, or create your own meal plan from any of my recipes.

Prepare extra portions at dinner time for lunch the next day. This will make it far easier to stick to the program and save you time too.

After a big shop at my local farmers market, or on a Sunday afternoon, I like to cook up a few snacks and soups, or meals that freeze well, to save time in the kitchen during the week.

Make sure you're fitting in some exercise and time out for you. This is SUPER important and all part of your journey towards overhauling your gut and overall health.

Weeks 3-4 Meal Planner
(MAINTENANCE PERIOD)

MEALS	SUNDAY	MONDAY	TUESDAY
ON WAKING LEMON JUICE, APPLE CIDER VINEGAR & WARM WATER GREEN GODDESS VEGETABLE JUICE PG. 163 METABOLISM BOOSTER PG. 317			
BREAKFAST QUINOA COCONUT PORRIDGE PG. 150 CHOC COCONUT SMOOTHIE PG. 157 GOATS FETA AND AVOCADO HERB OMELETTE PG. 146 BERRY DELICIOUS SMOOTHIE PG. 144 GREEN GODDESS POWER SMOOTHIE PG. 153 GRAIN FREE GRANOLA PG. 149 BAKED EGGS W/ SLICED AVOCADO PG.132			
LUNCH HALOUMI AND PAN FRIED WHITING PG.261 CHICKEN QUINOA RISSOLES W/ AVOCADO PG.244 SALLY'S SUPER FOOD SALAD WITH QUINOA PG.273 SPINACH AND FENNEL SOUP PG.254 SIMPLE QUINOA PG.186 QUINOA MINESTRONE SOUP PG.205 CHARGRILLED TUNA NICOISE PG.216			
DINNER ZUCCHINI NOODLES WITH HOMEMADE BOLOGNAISE SAUCE PG.238 HALOUMI AND PAN FRIED WHITING PG.267 LEMON GARLIC AND HERB CHICKEN PG.257 ZUCCHINI AND COCONUT CREAM SOUP PG.196 CAULIFLOWER RICE VEGETABLE AND CHICKEN STIR FRY PG.264 ROAST CHICKEN WITH FIG & STUFFING PG.235 SLOW COOKED LAMB SHANKS PG.223			
SNACKS KALE CHIPS PG. 179 ALMOND HUMMUS W/ CELERY STICKS PG.134 ACTIVATED NUT TRAIL MIX W/ FRESH GINGER LEMONGRASS TEA PG. 172/313 2 TABLESPOONS OF FERMENTED VEGETABLES PG. 288 ALMOND NUT BUTTER WITH CELERY STICKS PG. 175 1 CUP OF BONE BROTH PG. 189 1 BELLISIMO BALL PG.307			

Weeks 3-4 Meal Planner
(MAINTENANCE PERIOD)

WEDNESDAY	THURSDAY	FRIDAY	SATURDAY

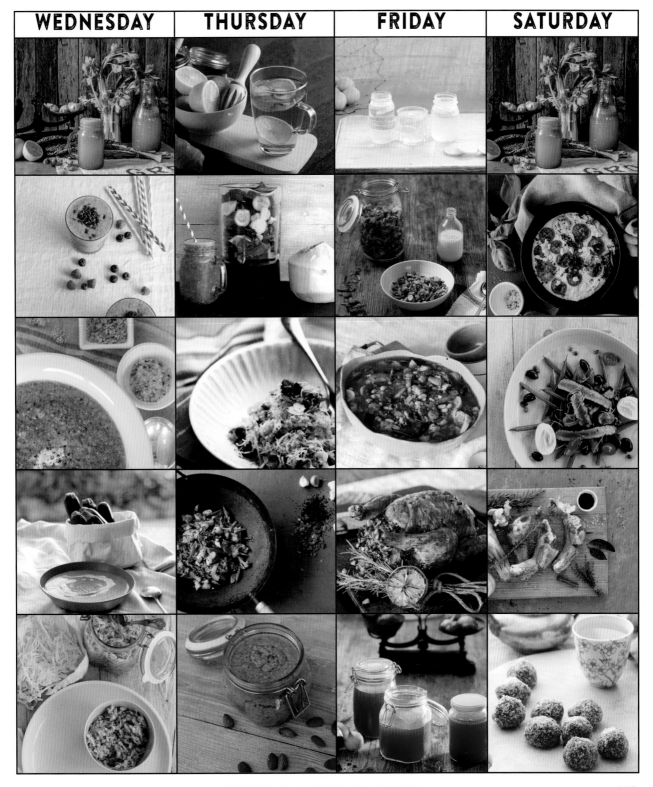

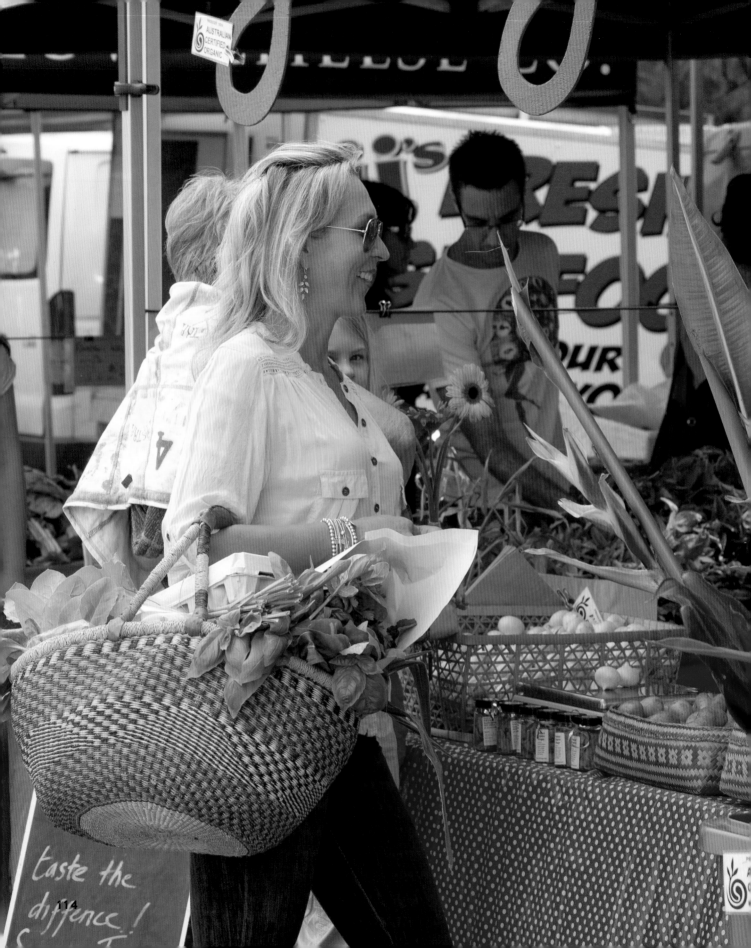

taste the
diffence !

Do I need to panic
if it's not organic?

There's plenty of debate surrounding organically produced food and whether it is all it's cracked up to be and although I don't think it's necessary to ensure 100 percent of your food is certified organic, there are a few simple guidelines you can follow that will help to minimize your exposure to chemicals, enhance the nutritional quality of your food as well as sustain Mother Earth and the nutrient content of the soil.

The main aim for eating organic food is to avoid chemical pesticides, herbicides and fungicides as well as GMOs – genetically modified organisms, because any food that has been contaminated with chemicals or has been genetically modified, may pose a risk to your health. But some foods are more heavily contaminated than others - The Environmental Working Group (EWG), compiles a list every year of the foods most heavily contaminated with chemical residue, referred to as 'The Dirty Dozen'.

So if your budget does not allow for buying organic varieties for all your fresh fruit and veg, at least avoid those from the Dirty Dozen with the highest levels of chemical residue.

THE DIRTY DOZEN

1. Apples
2. Celery
3. Tomatoes (including cherry tomatoes)
4. Cucumbers
5. Grapes
6. Bell Peppers / capsicum
7. Nectarines (imported)
8. Peaches
9. Potatoes
10. Spinach
11. Strawberries
12. Cherries

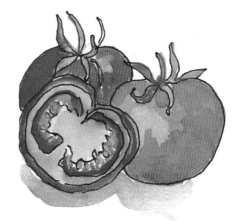

DIRTY DOZEN PLUS:

Kale/collard greens and Summer squash

Personally I would recommend avoiding all non organic berries, like raspberries, because they contain high levels of chemical pesticides and considering kids love eating berries, I think it's especially important to reduce their exposure to as many chemicals as possible. Berries tend to be very expensive at the best of times, so if you can't afford fresh organic berries, I recommend buying frozen organic brands, as this can be a more economical way to consume them.

The EWG have also released a list of fresh fruit and veg with the lowest levels of chemical residue referred to as 'The Clean Fifteen'. So you could compromise on buying non-organic varieties from this list if you're trying to stretch the budget, or find it difficult to access organic fruit and vegetables.

THE CLEAN FIFTEEN

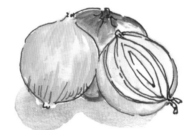

1. Asparagus
2. Avocados
3. Cabbage
4. Cantaloupe
5. Eggplant
6. Kiwi
7. Mangoes
8. Sweet corn – check it's non GM though
9. Mushrooms
10. Grapefruit
11. Onions
12. Papayas
13. Pineapples
14. Sweet peas (frozen
15. Sweet potatoes

I also tend to purchase other non-organic varieties of citrus, like lemons and limes, when my citrus orchard is not bearing any fruit, because you are removing the skin, making citrus a pretty safe bet to consume.

As far as organically produced food having a superior nutrient content compared to non-organic varieties, numerous studies are now revealing organic food does in fact come out on top, compared to many conventionally grown crops. A 2014 study published in the British Journal of Nutrition revealed that organically produced food contains anywhere from 18-69 percent more antioxidants than conventionally grown varieties, and higher levels of trace minerals such as zinc and magnesium.

But it's also what you're NOT getting when you buy organically produced food, that puts your health ahead – all those nasty chemical pesticides, herbicides and fertilizers

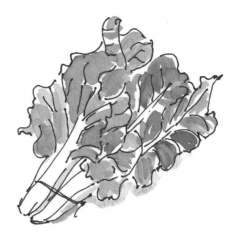

for a start! A recent study from RMIT University revealed eating organic food for just one week dramatically reduces your exposure to organophosphate pesticide residues by 90 percent.

Organic food production also leaves a much smaller footprint on the environment as well as the food, as the food is generally produced using more sustainable farming practices that also maintain the essential trace mineral content of the soil, making it more nutritious.

BUT WHAT ABOUT THE COST OF ORGANIC PRODUCE?

Many of us struggle to justify the extra cost of organic food, yet we can easily justify spending thousands of dollars a year on alcohol, cigarettes, house and car insurance, even health and life insurance premiums! Personally, I rationalize paying a little extra for organic varieties of certain foods as taking a preventative approach to my health, by reducing exposure to the chemicals and antibiotics that increase the risk of illness and disease.

The reason organic produce costs more compared to non-organic food comes down to the difference in economies of scale in production. Organically grown food is more labor intensive than mass produced monoculture farming, which relies on bucket loads of chemicals to keep the pests and weeds under control versus hand weeding or using non chemical sprays.

If you can't always afford or access fresh organic fruits and vegetables, then at the very least remove the skin where possible, or soak them in water and white vinegar for 20 minutes or longer, before refrigerating to reduce the chemical residue.

At the end of the day, the more you minimize your overall exposure to antibiotics, hormones and chemicals in your food, as well as in your personal care and cleaning products, and your environment, the healthier you will be and less at risk of disease. At a bare minimum, avoid non-organic varieties of the foods on the dirty dozen list, along with non-organic chicken and eggs, farmed varieties of seafood and stick to free range pork and 100 percent grass fed beef and lamb to avoid added hormones, antibiotics and GMO soy and corn.

ORGANIC LABELLING

Many folk are skeptical about the authenticity of organically labelled foods, so when in doubt, look for your country's government certified organic label. In Australia, look for the 'Australian Certified Organic' logo. This organic logo verifies the food is:

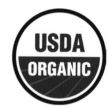

- pasture-fed
- socially responsible
- free range
- biodiversity friendly
- non GMO
- free from synthetic pesticides, herbicides, hormones and antibiotics.

Australia has some of the strictest standards when it comes to organic certification, and products carrying the Australian Certified Organic logo are audited annually to ensure they comply with an industry-agreed set of standards.

In America, the USDA have the strictest standards of organic certification, but be sure to choose organic foods labelled "100 percent organic" as foods simply labelled "organic" contain only 95 percent organic ingredients, and labels stating "made with organic ingredients" only contain between 70 to 95 percent organic ingredients.

Other foods I recommend buying either organic or chemical free include:
- Dairy - milk, cheese, butter, yoghurt
- Nuts
- Baby food

A WORD ON GENETICALLY MODIFIED FOODS

There's been a lot of debate surrounding the consumption of genetically modified foods, such as corn, soy and canola oil. The US is the biggest producer in the world of GM crops, but to help you understand the controversy over GM foods, let me start by explaining what 'genetic modification' is and why farmers are choosing to grow GM crops. The DNA of GM crops like soy and corn has been modified with the aim of making them more resistant to insects and disease, as well as to the chemical herbicide, RoundUp.

THERE ARE TWO MAIN ISSUES WITH GM FOODS

GM crops are designed to be resistant to the Herbicide RoundUP. The original purpose of these RoundUp resistant crops was to reduce herbicide use, which was the case in the first few years of use. However over-reliance led to the emergence of resistant weeds, forcing farmers to spray more often with RoundUP and add new herbicides, in an effort to combat these 'Super Weeds'. French scientists at the University of Caen found the combination of chemicals contained in RoundUp to be neurotoxic and carcinogenic, and capable of killing human cells, particularly embryonic, placental and umbilical cord cells.

The second major issue with GM crops like corn, is that they contain their own 'inbuilt pesticide', known as Bt-toxin, a protein that's been isolated from a soil bacteria called Bt - Bacillus thuringiensis. The purpose of the inbuilt Bt-toxin is to protect GM crops from insects by killing them - essentially by punching holes in their digestive tract. Although science knows very little about the long term effects Bt toxin has on human DNA and health, we do know that BT toxin is able to survive human digestion, transferring into the bloodstream. A study by doctors at Sherbrooke University Hospital in Quebec, confirmed that Bt-toxin was detected in pregnant women, their fetuses and non pregnant women, implying it could pass on to the next generation.

As yet, scientists have not been able to prove that Bt-Toxin has the same effect on the human digestive tract as it does on insects. However if Bt genes are able to colonise the bacteria living within the human digestive tract, could our intestinal flora be converted into living pesticide factories, possibly producing Bt-toxin inside of us year after year? Could this phenomenon also go a long way to explaining the increase in gastrointestinal problems, autoimmune diseases, food allergies, and childhood learning disorders, including autism, since Bt crops were introduced in 1996?

My stance on genetically modified foods is to avoid them at all costs, because science is a long way from fully understanding the long-term effects they have on our health.

Although no human studies have been conducted into their long term safety, several animal studies indicate serious health risks associated with GM food consumption, including infertility, immune dysregulation, accelerated aging, dysregulation of genes associated with cholesterol synthesis, insulin regulation, cell signalling and protein formation, and changes in the major organs and the gastrointestinal system.

My advice is to stick to foods produced using natural farming methods, free from chemical sprays and additives as much as possible.

And if you think you are safe from exposure to GM foods because you live outside the US, think again, because the US is the biggest producer of GM foods like corn and soy in the world, which are also exported globally and added to thousands of processed foods.

Thankfully, in Australia, food manufacturers are required to state when a product contains GM ingredients, so be sure to always read your labels. However, in the US there is no such legislation and many people are consuming GM foods without realising. If you choose to eat corn, I recommend only consuming fresh organic corn, and avoid it all together if it upsets your gut, or at least during the first –four to six weeks of avoiding gluten, to help eliminate any sensitivity.

LIST OF CURRENT GM FOODS IN US

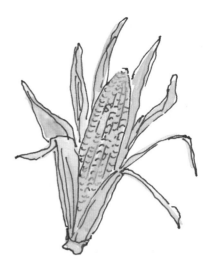

- Corn
- Soy
- Silver beet
- Alfalfa
- Papaya
- Squash
- Canola

COMMON INGREDIENTS DERIVED FROM GMO RISK CROPS

Amino Acids, Aspartame, Ascorbic Acid, Sodium Ascorbate, Vitamin C, Citric Acid, Sodium Citrate, Ethanol, Flavourings ("natural" and "artificial"), High-Fructose Corn Syrup, Hydrolyzed Vegetable Protein, Lactic Acid, Maltodextrins, Molasses, Monosodium Glutamate, Sucrose, Textured Vegetable Protein (TVP), Xanthan Gum, Vitamins, Yeast Products.

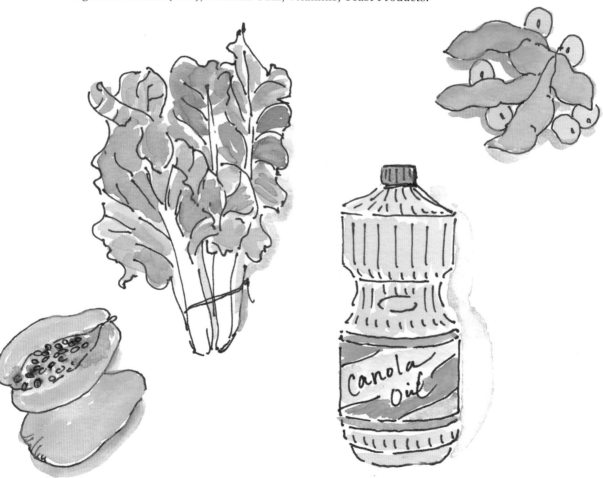

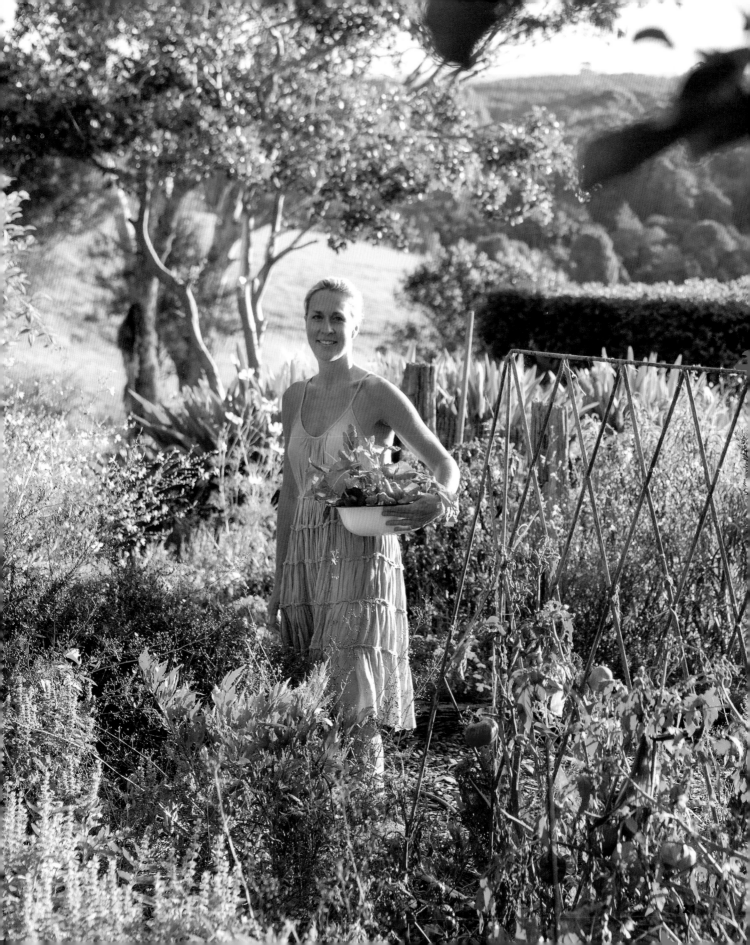

Tips for eating out on the LYG program

Now there is no need to lock yourself away and turn down invitations to go out with friends just because you're on the LYG program, because the aim of this program is to adopt the principles into your everyday lifestyle, as much as possible, for life! Although I do recommend adopting a 90 percent compliance for the initial 28 days, in order to experience the full health benefits and give the gut healing process a decent kick start, and to reduce chronic inflammation.

When you head out to eat, it's just a case of learning the best meal options to choose from and what to look for on the menu! I have to eat out a fair bit for work and it really is a rare occasion that I can't find something on a menu that not only tastes delicious, but enables me to stick to the principles of the LYG program. Stick to the following tips and you won't go wrong.

HANDY HINTS WHEN EATING OUT

- Say no to the bread - allowing the waiter to leave the bread basket will only tempt you, so ask for a serving of olives instead if you want to snack.

- Replace a side of chips with a side of steamed vegetables.

- Swap alcohol for soda water and bitters with fresh lime or lemon.

- Always order a side of greens to leave you feeling satiated.

- Avoid buffets - these are usually a haven for hidden sources of sugar, gluten and artificial additives, as well as being a major temptation to over eat, because you can!

- Skip dessert and, if you must indulge, go for a goat's and sheep's cheese platter, but avoid the crackers and biscuits or go for fresh fruit.

- Order two entrees/appetisers instead of an entrée and a main, that way you'll be at less risk of over eating.

- Ask for a simple salad dressing of lemon juice and olive oil to avoid balsamic vinegar or high sugar dressings that may also contain hidden gluten.

- Avoid high starch carbohydrates, even if they are gluten free eg: pasta, rice, pizza, potato and sandwiches, as grains can impair weight loss.

- Request a side of avocado to add to salads or eggs for breakfast, to help fill you up.

- Order a pot of fresh herbal tea after meals, you will feel less inclined to crave dessert and it will help to fill you up.

FOODS TO AVOID WHEN EATING OUT

- Thai & Vietnamese – generally packed with hidden sugars, gluten & artificial additives.

- Pizza – even gluten free pizza is not a great option, especially if you are trying to lose weight as they are high in starch and generally contain cheese and tomato paste.

- Pasta – same goes!

- Risotto –high in starch and usually made with cream or cheese, which can leave you bloated. Not a great option if you're trying to lose weight.

- All fast food take away chains.

HEALTHIEST OPTIONS WHEN EATING OUT

- Choose wild seafood, 100 percent grass fed meat, or organic chicken.

- Japanese – only go for organic miso soup and sashimi and avoid teriyaki and sushi as these are high in sugar and fast burning carbs from rice. Beware that soy sauce and teriyaki sauce also contain gluten. Tamari sauce is a gluten free option.

- Turkish and Greek food is usually clean and lean – although you may want to dodge the cow's yoghurt and feta in the tzatziki dip and Greek salad if you are particularly sensitive to cow's dairy, and avoid moussaka as it contains milk, cheese and flour.

- Look for a salad bar and load up on a variety of salads, but avoid those with pasta and rice and creamy sauces, and avoid the croutons and cheese in Caesar salad.

- If you only have the option of a sandwich bar, ask for a container or plate so you can make a breadless sandwich - load up with heaps of fresh salads, avocado and some clean protein like roast turkey or roast beef and avocado and avoid any cured meats like ham or salami.

- Italian is ok if ordering things like meat with salad but avoid dishes with pasta, cheese, tomato paste or tinned tomatoes.

- Tapas - be sure to choose lean protein options like seafood, chicken or meat, but enquire with your waiter about the sauces in case of high sugar and gluten.

My thoughts on exercise

Do you want to know my top tip when it comes to exercise? I'll give you a hint. It doesn't involve thrashing yourself at the gym, pounding pavements 'til you drop to the floor in a heap of sweat, weighing yourself each day and stressing over whether you've lost the 400 grams you gained overnight, because you ate too much out to dinner. No my secret tip for losing weight and functioning at your best, aside from eating healthy whole foods, is two words...DON'T STRESS.

Do you remember how my health journey began? Exactly that way; thrashing myself at the gym; and pounding pavements in training for a marathon. I was always trying to be very precise about what I did for exercise and not over eating, yet I was often hungry because I was eating too much of the wrong foods that failed to fill me up. Well if you recall, that approach didn't turn out so well for me and when my thyroid spiralled out of control, following a period of chronic stress, I ended up packing on the pounds, despite the fact I was exercising like crazy.

Today I enjoy a different approach to exercise. It's all about listening to my body vs my mind and giving myself permission to enjoy myself first and foremost. I don't exercise out of guilt or fear and I certainly don't exercise to control my weight. I do that through my food and maintaining a healthy gut, and exercise is just the icing on the cake when it comes to maintaining my muscle mass and fitness.

Like everything in life, if you don't enjoy it, it's unlikely to bring you happiness. Whether it's your food, your job, your relationships, where you live, or how you exercise. But guess what? YOU have the power and the choice to change it, so that you do enjoy good health.

When you do things with joy in your heart, your body will respond in a positive way, compared to if you are stressed or do something out of fear – which is how I see so many people exercise. Exercising out of fear – whether it's fear of putting on weight, or not looking good, or being attractive to your boyfriend – will eventually work against your health. In some cases you may find exercise makes no difference to your weight, or you may even start to gain weight if you over-exercise when your body is chronically stressed.

If you don't have the adrenal reserve to spend your 'energy dollars' on high intensity exercise, then I recommend pulling right back and focus on restorative forms of exercise like yoga, pilates, Qigong, stretching, even

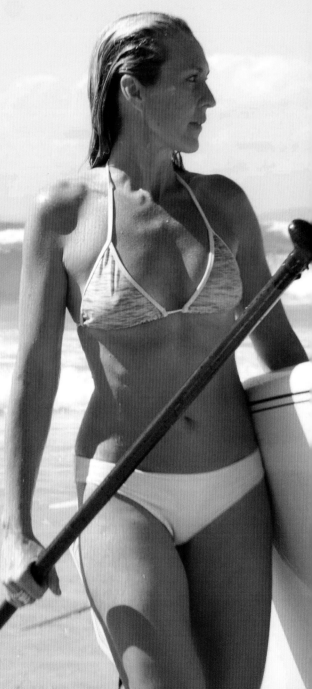

walking in nature. As you restore your adrenal function and heal your gut, you'll be able to build up your exercise routine to a point where it's the equivalent of a 'deposit' towards your health vs a 'withdrawal'.

LEARN TO MEDITATE

Meditation is simply a practice to quieten your mind, to create gaps in your thinking and feel the spaces between. The purpose of meditation is to experience a deeper level of consciousness, resulting in a greater sense of calm and mental clarity. On a physical level, meditation works to balance the function of every cell in your body, helping to reduce inflammation, boost your immune defences and balance your hormones.

It's as simple as focusing on your breath and allowing it to take over from your thoughts. But the number one rule with meditation, is...there are no rules, there are no restrictions or boundaries, or 'right' or 'wrong' ways to meditate. All you have to do is focus on your breath and the rest will take care of itself, as long as you are consistent with your practice. It's natural for thoughts to wander in and out of your mind, even for your mind to race at times, this is all part of the practice. All you need to do in this instance, is be aware of your thoughts, rather than engage with them, and go back to focusing on your breath. The more you meditate the quieter your mind will become.

In conjunction with restoring my gut health and eating the right foods, meditation was the missing link that enabled me to recover when I was chronically ill.

HERE ARE MY TIPS FOR EXERCISING SMARTER NOT HARDER

- Choose something you enjoy

- Listen to your body, not your mind - it will never lie

- Scale back if your adrenals are flagging

- Move EVERY day – even if it's just gentle stretching or a walk in the park, or by the ocean.

- Schedule some form of exercise into your daily routine the same way you do anything else in your life, but don't bite off more than you can chew

- Get your daily dose of sunshine – your body needs vitamin D

- Walk or take a bicycle vs the car, you'll be amazed at how much more movement you will get into your day when you do.

LYG Recipe Symbols Explained

It goes without saying that all of my recipes are free from gluten and cow's dairy and when it comes to sugar, the majority of my recipes are either sugar free, or low sugar, and all of them are free from processed forms of sugar. The only fructose you'll find in my recipes is naturally occurring in fruit or vegetables. I do not recommend using any natural fructose sweeteners such as honey, maple syrup, rapadura, coconut sugar, agave or dates, because one of the main aims of the LYG program is to break your addiction to fructose. Instead I only recommend using stevia or sweeteners containing 100% glucose, but even then, these must be used sparingly, in order to heal your gut, balance your hormones and lose any excess weight.

 GLUTEN FREE

All of my recipes on the LYG program are 100% gluten free so they are suitable for celiac sufferers, or those suffering gluten sensitivity. Even if you feel you are not sensitive to gluten, many people find they lose weight and have far more energy avoiding all forms of gluten for at least 4 – 6 weeks.. This will enable you to get a true gauge of your tolerance for gluten.

 DAIRY FREE

All of my recipes are free from cow's dairy. The only form of dairy I have included in some recipes is from sheep or goat's dairy. This is usually far better tolerated than cow's dairy, because sheep and goat's dairy predominantly contain the 'A2' protein. This is far less inflammatory than cow's dairy, which predominantly contains the 'A1' protein. Although goat and sheep's dairy also contain lactose, many people with lactose intolerance find they do not react to goat or sheep's dairy. If you wish to avoid goat or sheep's dairy, you can of course substitute with nut or coconut milk or yoghurt.

 LOW SUGAR

Many supposedly 'healthy' recipes claim to be 'sugar free' when in reality they have just swapped out refined forms of sugar for unrefined forms, such as raw honey, maple sugar or dates. These are still sugar! Many of my recipes are sugar free and any that recommend a little sweetener are low in sugar and free from added fructose. I have used fructose free sweeteners in all of my recipes, either in the form of rice malt syrup, stevia, or xylitol. I have also ensured my 'Nothing Naughty Treats' are low in sugar to help you wean off the sweet stuff and reduce any cravings. If you have a particularly sweet palette, you may find these recipes don't taste very sweet at first, but as your palette adjusts to less sugar, these nothing naughty treats will begin to taste sweeter.

PALEO

The majority of recipes on the LYG program are suitable for lovers of the Paleo diet. I only recommend using whole, fresh ingredients that are free from gluten and cow's dairy, as well as being low in sugar. Although some of my recipes recommend a little sheep or goat's dairy, this can easily be left out or substituted. The majority of my recipes are also grain free, although a few include pseudo grains like quinoa, or a little rice flour to coat fish or meat. Of course this is optional. Some recipes contain lentils and legumes, however small servings, pre-soaked and consumed occasionally, should be tolerated by most people, or can be avoided.

 DIABETIC

This symbol indicates a recipe is suitable for type 1 and 2 diabetics or anyone suffering insulin resistance. Many supposed diabetic friendly recipes are too high in sugar and starchy carbohydrates like grains. I have designed my recipes to promote healthy blood sugar and insulin levels to help reduce inflammation and stimulate healthy weight loss.

  VEGETARIAN/VEGAN

Many of my recipes are suitable for vegetarians and or vegans, or can be adapted to suit. If you are vegetarian or vegan, I highly recommend supplementing your diet with an organic pea or hemp seed protein powder to ensure you are getting a balance of the essential amino acids. It is also important to consume enough protein for muscle growth and repair and healthy immune defences. Consuming enough protein will also leave you feeling more satiated at meal times. I recommend vegetarians and vegans supplement with B12, Iron and vitamin C in particular, to prevent anemia and boost energy.

 LOW FODMAPS

The FODMAPS diet can be a complex one to follow, and whilst many of my recipes are low FODMAPS and free of processed fructose, I recommend consulting with a health practitioner experienced in the FODMAPS diet for further advice and guidance, or swap out any high FODMAPS ingredients where possible. If you suffer from bad IBS and or fructose malabsporption syndrome, consult my list of HIGH FODMAPS foods on page 100.

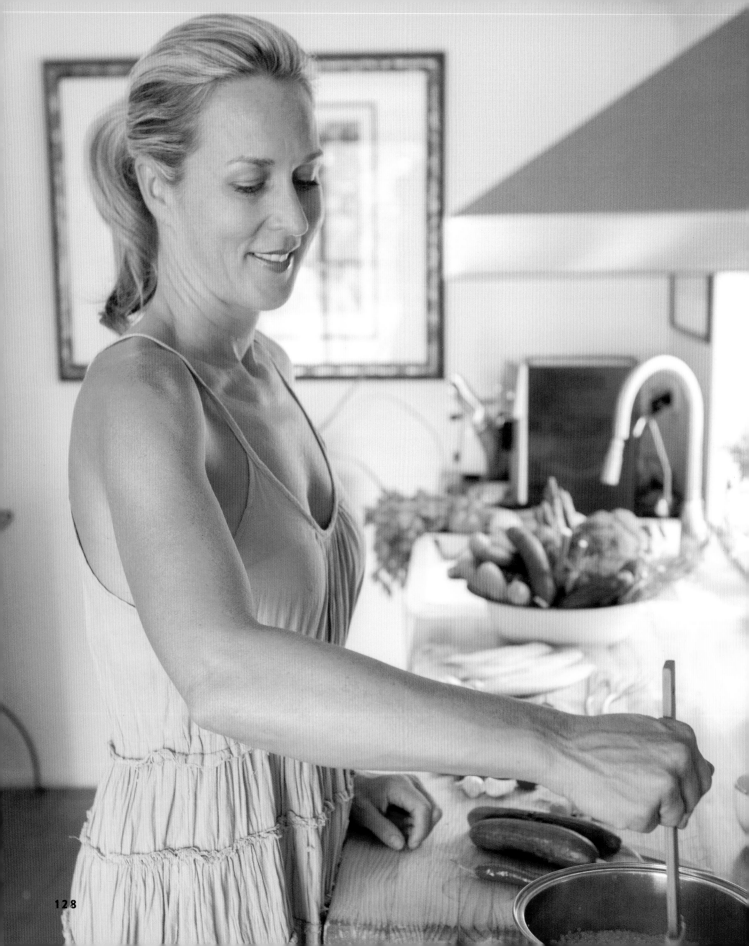

Recipes

Breakfast

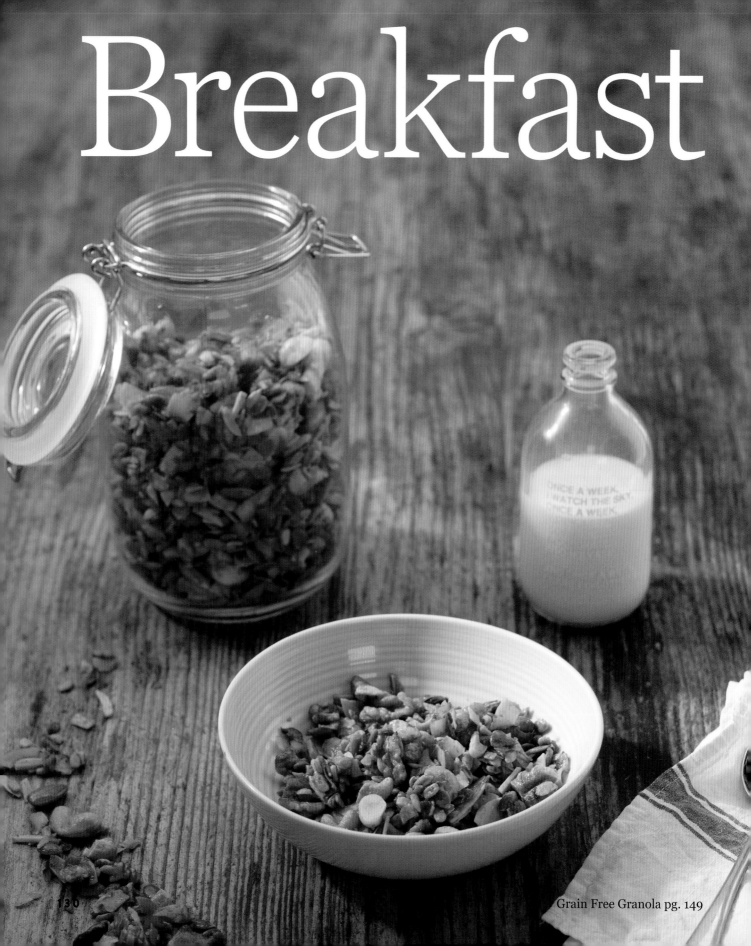

Grain Free Granola pg. 149

BREAKFAST

If skipping breakfast has become a habit, either because you're 'too busy', or not hungry, then it's time to get your priorities straight and your gut sorted out, so that you are naturally hungry when you wake up.

Your breakfast choice will influence your metabolic rate and blood glucose and insulin responses throughout the rest of the day, so it's essential to make a good choice. It will also impact on your serotonin levels for the day – the happy hormone that influences your mood, sleep and appetite. Have you ever noticed those people who are grumpy when they wake up, at least until they get some food into them?

Skipping breakfast may initially cause you to lose weight, but eventually this will catch up with you and the reverse will happen: You will feel grumpy, have trouble focusing and crave sugar!

If you often wake still feeling full from last night's dinner, this can be a sign that your body is still digesting food, either because you ate too much and/or too late, or you're not completely emptying your bowel each morning.

HERE ARE MY ESSENTIAL TIPS FOR GETTING YOUR DAY OFF TO A GOOD START

- Hydrate on waking. It's been eight or more hours since you drank any water, so it should be the first thing you put into your body when you wake. Drink it preferably warm with the juice of half to one lemon and maybe add a splash of apple cider vinegar to really crank up that digestion!

- Ideally wait 20 minutes before eating, or start your day with my Green Goddess veggie juice or one of my smoothie recipes.

- Always choose a nutrient dense breakfast, that includes healthy fats, clean digestible protein and slow burning, low sugar carbs.

I've ensured these breakfast recipes are super low in sugar and fast burning carbs, whilst being high in clean, quality protein and packed with healthy fats, so that you'll feel fuller for longer. They are of course gluten and cow's dairy free – so you won't feel tired, bloated or have cotton wool brain after eating them.

Baked Eggs

Eggs are a rich source of protein and Omega–3 fatty acids and baked eggs make a delicious change to the usual boiled, scrambled or poached. Feel free to experiment with other healthy ingredients, like naturally smoked salmon or trout, home-made baked beans or extra greens such as English spinach or kale. Use individual ramekins or a small ovenproof casserole dish or fry pan.

Ingredients

2 eggs (per person)

Small handful of baby tomatoes, halved

Goats feta, to taste – approximately 1 desert spoon per 2 eggs

1 tbsp fresh chives, basil or flat leaf parsley, roughly chopped

Himalayan or Celtic Sea Salt and cracked pepper to taste

1 tbsp of extra virgin olive oil

Method

Preheat oven to 180°C / 350°F

Grease ovenproof dish with the olive oil.

Warm your dish in the oven for around 10 minutes, then while still warm, break the eggs into the dish, then add the tomatoes, goats feta and fresh herbs. Season with salt and pepper to taste and place back in the oven for another 15 – 20 min

SALLY'S TIP
To supercharge your brekkie, serve with a side of sliced avocado or steamed baby spinach.

GF DF P V LF

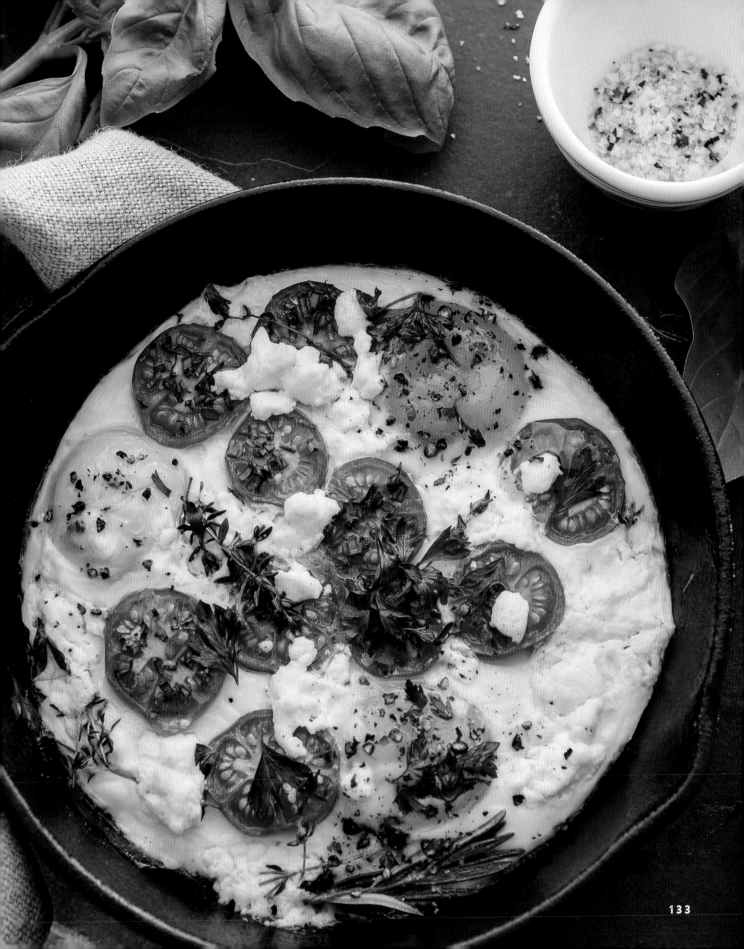

Grain Free Bircher Muesli

Ingredients

1 small green apple, peeled, cored and grated

1 tbsp chia seeds

1 tbsp coconut flakes, toasted

1 tbsp slivered almonds (raw or toasted)

1 tbsp pepitas

1 tbsp sunflower seeds

1 tbsp flax seeds

1 tbsp goji berries (optional)

1 tsp vanilla essence or 1/2 tsp vanilla powder

1 tsp buckwheat kernels (optional)

1/2 - 1 tsp ground cinnamon to taste

2/3 cup unsweetened coconut, almond or cashew milk

Finely grated rind and juice of half a lemon (optional)

Bircher muesli brings back memories of friends coming to stay growing up. Mum would always whip up a fresh batch for breakfast and although her recipe was super-delicious, it was made the traditional way - with lots of not so gut- friendly ingredients like sugar from the honey and dried fruit, cow's milk and yoghurt and oats that weren't necessarily gluten-free. So this is my low-sugar, gluten-free, grain-free and dairy-free take on my Mum's Bircher muesli. This recipe can be prepared in minutes and soaked overnight ready for the next day, making it a great option for a healthy breakfast on the run.

Method

Combine all the dry ingredients in a mixing bowl then stir in the milk. Add lemon rind and juice if using. For best results, cover and soak overnight in the fridge and enjoy the next day, or if short on time serve straight away..

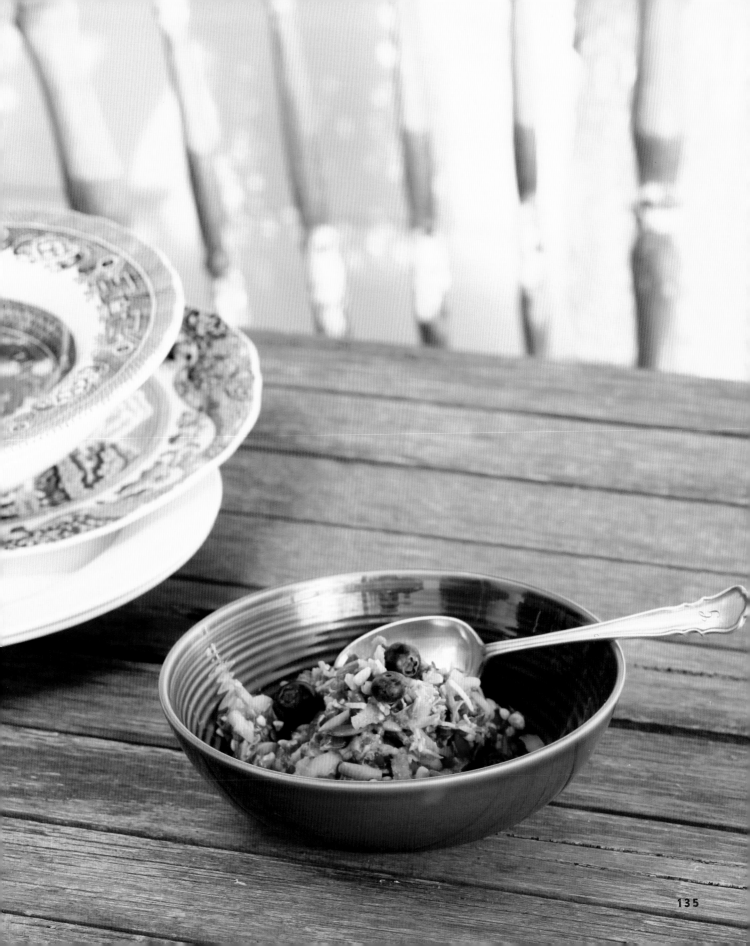

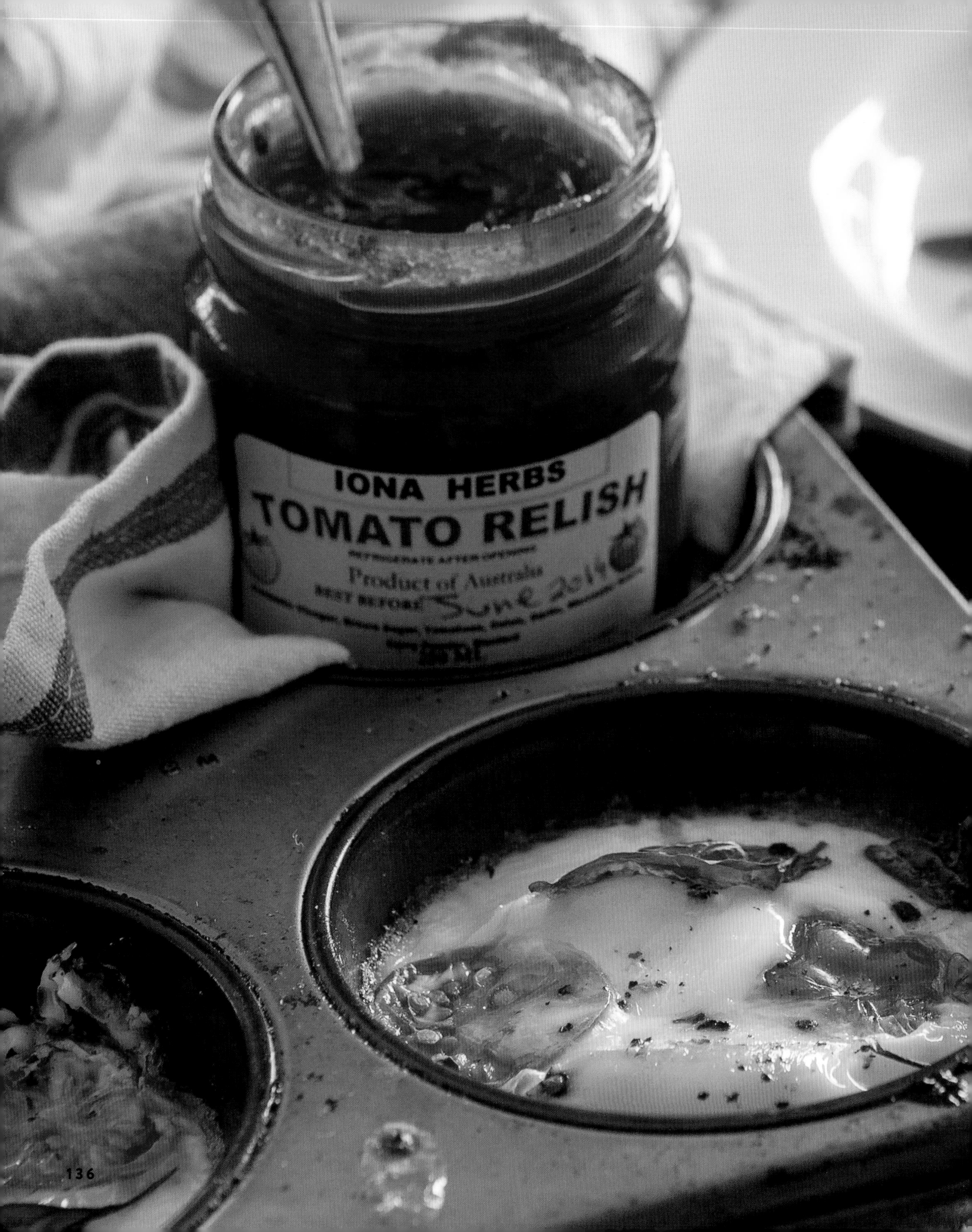
IONA HERBS
TOMATO RELISH
Product of Australia
BEST BEFORE June 2014

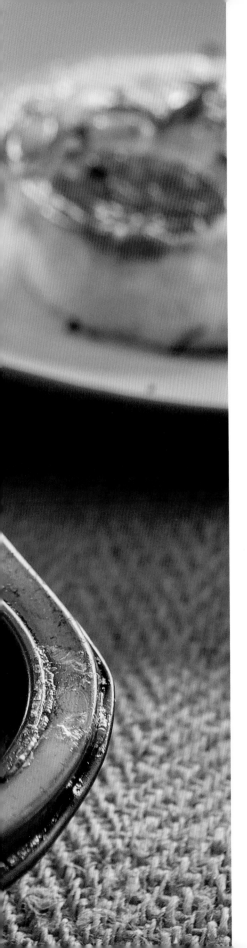

Herb Tomato & Egg Muffins

These breakfast muffins are easy to make and even easier to eat! There's no excuse for skipping breakfast when you're busy, because you can prepare these in advance and store them in the fridge for up to three days. These muffins are a healthy, high-protein snack or light lunch for those times when you are on the go or find accessing healthy food is difficult. They also make a handy addition to kids' lunch boxes or the picnic basket.

Method

Preheat the oven to 180°C/350°F. Lightly grease a 6-pan deep muffin tray.

Crack 2 eggs into each muffin unit and add 2-3 tomato halves. Press a couple of basil leaves into the egg white, making sure they are submerged so they don't burn. Season with salt and pepper.

Bake for 20 minutes or until whites are set and opaque. To remove, run a non-serrated knife around the edge of each muffin and ease out of the tray.

Ingredients

Ghee/coconut/macadamia oil, to grease pan

12 organic eggs

6-9 cherry tomatoes, halved

Fresh basil leaves

Himalayan or Celtic Sea Salt and freshly ground black pepper, to taste

Optional

You could add some nitrate free bacon to each muffin after week 2 on the program

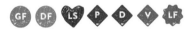

Packaged coconut milk has become all the rage as an alternative to cow's milk. Remember though, these products have been pasteurized which destroys a lot of the nutrients, and many brands contain added sugar and/or carrageenan, which is used as a stabilizer and thickener. Consuming too much canned coconut milk will expose you to the toxic chemical BPA, contained in the lining of food cans, which can leach into acidic, salty or fatty foods such as coconut milk, tomatoes, soup and vegetables. So where possible, fresh is always best. If you choose to use packaged coconut milk in your smoothie, be sure to choose a brand that is unsweetened and carrageenan free.

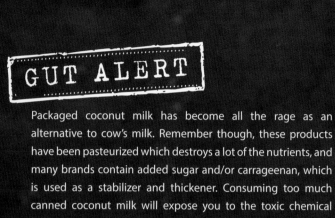

Fresh Coconut Milk Vanilla Smoothie

I recommend going to the effort of making this smoothie using fresh coconut milk, not just because it is a rich source of essential minerals like magnesium and potassium and one of the healthiest sources of fat you can feed your body for beautiful skin and a healthy metabolism, but also because once you experience the flavour, you will understand why fresh coconut milk is called 'nectar of the gods'!

Method

Using a meat clever cut a triangle into the top of the coconuts, large enough to fit a tablespoon into (or use a coconut opener).

Pour the water from the coconuts into a blender. Scoop the flesh from the inside of the coconuts and add to the blender. Add the remaining ingredients. Blend on high speed for 2-3 minutes or until smooth and creamy.

Sprinkle with ground cinnamon if using.

Serve immediately or store in the fridge in an air-tight container for up to 3 days.

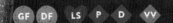

Ingredients

2 young green coconuts (available in the fruit and vegetable section of most supermarkets)

Juice of 2 fresh limes (optional)

2 tbsp coconut oil

1 tsp natural vanilla powder, essence or paste

2 tbsp organic collagen/pea/hemp seed protein powder (optional)

2 tsp of rice malt syrup or xylitol, or 4 drops of stevia (optional)

Handful of ice cubes

1 tsp ground cinnamon (optional)

Homemade Baked Beans

There's nothing quite like homemade baked beans for breakfast or a light meal or snack but the reality is most processed brands contain lots of sugar, hidden gluten and artificial additives. I recommend using navy beans because they are better tolerated by the gut than other legumes like cannellini beans.

Ingredients

300 - 330 gm dried or canned navy beans. If using dried, soak them in cold water overnight. Otherwise rinse and drain if using canned.

1 brown onion, peeled and diced

75 ml extra virgin olive or macadamia oil

2 cloves garlic, crushed

2 thyme sprigs or 1 tbsp fresh basil leaves

1 fresh bay leaf

400 gm fresh ripe tomatoes, preferably organic Roma or vine ripened

Cracked pepper and Himalyan or Celtic Sea Salt to taste, or 1 tsp smoked paprika (optional)

60 ml (1/4 cup) rice malt syrup or xylitol, or 4 drops of liquid stevia

Method

Drain and rinse beans in cold water. Set aside.

Add onion and garlic with oil to a medium saucepan and cook on a low to medium heat until onion becomes soft and transparent–being careful not to burn the garlic.

Add the herbs and tomatoes to the saucepan and season with salt and pepper to taste.

Allow to simmer for 5 minutes or until tomatoes are soft, then add the beans and stir through with the rice malt syrup.

Allow to simmer on low heat for a further 3 – 5 minutes.

Serve with poached eggs and sautéed baby spinach for a delicious breakfast, or eat cold on its own for a healthy snack. This dish makes a healthy addition to the kids' lunch box

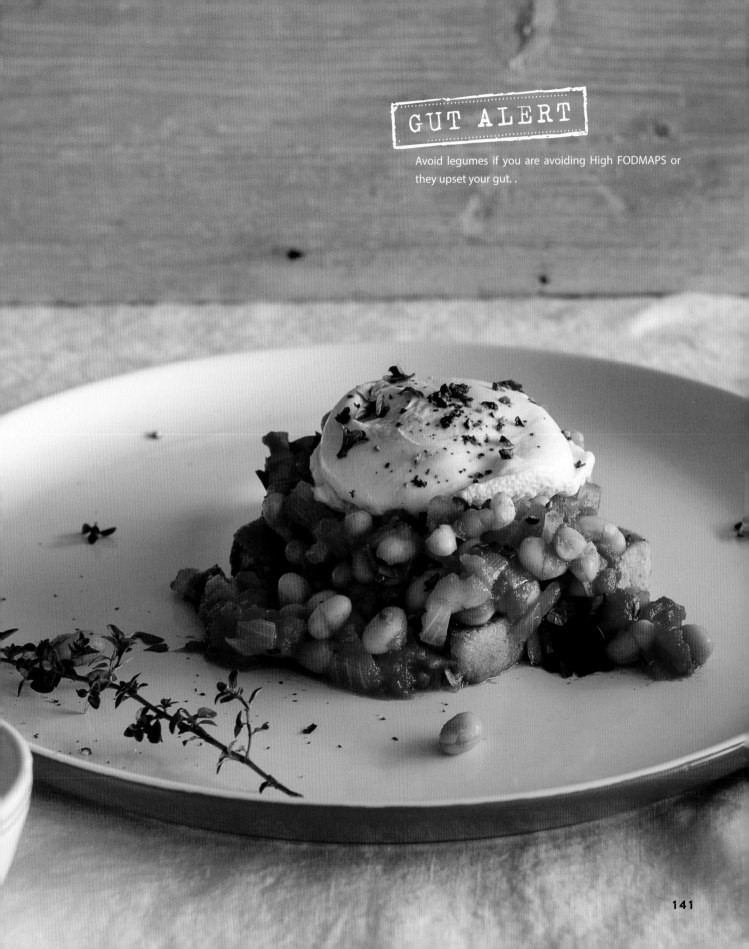

GUT ALERT

Avoid legumes if you are avoiding High FODMAPS or they upset your gut. .

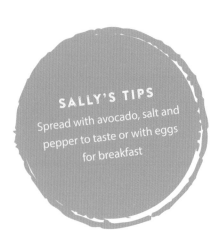

SERVING SIZE 1 SLICE · MAKES 1 LOAF

Grain Free Bread

I love my gluten free bread, but back in the days when I was diagnosed with a pretty severe intolerance to gluten, I think I would have found more flavour in a cardboard box than most brands on the market! Nowadays gluten free bread is far easier to find and the quality and flavour has improved dramatically, although many brands still contain soy flour, vegetable oil, sugar and preservatives. Because I am not a fan of eating many grains, (even gluten free varieties) because of the effect they have on the gut and because they can inhibit weight loss, I created this delicious grain-free bread recipe - perfect for those times you feel like a piece of toast. I love to top it with fresh avocado and a little goat's feta, or a couple of poached eggs, or even coconut oil and a sprinkle of cinnamon... yum!

Ingredients

2 cups almond flour

2 tbsp coconut flour

1/4 cup flax meal - ground flax seeds

1/4 tsp Celtic Sea Salt

1/2 tsp baking soda

5 large eggs

1 tbsp coconut oil, melted

1 tbsp rice malt syrup

1 tbsp apple cider vinegar

Method

Grease and line a loaf tin with baking/parchment paper - approx 7.5 x 3.5inches.

Place almond and coconut flour, flax meal, salt and baking soda in a food processor. Pulse ingredients together.

Add the eggs, oil, rice malt syrup and vinegar and pulse to gradually combine.

Transfer the batter to the loaf tin lined with grease proof paper. Bake at 180C or 350F for 30 minutes. Cool in the pan for 2 hours

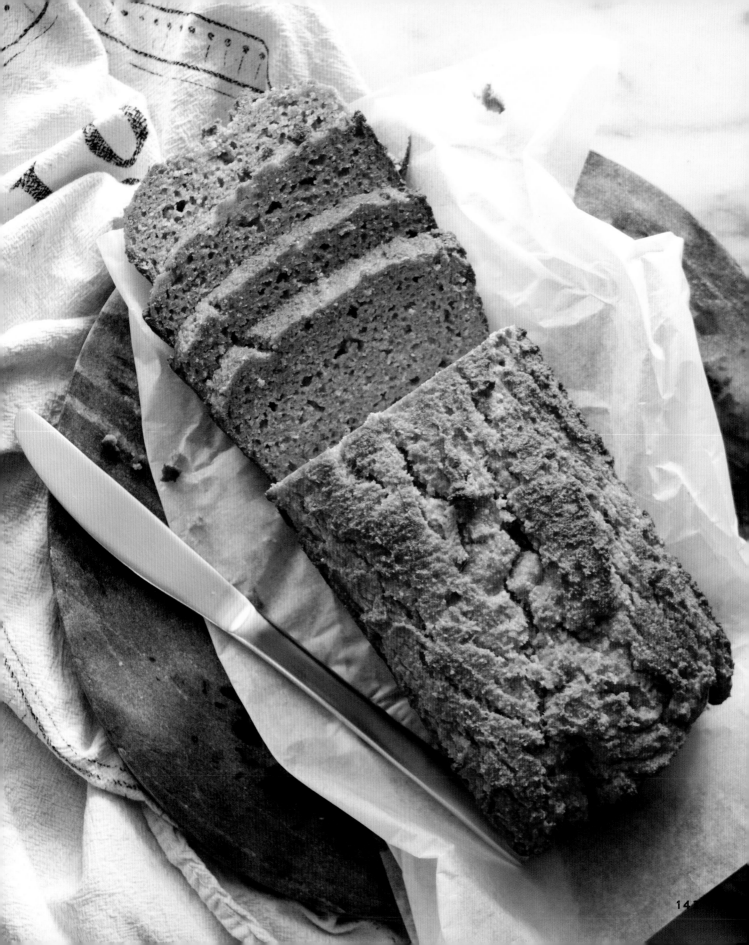

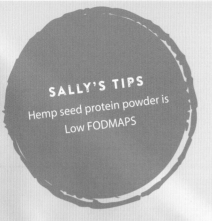

SERVES 1-2

Berry Delicious Smoothie

This is one of my absolute favourite breakfast smoothies, second only to the Green Goddess power smoothie. Berries are a powerful source of antioxidants, but it's important to buy organic berries to avoid the chemical sprays, especially if you or your kids are consuming them regularly. This recipe is a great high-protein breakfast choice if you're intolerant to eggs, or always in a rush around breakfast time but want to ensure you are getting all your essential nutrients.

Ingredients

1 cup frozen organic berries, such as blueberries, raspberries, strawberries or blackberries

2 tbsp organic collagen, pea or hemp seed protein powder

2 tsp virgin coconut oil

2 tsp organic or chemical-free chia seeds

200ml unsweetened almond, cashew or coconut milk

100ml filtered water

Handful baby spinach leaves or 1 tsp spirulina powder (optional)

Method

Place all the ingredients into a blender and blend on high speed until well combined. Pour into a tall glass and garnish with a couple of raspberries, ground cinnamon or a sprinkle of cacao nibs..

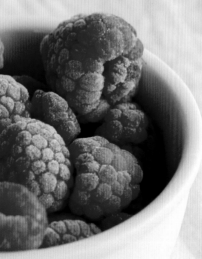

144   **BREAKFAST**

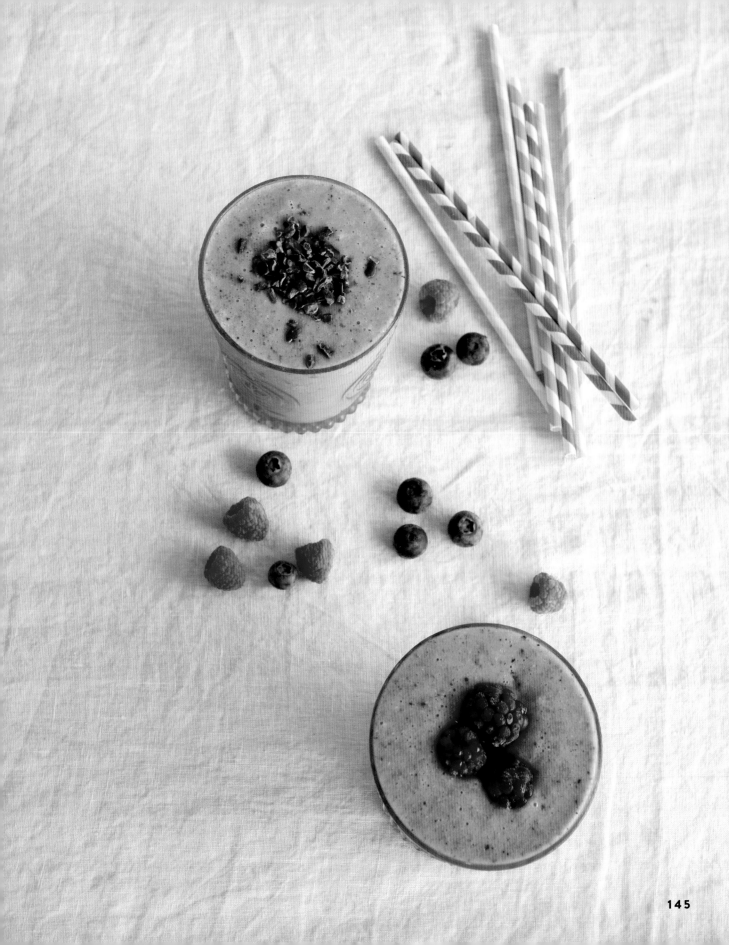

Goat's Feta, Avocado & Herb Omelette

Ingredients

1 tbsp ghee / coconut / macadamia oil

2 organic eggs, lightly beaten

1/4 cup roughly chopped basil

1/4 cup roughly chopped flat-leaf parsley

1/4 avocado, thinly sliced

1 tbsp goat's feta, crumbled

Himalayan or Celtic Sea Salt and freshly ground black Pepper to taste

Omelettes can be enjoyed for lunch, brunch or even a light dinner if you're running low on supplies! By combining protein with fats, you will feel fuller for longer and are less likely to crave sugar or snack in between meals.

Method

Heat oil in a small frying pan on medium heat.

Pour eggs into the pan and tilt to spread evenly across the base. Sprinkle herbs over half the omelette and top with avocado and goat's feta. Season with salt and pepper to taste.

When the egg has just set and the underside is lightly golden, flip the bare half of the omelette over the filling to enclose.

Serve immediately and garnish with extra fresh herbs.

AVOCADO

Avocados are an excellent source of monounsaturated fats as well as Omega–3, making them are particularly effective in lowering cholesterol and blood pressure, and reducing inflammation, especially in the joints. The monounsaturated fats in avocados can also help to prevent insulin resistance and Type 2 diabetes, while the high soluble fibre content helps to prevent blood sugar spikes and sugar cravings. Avocado contains 30 percent more blood-pressure-busting potassium than bananas. Avocados are a great pregnancy food because they are a natural source of folic acid, the number one supplement that pregnant women are advised to take.Specific nutrients and enzymes in avocados help to reduce inflammation in the stomach and lining of the small intestine, making them effective for aiding digestion. The nutrients in avocados are also known to help protect against prostate and breast cancers. Try to include some avocado with your meals each day, if you can.

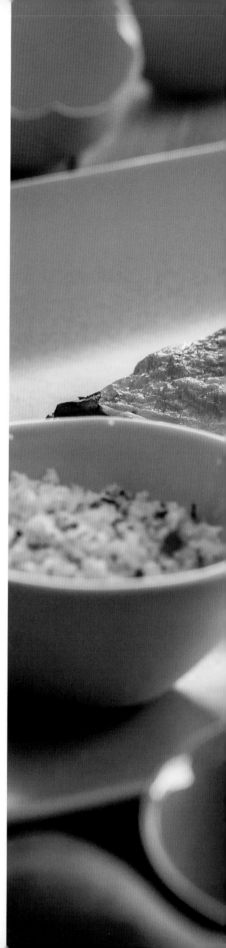

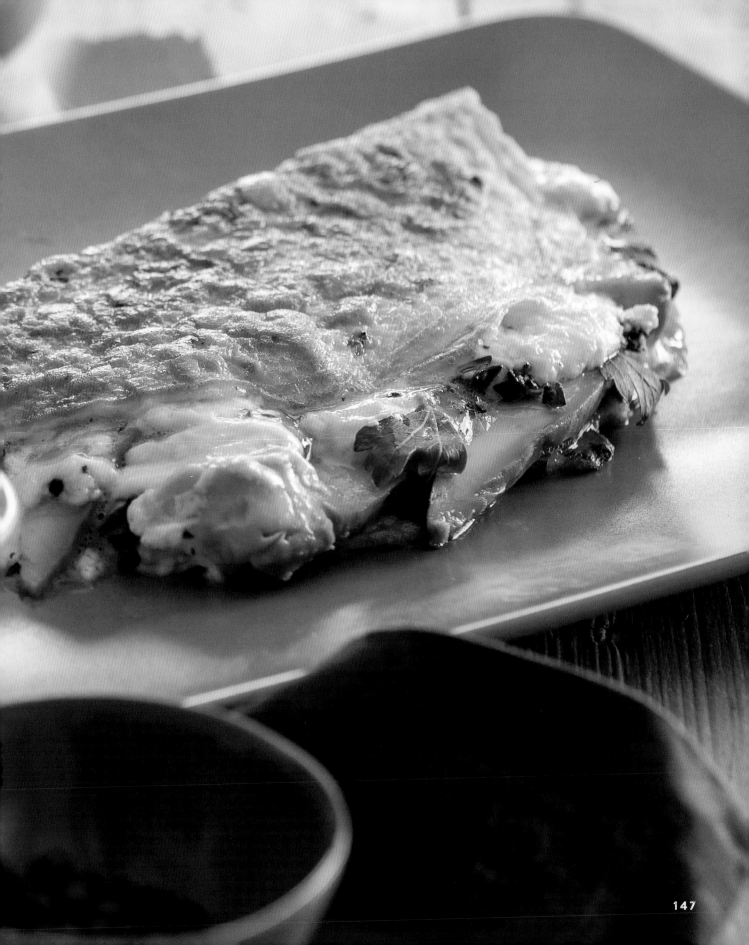

Almond Milk

Almond milk is a delicious tasting, dairy free alternative you can add to your morning muesli in smoothies, tea or coffee, or recipes in place of cow's milk. Aside from saving money, I recommend making your own almond milk because the majority of store bought brands contain as little as 2-2.5% almonds and the rest is water and added thickeners like carrageenan – which can upset your gut. You can substitute any nut in this recipe, including pumpkin seeds! Just ensure they are raw and unsalted. A word of caution if you live in the US - since 2007, the USDA require all nuts be pasteurized, either by steaming, roasting or blanching them, or using a controversial ionization process, or propylene oxide (PPO) - a known carcinogen. Pasturiation also destroys the valuable nutrients found in nuts. Despite being heat treated, many nuts in the US are still labeled "raw." There is also no requirement to specify what kind of pasteurization treatment was used. The best way to avoid pasteurized, or chemical treated nuts in the US is to either purchase them directly from the farmer - either at farmer's markets - or online from suppliers like Bremner Farms, Blue Mountain Organics or from Sunfood on Amazon, or try to purchase imported nuts from your local grocery store. If you do choose to buy US grown almonds, at least stick to organic varieties to avoid the chemical pasteurization process.

Ingredients

1 cup organic raw almonds (soaked for 12 hours or overnight (optional, but recommended to reduce the phytic acid levels)

4 cups of purified /filtered water

Pinch of Himalayan or Celtic Sea Salt (optional)

1 tsp natural vanilla extract (optional)

Method

Place the almonds in a bowl or large jar and cover with filtered water and one teaspoon of salt and soak for 8- 12 hours.

Rinse the nuts thoroughly - If soaking for the full 12 hours, make sure you rinse and soak a few times within the 12 hrs. Any nuts that float to the top indicate they are rancid, so be sure to throw these out.

Place almonds and water in a blender and set at low speed, before increasing to high speed until all the nuts are completely pulverized. If you don't mind a bit of texture to your milk, or if you're in a hurry, avoid straining. This will also retain more of the calcium. Just be sure to blend thoroughly.

To achieve a smooth and creamy texture strain the milk by placing a nut milk bag or cheesecloth over the opening of a glass jug or bowl. Pour the milk into the bag or cloth in small quantities and then squeeze the bag or cloth tightly with your hands until every last drop of milk is extracted. Alternatively you could pour the milk through a fine sieve, although this is not as effective. Remove the left over almond meal and freeze or refrigerate to use for baking some of my Nothing Naughty Treats. Nut milk bags are available from my website or from health food stores.

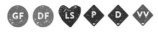

Grain Free Granola

Toasted muesli and granola are often promoted as a 'healthy' breakfast option, but in reality they're typically loaded with sugar - thanks to being baked in honey and chock full of dried fruit. Toasted muesli and granola are also typically baked at high heat, destroying the goodness of the healthy fats in the nuts and seeds and they usually contain oats, which can be a source of gluten. The idea of eating a grain free granola, is to promote better gut health and weight loss. So if you're someone who can't live without your morning muesli, my grain-free granola recipe is here to save the day and your hips! It's baked in virgin coconut oil at a really low temperature to preserve the healthy fats found in the nuts and seeds, and it's also super low in sugar. Your breakfast won't ever taste the same when you whip up a batch of this deliciousness!

Method

Pre-soak all the nuts and seeds (except the chia seeds) for 4 – 6 hours the day before. Pre-heat oven to 120° C / 215° F.

Place all the dry ingredients in a large mixing bowl & combine well. Melt the coconut oil and rice malt syrup on low heat in a saucepan, stirring to combine.

Transfer dry mix to a baking tray lined with greaseproof/parchment paper and spread evenly across the tray. Pour the melted rice malt syrup and coconut oil evenly over the granola and mix with your hands until evenly coated.

Place in the oven for around 1-2 hours to bake, or until a light golden brown and crunchy. Give the mix a toss halfway through to ensure it bakes evenly.

Remove from the oven when coconut is lightly toasted. Allow to cool before storing in an airtight container, such as a large glass jar. Serve with unsweetened coconut or almond milk, topped with a few fresh berries or strawberries & a dessert spoon of plain sheep or coconut yogurt.

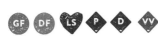

Ingredients

2 cups unsweetened coconut flakes /chips

2 cups mixed raw nuts - pecans, walnuts, cashew, brazil nuts

1 cup slithered almonds - or you can use a food processor to chop up whole almonds

1 cup sunflower seeds

1 cup pumpkin/pepita seeds

1 cup buckwheat (optional - this is a pseudo gluten free grain and more like a seed)

3 tbsp. chia seeds

1/2 cup coconut flour

1/4 -1/2 cup virgin coconut oil, melted

1-2 tbsp. brown rice malt syrup (optional)

2 tsp. ground cinnamon, or to taste

2 tsp. ground nutmeg, or to taste

Coconut Quinoa Porridge

Ingredients

1 ½ cups quinoa, soaked in water overnight

1 ½ cups unsweetened almond or coconut milk, plus extra to serve

1 ½ cups filtered water

2 tsp rice malt syrup or 1/4 tsp stevia, if desired (I find the coconut milk makes it sweet enough)

2 tsp virgin coconut oil

1 tsp ground cinnamon, or 1 cinnamon quill

3 cardamom pods, optional

1 tsp natural vanilla essence, or vanilla bean paste or powder

1 dessert spoon coconut oil

Fresh or frozen berries, toasted coconut flakes, pepitas and chia seeds, to serve

Traditional porridge is made from cooked oats, but as the 'Love Your Gut' program is grain and gluten-free, quinoa makes a great alternative. Being a seed, quinoa does not contain as much starch as grains and is usually well tolerated by sensitive tummies. If you're looking for something to warm your cockles in the cooler months or you need a bit of extra energy, this breakfast recipe is the go! Just remember if you suffer acute IBS, insulin resistance, Type-2 diabetes or you are just struggling to shift that spare tyre, you may want to hold off on eating quinoa until after your gut has healed a little more or your body starts to burn fat and you are nearing your goal weight. Otherwise... tuck in!

Method

Drain and rinse the pre-soaked quinoa in a sieve under running water.

Place the quinoa into a saucepan with the milk, water, rice malt syrup, cinnamon, cardamom pods and vanilla. Stir to combine.

Bring to the boil over medium heat, then reduce to low and simmer for about 15 minutes or until the milk has been absorbed and the quinoa is tender. You may need to add a little more milk if the mixture becomes too dry which means the quinoa needs to cook for longer. It is cooked when it's soft and fluffy like rice.

Stir in the coconut oil. Divide between bowls and drizzle with a little extra almond or coconut milk. Top with berries, toasted coconut flakes, pepitas and chia seeds. Sprinkle with extra cinnamon if desired.

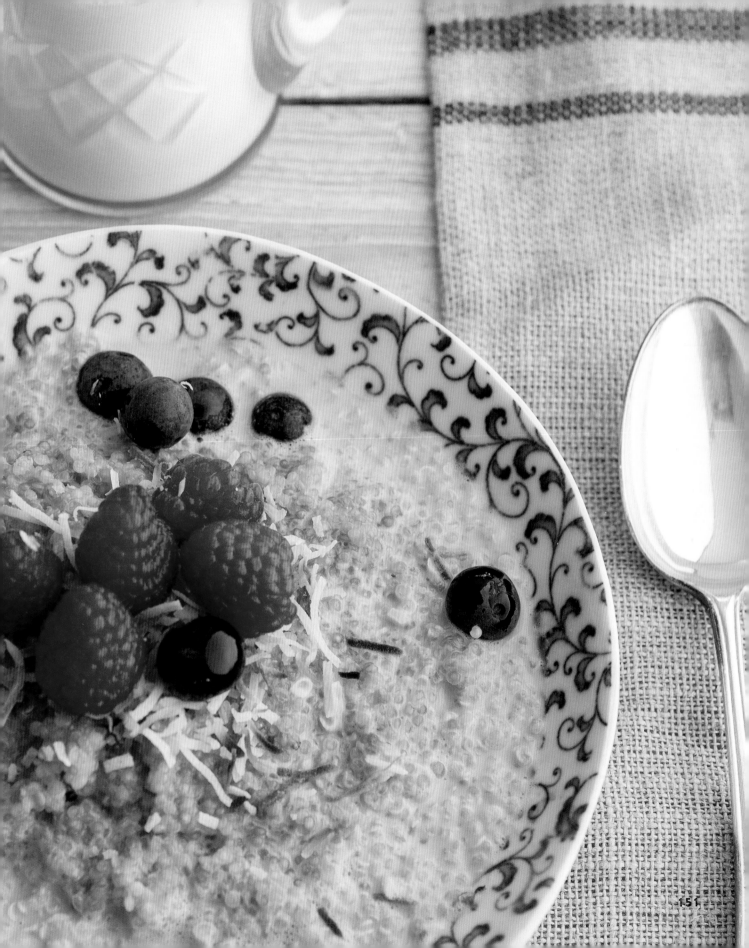

SALLY'S TIPS

If you are using fresh coconut water, scoop out the coconut flesh and add it to the blender for a dose of healthy fats. Be sure to use organic green vegetables to avoid chemical sprays.

Green Goddess Power Smoothie

The ingredients in this recipe are the ultimate anti-inflammatory concoction, packed with superfoods and easily digestible sources of protein. This smoothie is also super alkalizing and makes a great alternative to the Green Goddess if you are short on time, or don't have a juicer. Feel free to add any additional superfoods of your choice, including acai powder, aloe vera, spirulina, or my gut repair formula.

Method

Combine all the ingredients in a blender and blend until smooth.

Serve in a large glass and drink immediately to maintain freshness and optimal nutrient content.

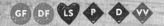

Ingredients

1 handful baby spinach leaves

1 medium cucumber

Juice of 1 lemon or grapefruit

2 tbsp fresh mint leaves

1 tbsp fresh parsley or coriander / cilantro leaves

1 knob ginger and/or turmeric, peeled (or 1 tsp of ground ginger and/or turmeric if you can't get fresh)

1 tbsp virgin coconut oil

1 tbsp organic or spray free chia seeds

1-2 tbsp organic collagen/ pea/hemp seed protein powder

1/4-1/2 avocado, depending on size (optional)

1 tsp maca root powder (optional)

300 ml coconut water (preferably fresh)

Handful of ice cubes

Scrambled Eggs with Smoked Trout

Ingredients

4 eggs

200 grams of naturally smoked trout, flaked

2 tsp macadamia or coconut oil

1 tsp pure butter or ghee

Himalayan or Celtic Sea Salt and freshly ground black pepper, to taste

Chopped fresh dill or flat-leaf parsley, to serve

Method

Crack the eggs into a glass mixing bowl and beat until they turn a pale yellow.

Preheat a heavy-based non-stick frying pan over medium-low heat. Add the oil and butter and let it melt and start to bubble.

Add the egg to the pan. Cook without stirring for about 30 seconds or until it just starts to set.

With a heat-resistant rubber spatula, gently push one edge of the egg into the centre while tilting the pan to allow the liquid egg to flow underneath. Repeat with the other edges, until there's no runny egg left.

Turn off the heat and continue gently stirring and turning the egg until all the uncooked parts become firm. Don't break up the egg though. Try to keep the curds as large as possible. Gently fold the trout through.

Transfer to a plate when the eggs are set but still moist and soft. Sprinkle with dill or parsley and serve immediately.

GF DF LS P D LF

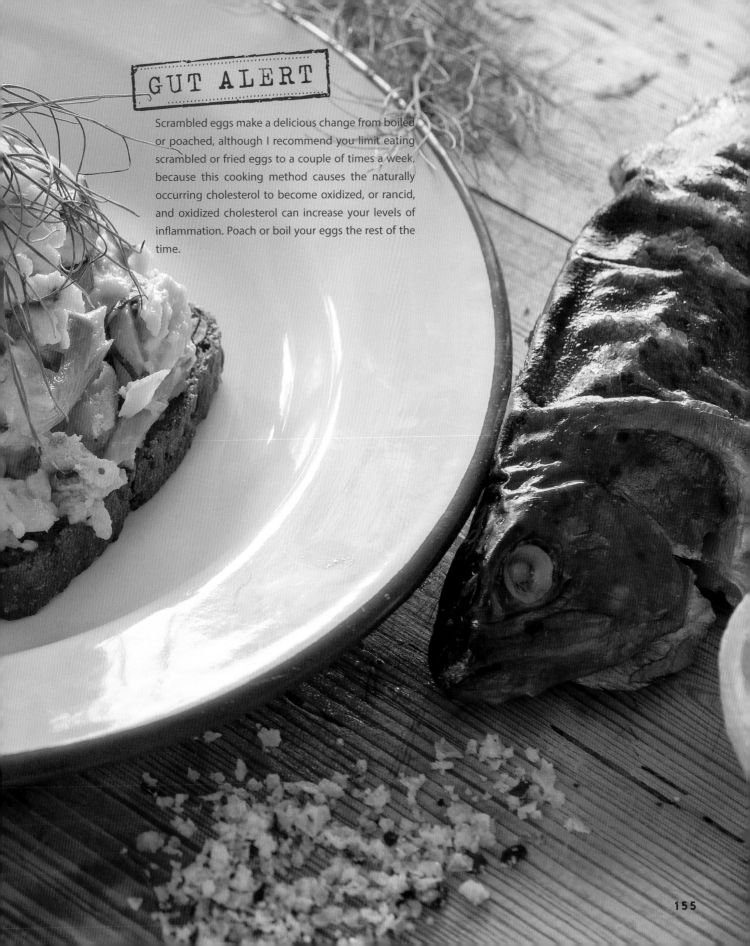

GUT ALERT

"being a lectin, Cacao can cause an upset gut in those who are sensitive, however once digestive symptoms have eased, it's ok to reintroduce, just observe any reaction"

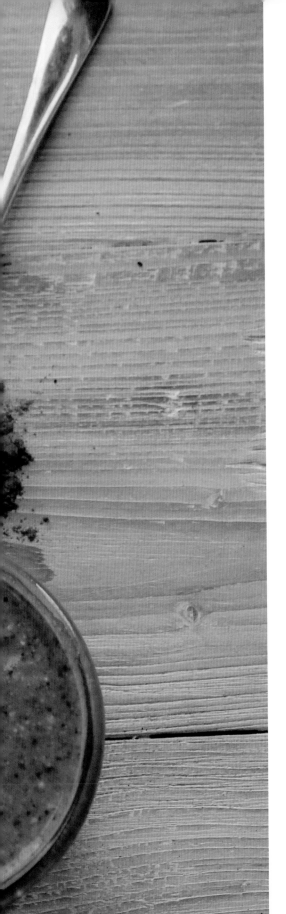

Choc Coconut Smoothie (aka Messy Daddy Drink)

One of my oldest and 'bestest' friends, Jack, christened this smoothie the 'Messy Daddy Drink' after I passed on the recipe to make with his little boys for a healthy, nutrient-packed breakfast! I think this tastes like a cross between a chocolate crackle and Milo, only it's much, much healthier. Little kids love it as much as the big kids, thanks to the natural chocolatey flavor.

Ingredients

1 young green coconut (alternatively you could use unsweetened nut milk)

2 tbsp organic collagen/pea/hemp seed protein powder

2 tsp virgin coconut oil

2 tsp raw cacao powder

2 tsp raw cacao nibs

1 tbsp organic or chemical-free chia seeds

Handful of ice cubes

1 dessert spoon rice malt syrup/xylitol/1 banana (optional)

Method

Cut a triangle into the top of the coconut using a meat cleaver, large enough to fit a tablespoon into (or use a coconut opener).

Pour the coconut water into a blender. Scoop out the coconut flesh with a spoon and add to the blender.

Add the protein powder, coconut oil, raw cacao powder and nibs, chia seeds and ice. Blend on high speed until well combined and smooth. Pour into glasses to serve.

Grilled Sardines & Avocado on Grain-free Toast

Ingredients

2 whole sardines, cleaned and scaled

2 tbsp macadamia oil, butter or ghee

2 lemon wedges

Himalayan or Celtic Sea Salt and freshly ground black pepper, to taste

1/4 avocado, sliced

1 slice paleo-friendly bread, toasted (see page x))

Sprig of fresh dill

Sardines have a bit of a bad rep, thanks to their rather fishy smell, but if you have never tried freshly cooked sardines I challenge you to do so as you may be pleasantly surprised by how delicious they are! There is also good news on the health front: sardines are a particularly rich source of Omega-3 essential fatty acids and easy-to-digest protein, and they contain the lowest amount of mercury of all fish, making them safe to eat during pregnancy.

Method

Lightly score the skin of the sardines and drizzle with a little of the oil. Squeeze over juice from one lemon wedge and season with salt and pepper.

Heat remaining oil in a small frying pan on medium heat. Add the sardines and cook for 2 minutes each side, turning once only.

Spread avocado onto toast and top with the sardines. Drizzle with remaining lemon juice and garnish with fresh dill. Serve immediately.

GF DF LS P D

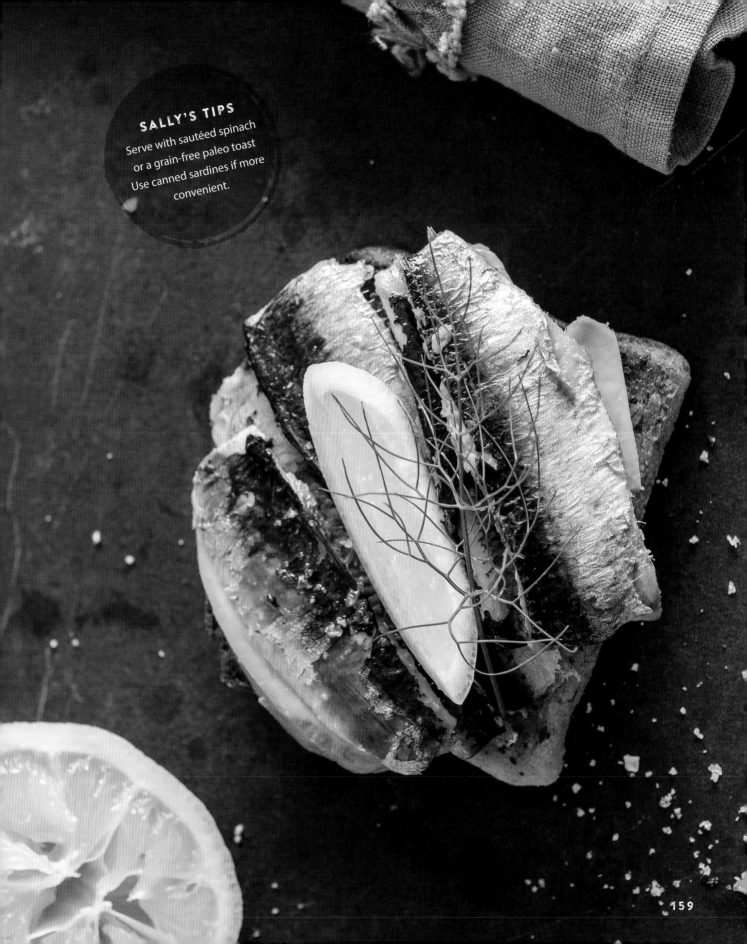

Grain Free Pancakes

Sunday mornings call for pancakes in my house, and pancakes never looked as healthy as this grain and gluten free recipe! They're also super filling, so one is usually plenty by the time you top it with the berry coulis and a dollop of plain coconut or sheep's yoghurt, drizzled with a little rice malt syrup and a sprinkle of toasted coconut flakes.

Method

In a large bowl, whisk the eggs and then add the almond milk, lemon juice, and vanilla. Whisk until well combined.

In a separate bowl, mix together the coconut/almond flour, cinnamon, baking soda, salt, and flax meal. Add the dry ingredients to the wet mixture, 1/4 cup at a time, while continuously whisking. Once combined, gently fold in the walnuts if using.

Grease a large fry pan with coconut oil or ghee and place over medium heat. Once the pan is hot, use a ladle to pour 3-inch pancakes onto the pan. Cook until bubbles appear, then flip. The pancake should cook on each side for about 2-3 minutes. Repeat with rest of the batter. Add more oil to the pan as needed.

To make the raspberry sauce, add 1-2 cups of frozen organic raspberries with 2 tablespoons of water to a saucepan and heat on low to medium, stirring until raspberries break up and turn to liquid. You may want to sweeten with a little bit of stevia, xylitol or rice malt syrup and a squeeze of fresh lemon juice, to enhance the flavour and brightness.

To serve, place 1-2 pancakes on each plate and top each stack with approximately 2 tablespoons of the raspberry sauce, dollop of plain coconut or sheep's yoghurt and sprinkle with some toasted coconut flakes or macadamia nuts and ground cinnamon.

Ingredients

3 large eggs

1 cup unsweetened coconut or almond milk

1/2 tablespoon freshly squeezed lemon juice

1 teaspoon vanilla extract

1/2 cup coconut or almond flour

1 teaspoon baking soda

Pinch of sea salt

1/4 cup roughly chopped walnuts (optional)

1/3 cup flax meal

1 teaspoon of cinnamon

Coconut oil or ghee for greasing the fry pan

200 grams frozen mixed berries

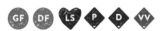

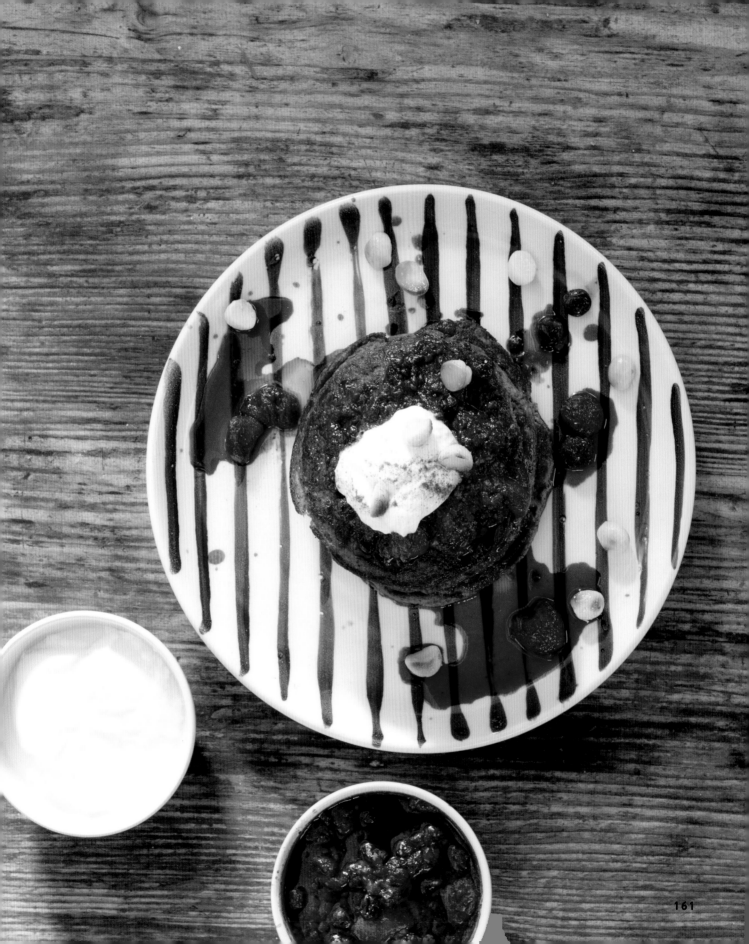

SERVES 1-2

Dukkah Poached Eggs with Roast Pumpkin & Avocado

If you're looking for a grain-free alternative to toast to eat with your morning eggs, then roast pumpkin is it. This recipe contains the perfect balance of healthy fats, slow burning carbs and clean protein, offset with the beautiful aromatic flavours of dukkah. This breakfast option is what I refer to as thinking outside the (cereal) box!

Ingredients

1 slice roast cinnamon pumpkin (see recipe page 245)

2 organic eggs, poached

1/4 large or 1/2 small avocado, sliced

1 small lemon wedge

Extra virgin olive oil, to taste

Dukkah, to taste (see recipe page 285)

Freshly ground black pepper and Himalayan or Celtic Sea Salt, to taste

Snow pea sprouts and fresh flat-leaf parsley, for garnish

Method

Place the roast pumpkin onto a plate and top with poached eggs and avocado. Squeeze juice from the lemon wedge over the avocado, and drizzle with a little extra virgin olive oil.

Sprinkle with dukkah and season with salt and pepper. Garnish with snow pea sprouts and fresh flat-leaf parsley if desired.

This dish can be enjoyed for breakfast, brunch or lunch. Feel free to add some sautéed baby spinach.

Green Goddess Juice

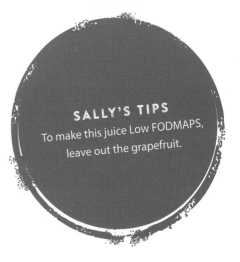

The Green Goddess juice has become one of the most popular recipes on my program, not only because of its powerful ability to cleanse and alkalise your body, but also because it is much lower in fructose than many other fresh juice combinations. I have specifically chosen the ingredients for their therapeutic and nutritional properties, as well as to minimize your fructose intake. You may find the flavour a little tart on your taste buds to begin with, but remember, as your gut health improves, your palate will become more sensitive to sugar, so you will not enjoy or crave sweet tasting foods as much. You may notice I have not included kale, which you will often find in other green juice recipes. This is because eating too many raw cruciferous vegetables like kale can block the absorption of iodine, an essential mineral necessary for a healthy thyroid and metabolic rate. Stick to consuming mainly cooked cruciferous vegetables or occasionally add raw to salads. If you really want to re-energize and achieve that healthy glow, then I recommend swapping your morning caffeine hit for the Green Goddess Juice and in no time your coffee cravings will switch to cravings for the Green Goddess!

Ingredients

2-3 sticks celery, depending on size

2 silverbeet leaves (exclude if it irritates your gut at first)

1 large cucumber or zucchini

1 whole lemon, peeled (see Tips)

1/2 pink grapefruit, peeled (see Tips)

1 knob ginger and/or turmeric, peeled (or 1 tsp of ground ginger and/or turmeric if you can't get them fresh)

Method

Add all ingredients one by one to your juicer, pour into a glass and drink immediately, as oxygen and light will oxidize and destroy the nutrients and enzymes in the juice after around 20 minutes. Be sure to follow your juice with a large glass of filtered water.

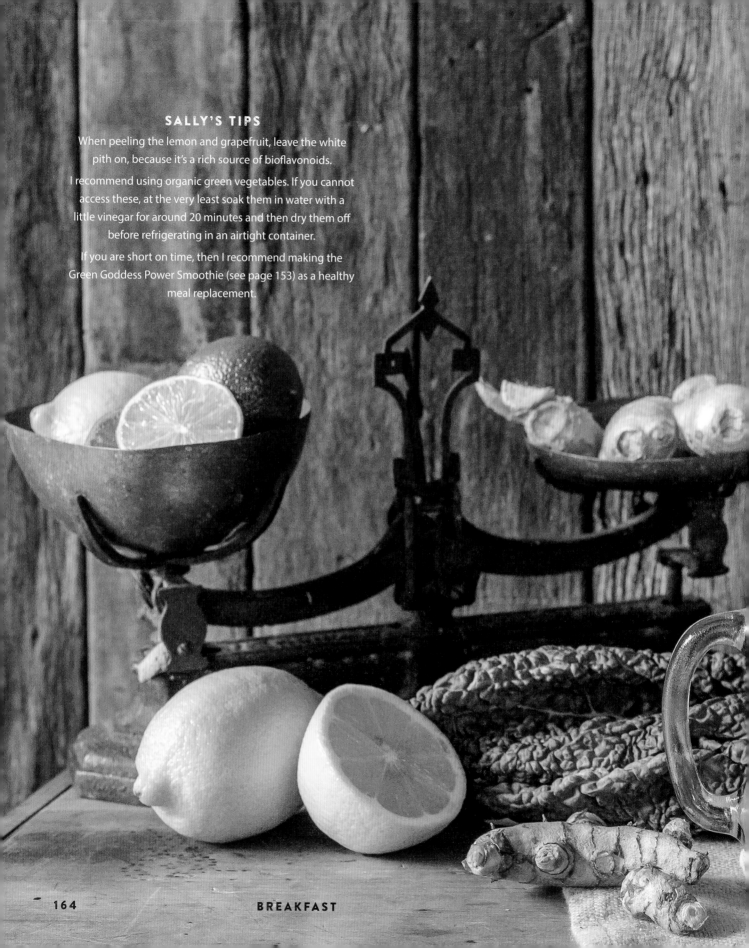

SALLY'S TIPS

When peeling the lemon and grapefruit, leave the white pith on, because it's a rich source of bioflavonoids.

I recommend using organic green vegetables. If you cannot access these, at the very least soak them in water with a little vinegar for around 20 minutes and then dry them off before refrigerating in an airtight container.

If you are short on time, then I recommend making the Green Goddess Power Smoothie (see page 153) as a healthy meal replacement.

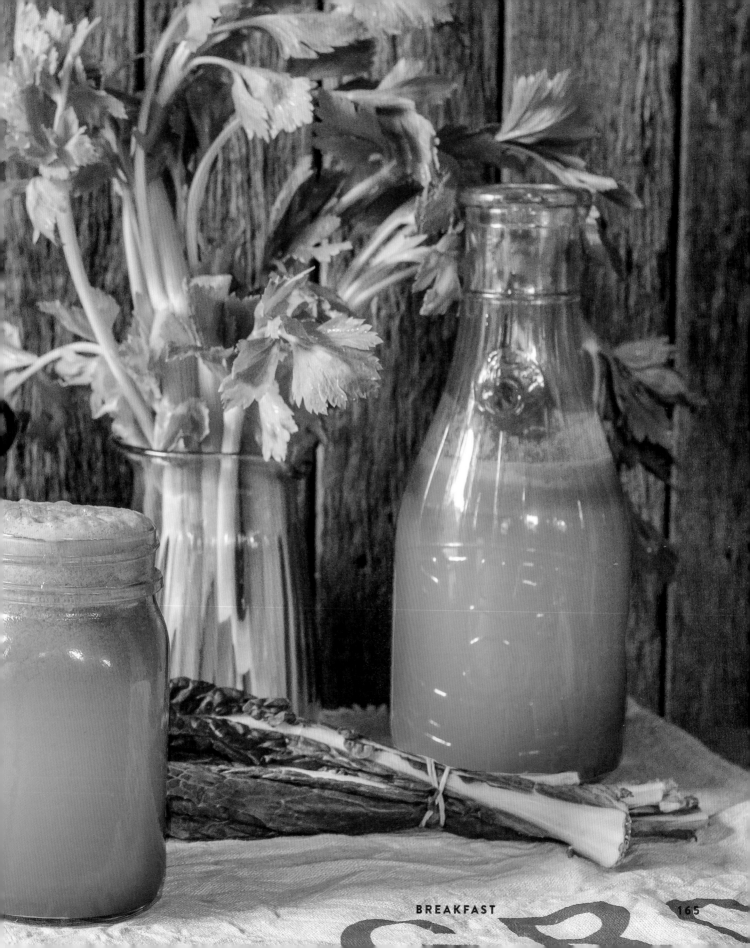

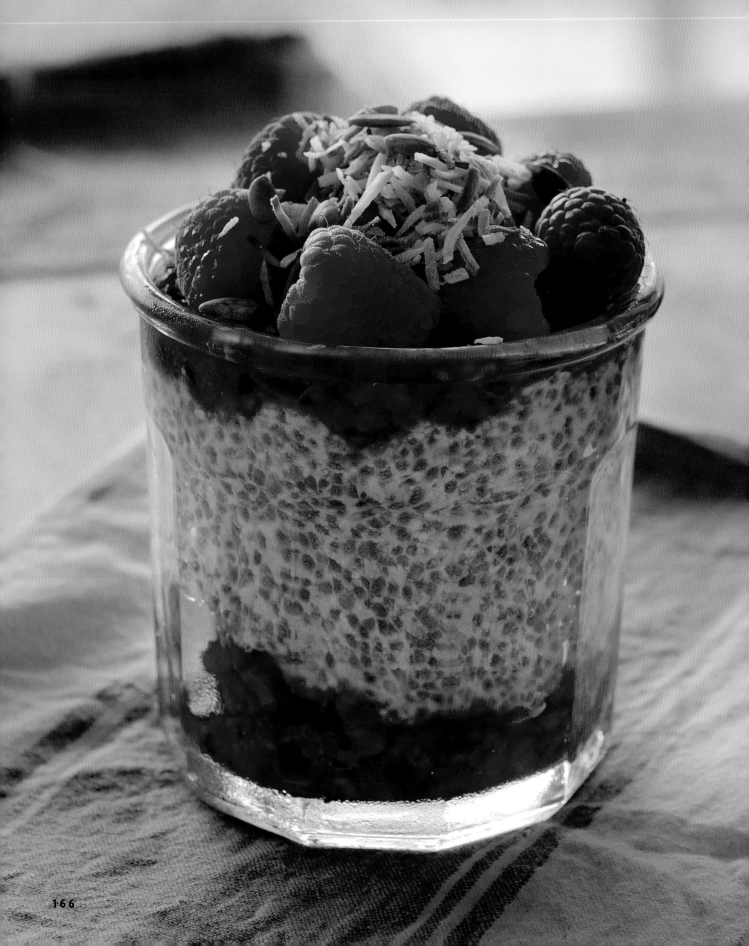

Raspberry Chia Pudding

If you fancy a change from eggs or smoothies for breakfast, then chia seed pudding is a great alternative! It's easy to make, but best prepared the night before or when you have an hour or so to allow it to set. Chia seeds are a rich source of fibre and combined with creamy coconut milk, make for a delicious healthy breakfast.

Method

Place the chia seeds, milk, cinnamon, rice malt syrup (or stevia) and vanilla in a mixing bowl. Stir with a wooden spoon until well combined. Refrigerate overnight, or for a minimum of 2 hours, until set.

Spoon a layer of the chia seed pudding into 2 glasses, followed by a layer of the mashed berries. Repeat with another layer of chia seed pudding and raspberries, then sprinkle with the raw cacao nibs, toasted coconut and pepitas.

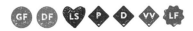

Ingredients

1/2 cup chia seeds

3 cups organic unsweetened coconut milk or almond milk

1/2 tsp ground cinnamon

2 tsp of rice malt syrup or 5 drops of stevia (optional)

1/2 tsp natural vanilla essence or powder

3/4 cup fresh or frozen organic raspberries, mashed

2 tsp raw cacao nibs (optional)

1 tbsp coconut flakes or desiccated coconut, toasted

2 tsp pepitas, toasted or raw

CHIA SEEDS

Chia seeds' main claim to fame is the fact that they are a great source of soluble fibre, the kind that feeds your gut flora and does not upset your gut like insoluble fibre can.

Chia is also claimed to be the highest source of Omega-3 fatty acids, with one tablespoon providing 2400 mg of Omega-3 fats, 3.5 g of protein and 5 g of fibre.

I add them to anything from soups or salads and many of my Nothing Naughty Treats recipes.

Be sure to buy a brand that is certified organic as some imported brands are heavily contaminated with nasty chemical sprays.

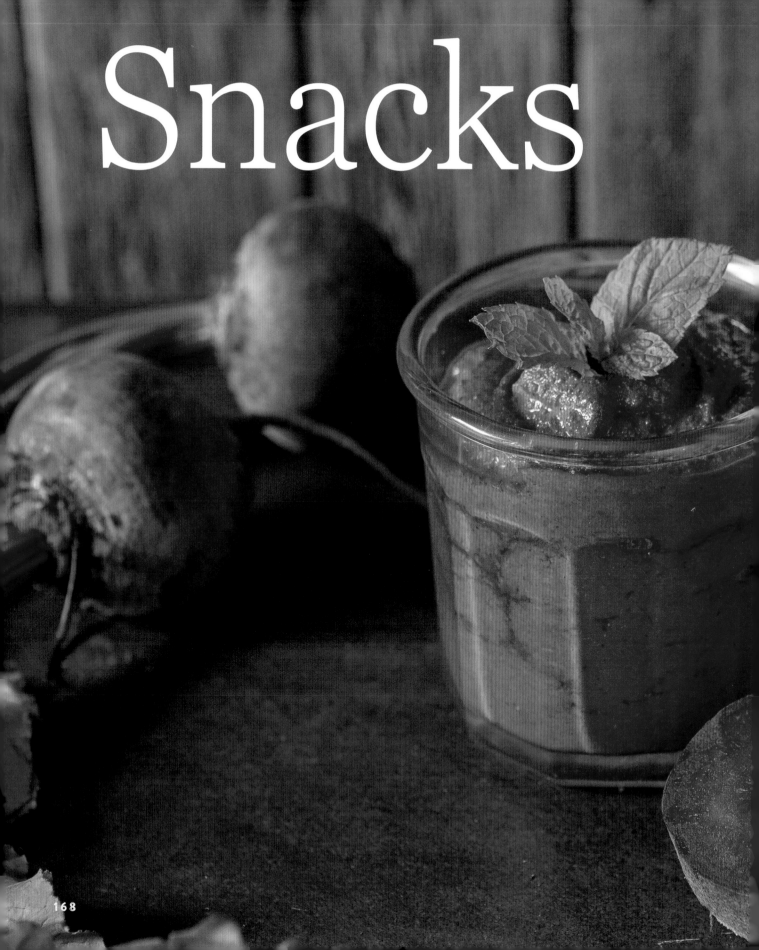

Snacks

Raw Beetroot & Mint Dip

I'm a big fan of preparing your own dips, because this way you know exactly what you're eating and can avoid all the artificial additives commonly found in packaged brands. This dip is a real winner, not only because it tastes delicious, but also because it can be used in so many dishes to add extra flavour, and makes a great accompaniment to salads.

Method

Place all the ingredients into a blender or food processor and blend until smooth and creamy. If too thick, add a little water to get the desired consistency

Store in an airtight container in the fridge for up to 3-4 days.

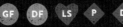

Ingredients

1 large beetroot, peeled

Juice of 1 lemon or 2 limes

2 tbsp extra virgin olive or macadamia oil

Himalayan or Celtic Sea Salt, to taste

3/4 cup raw cashew nuts

1/2 cup fresh mint leaves

SALLY'S TIPS
Serve a spoonful with salad, or as a side with lamb or chicken, or simply with some celery and cucumber sticks for a filling snack.

YOU CAN'T BEAT BEETROOT

Beetroot is a natural detoxifier and blood purifier and is rich in betaine, which can reduce inflammation and lower blood pressure. They also possess anti-cancer properties, thanks to the powerful phytonutrients that give beetroot its rich crimson colour. They are rich in fibre and nutrients such as vitamin C, potassium, manganese, folate and B vitamins. Be sure to keep your beetroot leaves as they contain many nutrients and can be juiced, sautéed with other vegetables or made into a tea simply by steeping in hot water for a few minutes with fresh turmeric.

Snacks

Who doesn't love a snack?! Snacking is something that can bring your weight loss efforts unstuck, mainly because we often go for the wrong choices. But if you make healthy snack choices, they can help to maintain your metabolism, balance your blood sugar and influence you to make healthier meal choices and better portion control. The key with healthy snacking is how much, how often, and what. Your tendency to snack is also influenced by your main meal choices and portion size.

Confusing "snacks" with "treats" Some snack foods can be confused with 'treats' offering little to no nutritional value, or they fail to leave you feeling satiated between meals and wanting to eat more. This is the case when you choose processed snacks which are typically loaded with sugar, gluten, soy, corn and artificial additives, not to mention processed vegetable oils.

If you're snacking on the office cookies, a can of soda, a chocolate bar, muffin or crisps, even a handful of 'fat free' pretzels or pop corn, then you are not snacking wisely and simply eating for pleasure vs nutrition. This type of snacking also puts you at high risk of overeating at meal times and weight gain.

A good way to gauge if you are making healthy snack choices is if you're eating smaller, healthier main meals and if your snack choice doesn't leave you wanting more. If you find yourself looking for sweet foods and feel you can't stop at just a few mouthfuls, this is a typical indicator that your snack choice is unhealthy.

TIPS FOR MAKING HEALTHY SNACK CHOICES

DON'T OVERDO THE FRUIT - While fruit is packed with vitamins and minerals, remember it also contains fructose so you may not find yourself feeling satiated from snacking on fruit alone, and be sure to choose low sugar varieties like berries, kiwi or grapefruit.

GO FOR PROTEINS AND FAT - foods containing protein and healthy fat fill you up! Snacks such as nut butter on celery sticks or sliced green apple, or healthy dips with celery or zucchini sticks, or even a few slices of roast turkey, or plain sheep or coconut yoghurt with cinnamon, will curb those sugar cravings and hunger pangs.

AVOID HIGH SUGAR AND HIGH STARCH - sitting on the couch or at your desk with a big bowl of crisps or biscuits is a sure fire way to put on weight, not just because you're sedentary, but because you're eating pure sugar which is more likely to convert to fat and fail to fill you up.

EAT SMART AT MEAL TIMES - Ensure you are eating enough of the right foods at meal times because this will influence your tendency to crave sugary snacks later in the day.

My advice is to make your own as often as possible, so why not try some of my simple snack recipes to get you on the right track.

MAKES 1 CUP (SERVING SIZE 3/4- 1 CUP)

Guacamole

Avocados are a rich source of monounsaturated fats and I recommend including a serve every day, either in your salads, breakfast smoothie or in this delicious guacamole dip which you can enjoy with a few zucchini , celery or carrot sticks.

Ingredients

2 ripe avocados, peeled, seed removed

Juice of 1 lemon

1/4 cup of extra virgin olive or macadamia oil

Himalayan or Celtic Sea Salt and freshly ground black pepper, to taste

1-2 tsp rice malt syrup (optional)

1/4 cup fresh coriander/cilantro leaves (optional)

Method

Place all the ingredients into a mixing bowl and mash with a fork to combine well. Add more lemon juice if you prefer a more tangy flavour.

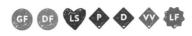

AVOCADO

Contrary to popular belief, avocados are not fattening and they certainly do not increase cholesterol, but in fact help to reduce bad cholesterol and inflammation and are great for healthy skin, hair and nails. Avocados are also a really good source of potassium, a mineral essential for a healthy heart function and fluid regulation.

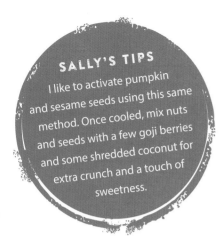

SALLY'S TIPS

I like to activate pumpkin and sesame seeds using this same method. Once cooled, mix nuts and seeds with a few goji berries and some shredded coconut for extra crunch and a touch of sweetness.

(SERVING SIZE 3/4-1 CUP)

Activated Nuts & Seeds

Now you may think it a little odd to go 'activating your nuts', but I'm talking about a process which enhances their nutritional benefits, by decreasing levels of a not-so-healthy compound known as phytic acid. Excess levels of phytic acid from eating too many raw nuts can block the absorption of essential trace minerals like magnesium, iron, potassium, zinc and calcium. So although nuts are a rich source of plant protein and slow burning carbohydrates, they are also high in Omega-6 fats. These type of fats need to be carefully balanced with your intake of Omega-3 fats. I recommend you don't overdo your nut consumption for this reason, and try to consume mainly activated nuts.

This recipe is simple to prepare and is a heck of a lot cheaper than buying activated nuts, but it does take all day to prepare, so I recommend making a big batch when you can be at home and can leave the oven on safely.

Soaking the nuts in water overnight, before putting them in the oven, will also activate specific enzymes, making them easier to digest. Using a low heat to roast them will prevent the Omega-6 fats from oxidizing.

Method

To make, place a batch of mixed raw nuts such as almonds, walnuts, Brazil or pecans and seeds like pumpkin and sesame, in a big bowl of water with a tablespoon of Himalayan or Celtic Sea Salt. Cover and leave to soak 4-6 hrs. Preheat the oven to 50°C - 60°C or 120-140°F. (too high and you will damage the delicate essential fatty acids in the nuts and seeds). Rinse and drain the nuts, then spread evenly onto baking trays. Bake for a minimum of 6 hours - up to 24hrs if desired.

Cool completely then store in an airtight container either in the fridge or in a cool dark pantry to maintain freshness and prevent oxidation from exposure to air.

Store in an air tight jar in the fridge to prevent from going rancid, for up to 6 weeks.

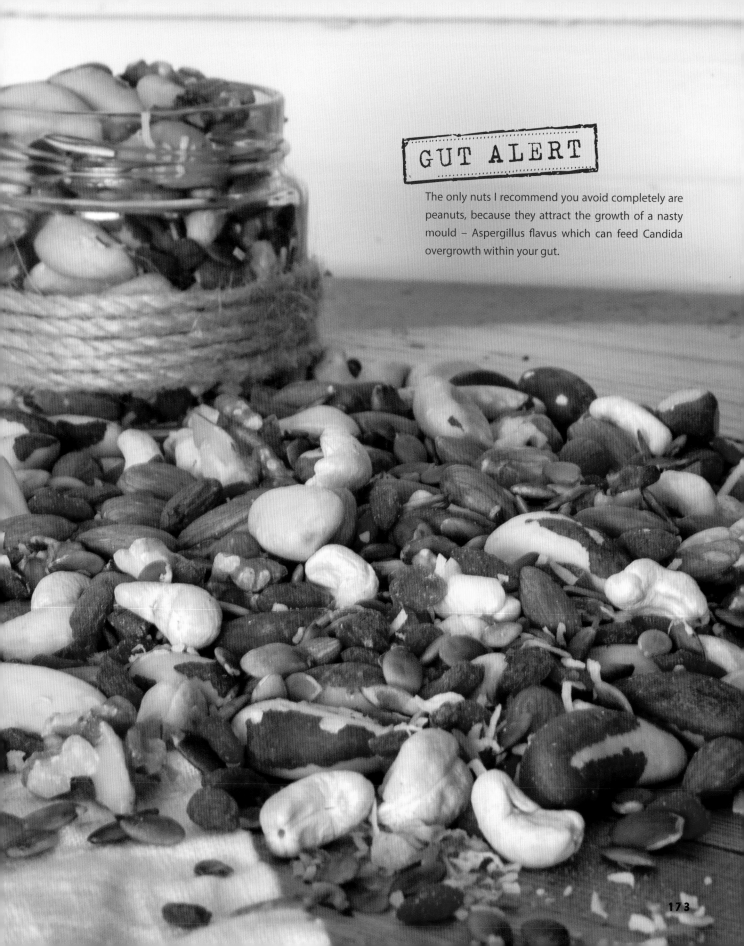

The only nuts I recommend you avoid completely are peanuts, because they attract the growth of a nasty mould – Aspergillus flavus which can feed Candida overgrowth within your gut.

Because hummus is made from chickpeas, which are a legume, they can cause an upset tummy for some people. If you find this is the case, hold off until after your gut has healed before introducing them back into your diet.

MAKES 2 -3 CUPS (SERVING SIZE 1/2-3/4 CUP)

Almond Hummus

I prefer to make my own hummus, as I do all dips, because it always tastes so much better, not to mention the money it saves! It only takes 5 minutes to make this and I like to whip up a batch each week for a healthy high-protein, low-carb snack.

Ingredients

400g tin organic chickpeas, rinsed and drained

1/2 cup water

Juice of 1 lemon, or to taste

1 tbsp hulled tahini

1/2 cup raw almonds

1 cup extra virgin olive oil or macadamia oil

1 tsp rice malt syrup

Pinch of Himalayan or Celtic Sea Salt, or to taste

1 garlic clove, crushed

1/4 cup fresh coriander or parsley (optional)

Method

Place all the ingredients into a food processor and blend until smooth and creamy. Feel free to adjust the flavour to taste, by adding more tahini, lemon juice or olive oil.

(GF) (DF) (LS) (P) (D) (VV)

SALLY'S TIPS
You can soak & cook chickpeas from scratch rather than using them from a tin. You will need 1 1/2 cups cooked chickpeas.

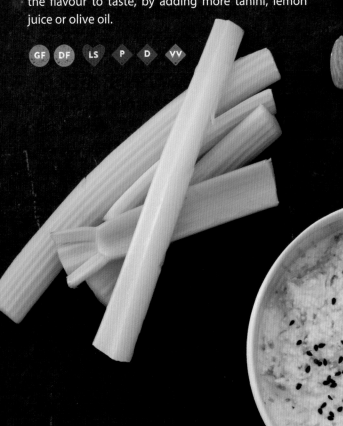

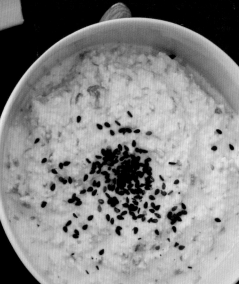

MAKES 1 CUP

Almond Nut Butter

Nut butter makes a great sugar-free snack for you or the kids, and you can make it using Brazil nuts, cashews, macadamias, hazelnuts or raw almonds — or a combination of nuts! Nut butter is quick and easy to make and a heck of lot cheaper than buying it. If you do choose to buy nut butter, look for a brand that is unsweetened and remember to moderate your consumption, because they are typically made with nuts that have not been pre-soaked so they will be higher in phytic acid. If you live in the US, you cannot buy raw nuts in most supermarkets.

Ingredients

3 cups raw almonds, soaked overnight

1 tbsp virgin coconut oil

1 tbsp olive, flax or macadamia oil

1/4 tsp Himalayan or Celtic Sea Salt

Method

Place the nuts into a food processer. Blend for approximately ten minutes (the time will vary depending on the strength of your food processor), until smooth. Scrape down the sides occasionally to ensure the nuts are crushed to the same consistency. The nuts will be powdery at first, but keep processing until they turn to a buttery paste. Add more coconut oil if required (be consistent with ingredients).

Transfer the mixture to a large mixing bowl and add the virgin coconut oil, salt and brown rice syrup or stevia and mix with a wooden spoon.

SALLY'S TIPS

Spread over a couple of sticks of celery or a few slices of green apple — but a word of warning, this snack is VERY moreish, so watch you don't overdo it!

Grain Free Granola Bars

I classify most muesli and granola bars as nothing more than high-sugar junk food, despite what the manufacturer may tell you! But there's no doubt that kids love the taste and Mums love the convenience, so I have created a recipe that contains none of the nasties and all of the goodies of this popular snack. It's very low in sugar and tastes delicious, I guarantee it! Feel free to leave out the nuts if your kids can't take them to school

Method

Preheat the oven to 180°C / 350°F and line a 28 x 18 cm slice tin with baking/parchment paper.

Place all the ingredients into a mixing bowl and use your hands to mix together thoroughly.

Transfer mix to the baking tray and, using your fingers or a spoon, firmly press the mixture evenly to cover the bottom of the tray.

Bake for about 20 minutes or until golden brown. Cool to room temperature, before cutting into slices around the size of your 3 middle fingers.

Ingredients

1 cup coconut flakes

1/2 cup of cashew nuts

1/2 cup slithered almonds

1/2 cup sunflower seeds

1/2 cup pepitas

1/2 cup sesame seeds

1/2 cup chia seeds

1/2 cup goji berries

1 tsp ground cinnamon

1 tsp ground nutmeg

2 tsp natural vanilla essence or powder

1 tsp Himalayan or Celtic Sea Salt

2 tbsp virgin coconut oil, melted

1/2 cup rice malt syrup

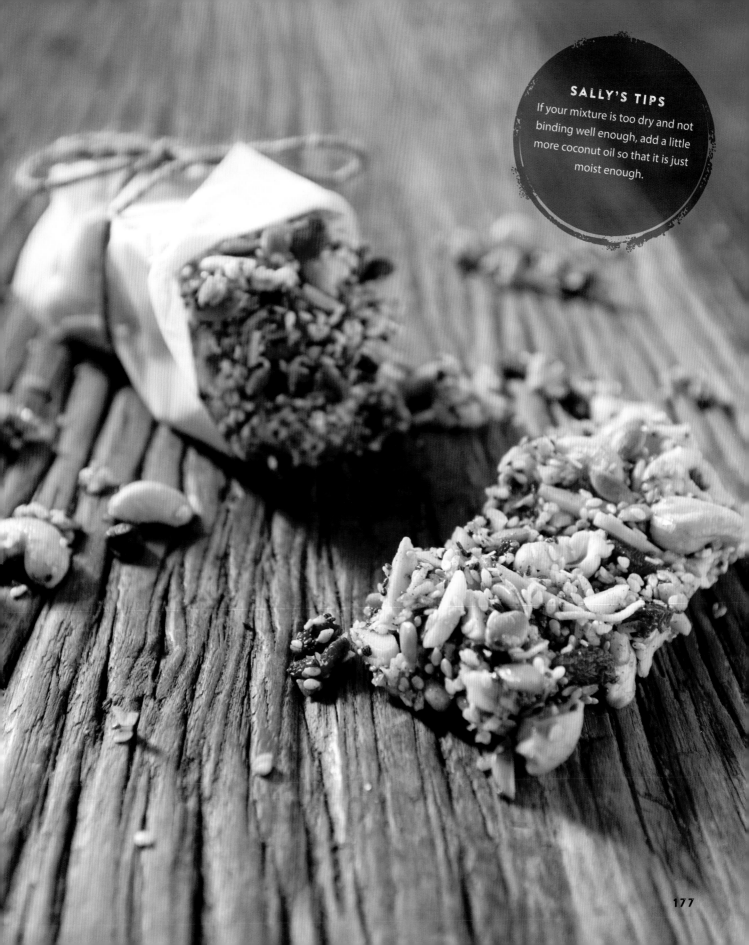

SALLY'S TIPS

If your mixture is too dry and not binding well enough, add a little more coconut oil so that it is just moist enough.

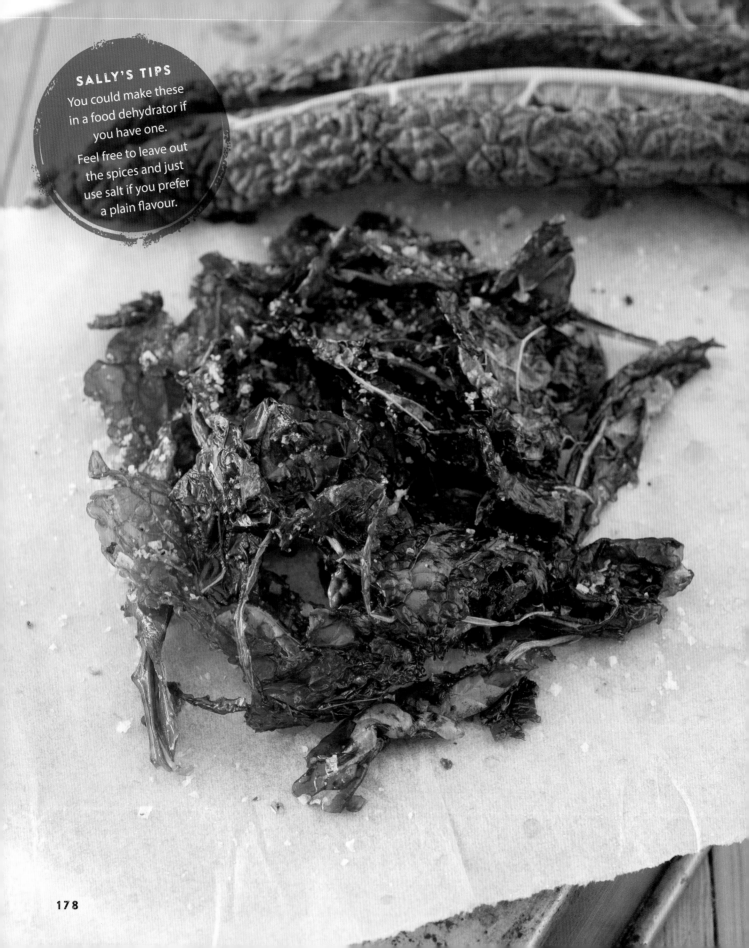

SALLY'S TIPS
You could make these in a food dehydrator if you have one.

Feel free to leave out the spices and just use salt if you prefer a plain flavour.

SERVES 2 (SERVING SIZE 1-2 HANDFULS)

Spicy Kale Chips

I fell in love with these a few years ago, when I was looking for a healthy snack, travelling in the US. When I got home I went on a mission to learn how to bake them myself. They are seriously delicious and a far healthier option than those standard high-starch fried potato or GMO corn chips, that are often cooked in vegetable oils and laden with artificial flavours and colours. Spicy Kale Chips are the perfect snack when you're on the run, or to pack in the kids lunch box. They might get some funny looks at first with their green chips, but they'll be converting their schoolmates before you know it!

Method

Preheat the oven to 120°C/250°F and line baking trays with baking /parchment paper. Tear or cut the kale roughly into pieces. Place the oil, salt and spices into a mixing bowl and stir to combine. Add the kale leaves and toss through the oil and spices to coat evenly.

Place the kale onto the prepared trays and place into the oven. Bake for 30 minutes or until crispy, turning them halfway through so they bake evenly.

Best served immediately, or store in the fridge in an airtight container.

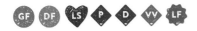

KALE ALERT

A word of caution. Because kale belongs to the brassica family of vegetables, it is a natural goitrogen. This means that eating too much raw kale, along with other cruciferous vegetables, can inhibit optimal thyroid function, especially if you already have an underactive thyroid. Like everything in life, moderation is the key!

Ingredients

1 bunch kale, removed from the stalk

2 tbsp ghee, coconut or macadamia oil

Pinch Himalayan or Celtic Sea Salt

1 tsp ground turmeric (optional)

1 tsp ground cumin (optional)

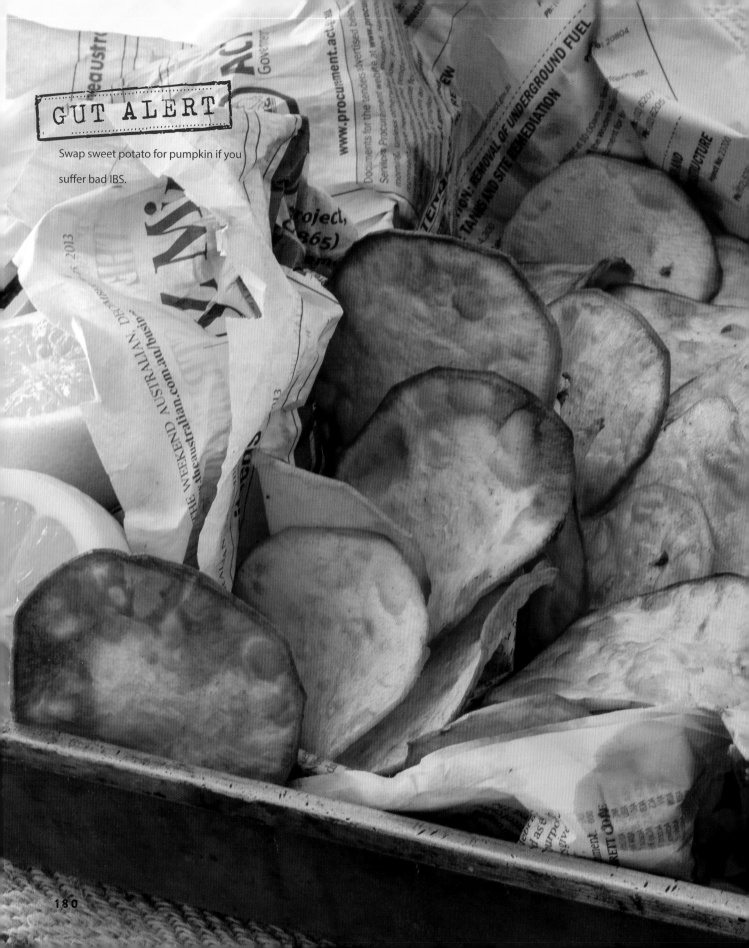

GUT ALERT

Swap sweet potato for pumpkin if you suffer bad IBS.

Sweet Potato Chips

Yes, even chips are on the menu! But these are baked, not fried, and made from sweet potato which is a healthier choice than higher-starch white potato. I find these are a great option for when you are weaning off sugar or craving some comfort food. I always bake in ghee or virgin coconut oil and season with Himalayan or Celtic Sea Salt, which is rich in essential trace minerals. Serve on their own or with a little homemade aioli mayonnaise (see page 283).

Ingredients

1 large sweet potato, peeled and into finger width slices

1 tbsp ghee or virgin coconut oil

Himalayan or Celtic Sea Salt

1 tsp ground cinnamon (optional)

1 tsp ground nutmeg (optional)

Method

Preheat the oven to 180°C/350°F and line a tray with baking/parchment paper. Place the sliced sweet potato in a mixing bowl and coat generously with the ghee or coconut oil, salt and spices.

Arrange sweet potato slices onto the prepared tray. Bake for about 20 minutes, or until crispy and cooked through.

Tzatziki Dip

I have replaced the traditional cow's milk yoghurt with sheep's to make a delicious healthy dip to serve with a few celery or cucumber sticks, or as an accompaniment to main dishes – especially lamb or pan fried fish! You will notice a lot of my recipes recommend serving with a dollop of plain sheep's yoghurt for a little extra fat and creaminess to leave you feeling fuller for longer.

Ingredients

1/2 cup sheep's milk yoghurt

1/3 cup cucumber, grated (I prefer the Lebanese variety)

1 garlic clove, crushed

1 tsp lemon juice

1 tsp roughly chopped fresh dill.

Method

Combine all ingredients in a bowl. Refrigerate until ready to use. Serve with fresh cucumber or celery sticks for dipping.

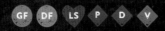

Zesty Herb Warm Olives

There's nothing quite like warm olives with herbs and the rind of fresh lemon and orange. Olives make a super healthy snack and are great to serve when friends drop by. I recommend always keeping olives on hand, as they are especially good for nipping those sugar cravings in the bud!

Ingredients

1 orange, I use a vegetable peeler and then cut the rind into thin strips

1/2 lemon

2 cups mixed olives

2 garlic cloves, crushed

2 tbsp fresh lemon juice

4 fresh bay leaves

1/3 cup extra virgin olive or macadamia oil

Fresh rosemary leaves, to serve

Method

Preheat the oven to 180°C or 350°F. Use a vegetable peeler to peel the rind from the orange and lemon, then cut into thin strips.

Combine the olives, garlic, orange and lemon rind, lemon juice and bay leaves in a small baking dish. Place into the oven for 5-10 minutes or until warm. Serve immediately, drizzled with a little extra virgin olive oil and rosemary leaves.

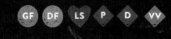

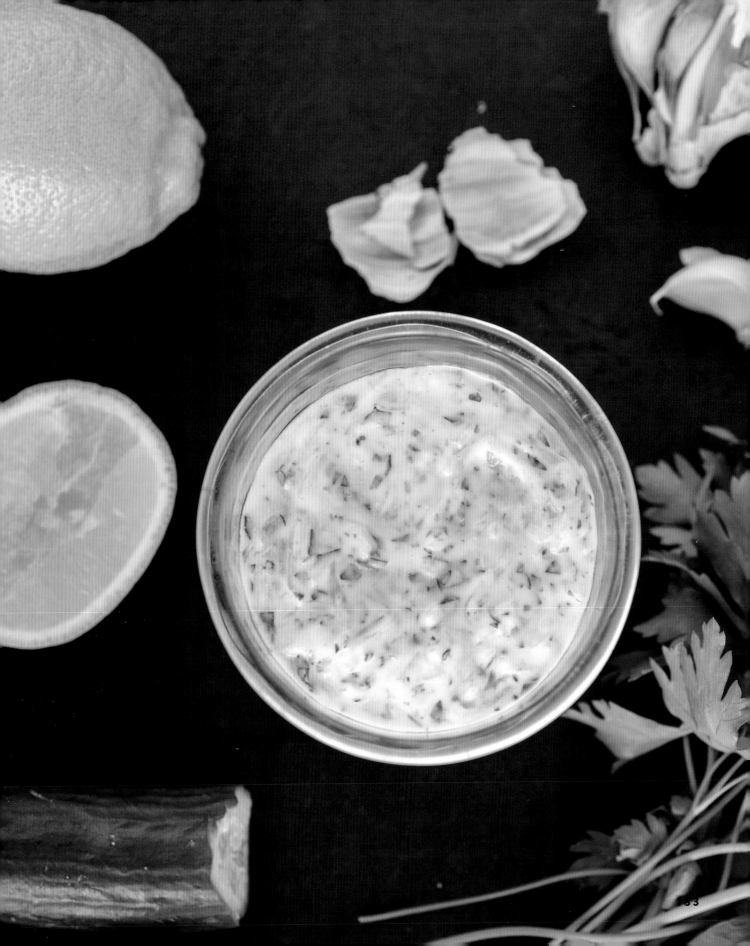

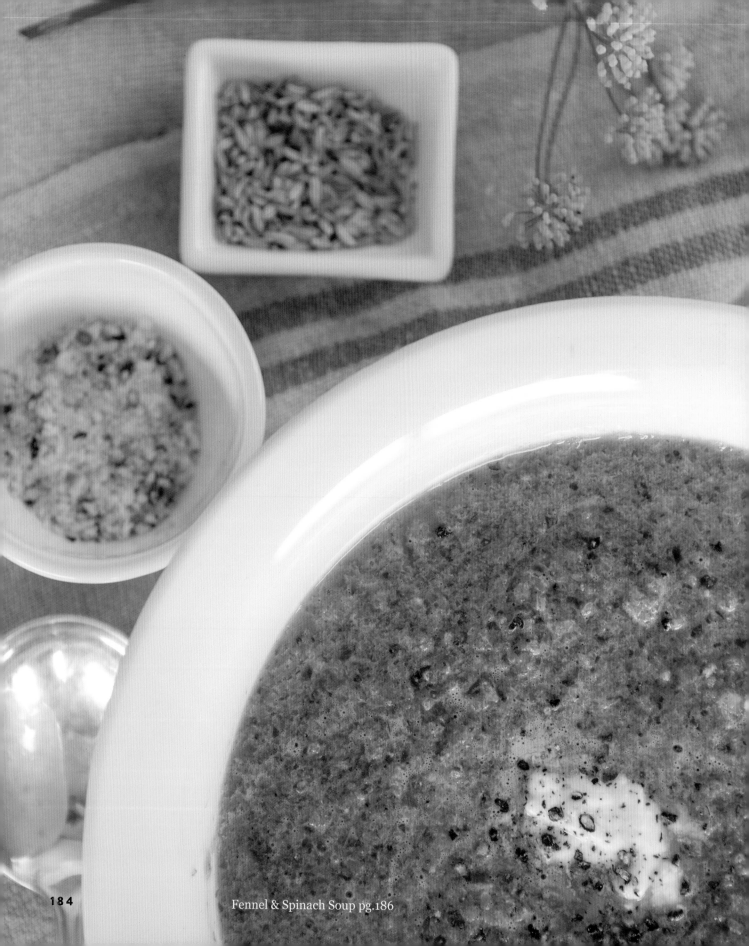

Fennel & Spinach Soup pg.186

Soups

Soups feature heavily on the LYG program and for good reason. First and foremost, soups are easy to digest, which translates to a happy gut; secondly, they are nutrient-dense, thanks to being rich in fibre from vegetables, which your gut flora also LOVE! But aside from all the nutritional benefits, soup also makes a super convenient meal choice. You can prepare it in advance and refrigerate or freeze it, so you will never have an excuse to say 'there's nothing healthy to eat'. Soups are also a perfect choice for dinner because, as soup is a liquid, your digestive system doesn't need to work nearly as hard to digest it, compared to animal proteins like chicken or red meat. Bottom line: eating a smaller, easily digestible meal at dinner translates to healthier digestion, better metabolism and more restful sleep.

Fennel and Spinach Soup

Ingredients

1 tbsp ghee, macadamia or coconut oil

2 fennel bulbs, sliced

1 brown onion, peeled and diced

Himalayan or Celtic Sea Salt and freshly ground black pepper, to taste

2 garlic cloves, crushed

3 cups chicken stock(see page 190) or vegetable stock (see page 187)

1- 2 cups baby spinach leaves

125g flat-leaf parsley, roughly chopped

Finely grated zest and juice of 1/2 a lemon

2 tbsp plain sheep's yoghurt or goat's feta

Method

Heat the oil in a large saucepan over medium heat. Add the fennel and onion, and season with salt and pepper. Sautee for 7-8 minutes, until the fennel and onion have softened, then add the garlic and continue cooking for a couple more minutes.

Add the stock and bring to the boil, then reduce heat to low and add the spinach and parsley. Stir until the spinach leaves have wilted. Transfer to a blender, or use a stick blender and blend until smooth.

Add the lemon zest and juice. Serve topped with a spoonful of sheep's yoghurt or goat's feta. Season with pepper.

This soup is delicious served hot or cold. Refrigerate in an airtight container for up to 3 days or freeze for up to 3 months.

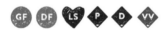

GUT ALERT

Fennel is great for digestive support and can relieve indigestion, heartburn, gas and bloating, unless you are sensitive to sulphur, in which case it may not agree with you. Sulphur is found in a range of other foods too including leek, garlic, onions, spring onions and shallots. If you have a sensitivity to sulphur, or if these foods cause gastrointestinal upset, I recommend avoiding them and substituting with other natural flavours from homemade vegetable or chicken stock, fresh herbs and lemon juice.

Alkalising Vegetable Broth

This broth is super alkalizing, which will help to reduce inflammation within your body and aid in natural detoxification. Be sure to use all organic ingredients to avoid any chemical sprays, but if these are difficult to access, then at least soakany vegetables in water and white vinegar for around 20 minutes.

Ingredients

3 carrots, peeled and diced

1/2 head celery, leaves included, chopped

1 cup of chopped spinach silverbeet, leaves and stalks

1 cup cabbage, chopped

1 cup zucchini, diced

1 bunch fresh flat-leaf parsley

1 tsp ground cumin

1 tsp ground turmeric

Himalayan or Celtic Sea Salt and freshly ground black pepper to taste

Method

Place the carrots, celery, cabbage and zucchini in a large stockpot or saucepan and cover with filtered

water – approximately 4 litres. Bring to the boil, then reduce the heat and simmer covered for 20 minutes.

Add the silverbeet and parsley and simmer for a further 5 minutes. Season with cumin, turmeric, salt and pepper. Strain the liquid and discard the vegetables as all the broth will now be jam-packed with all the nutrients. You can choose to double the recipe to make up enough for the next day.

Store in an airtight container in the fridge up to five days or freeze for up to three months.

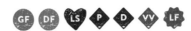

GUT ALERT

I recommend incorporating this broth during the 'strip back and alkalise stage' of the program, to fast track the detox process. Feel free to consume this broth any time your body needs a bit of a cleanse, or you're experiencing any symptoms of acute inflammation, like arthritis or skin rashes. I find this broth is also effective for helping to overcome sugar cravings.

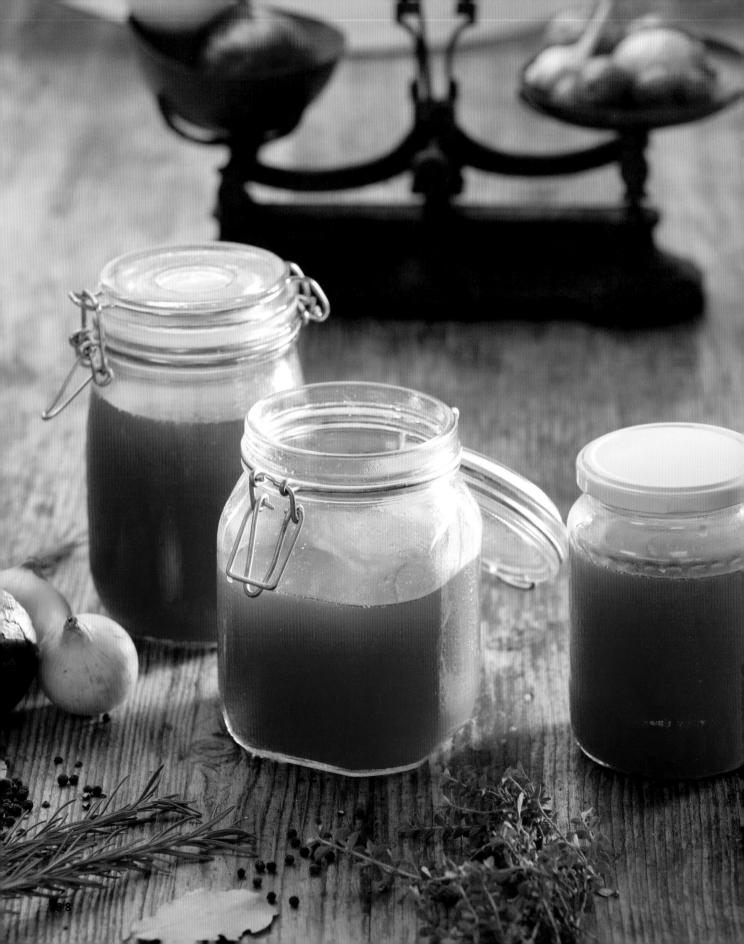

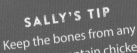

Bone Broth

SALLY'S TIP
Keep the bones from any recipes that contain chicken, beef or lamb bones, and freeze them to make bone broth.

Bone Broth is fine example of something old becoming new again, as the health benefits of this ancient tradition are rediscovered. There are endless nutritional benefits to drinking bone broth, including improving the absorption of nutrients. It is a rich source of essential minerals like magnesium, iron, calcium, phosphorus and the gut-healing amino acid glutamine. It's also a rich source of collagen and gelatine, which is fantastic for aiding skin, hair and nail growth and cartilage repair. If you suffer from any sort of gut or digestive problem, autoimmune disease or gluten intolerance, I particularly recommend including bone broth in your daily diet regularly. It has a soothing effect on the gut, making it ideal for calming any sort of inflammation and aids in the repair of the intestinal wall.

Ask your butcher for chicken, beef, or lamb bones – just ensure the chicken bones are organic, or at least chemical-free and the beef or lamb bones are from 100% grass fed animals - to avoid any nasty hormones and antibiotics. If you are making beef bone broth, ask your butcher to include a combination of knuckle and thigh bones and to cut any large bones in half to reveal the marrow, which is particularly nutritious.

Ingredients

4.5- 5.5kgs (10 - 12 pounds) organic chicken, beef or lamb bones

2 - 3 tablespoons of apple cider vinegar

1 large onion, peeled & sliced

1 head of garlic

1 celery heart

2 bay leaves

2-3 sprigs of rosemary

pinch of Himalayan or Celtic sea salt

Filtered water to cover

Method

If using raw bones, roast them in the oven at 200°C/400°F for 30- 45 minutes, or until golden brown, turning half way through. This will improve the flavour of the broth. Place the bones and remaining ingredients into a large stockpot or saucepan (or slow cooker) and add enough water to just cover the bones. Bring to the boil then reduce heat to low, and simmer for 12 - 24 hours. Top up with water to ensure the bones are kept covered at all times. Allow the broth to cool further so that any fat solidifies, then using a slotted spoon, skim any fat from the surface. Broth will keep in the fridge for 1 week, or you can freeze to use as a base for soups.

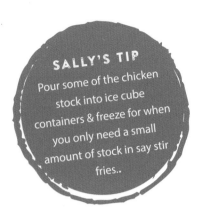

MAKES 2-3 LITRES

Home Made Chicken Stock

Chicken stock is a LYG healthy pantry essential on the LYG program, not only because it's super healthy for your gut, but also because it serves as the base for so many LYG recipes. Many folks are putting off making their own stock, thinking it is all too hard, but in fact nothing could be simpler and more nourishing. It tastes so much better than many packaged brands, which are often full of artificial ingredients and added sugar or yeast. If you choose to buy ready-made stock, be sure to look for an organic brand, free of antibiotics, yeast & addded sugar. Add the cooked chicken meat in this recipe to soups, or refrigerate and add to salads during the week.

Ingredients

1 whole organic or chemical free chicken

4-5 litres of water or enough to fill your soup pot

3 celery stalks, cut into chunks

2 carrots, peeled

2 tsp whole peppercorns

2-3 bay leaves

1 large handful mixed fresh herbs, such as tarragon, thyme, sage and flat-leaf parsley

1 onion, peeled and halved

4 garlic cloves

1/2 lemon

Method

Place all ingredients into a large stockpot and add enough water to cover the chicken (about 4-5 litres). Replace the lid and bring to the boil.   Remove the lid and reduce heat to low and simmer for 3-4 hrs (no less than 2 if you are in a hurry).

Remove the chicken from the pot when cooked and pull the meat from the bones and refrigerate in an air tight container to use in chicken soup or salads. Place a large strainer over a large soup pot and strain the remaining liquid into the pot.   Discard the solids and allow the stock to cool, before dividing between airtight containers. Refrigerate for up to 4 days, or freeze for up to 6 months.

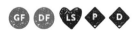

Parsley Oil

Prepare this recipe the day before to allow lentils time to soak.

Ingredients

2 bunches fresh flat-leaf parsley, leaves and stems, rinsed

1/4 cup extra-virgin olive oil or coconut oil

Method

Put parsley leaves and stems into a sieve and pour boiling water over. Hold under cold water to stop cooking, wrap in a paper towel and place in refrigerator.

Transfer parsley to a food processor and blend with the oil. Put mixture into cheesecloth, or a fresh, rinsed through "Chux" cloth or a coffee filter and allow to drain over a bowl. Add salt.

Store oil in an airtight container in refrigerator for up to 1 week.

Shake well before use.

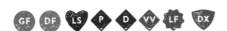

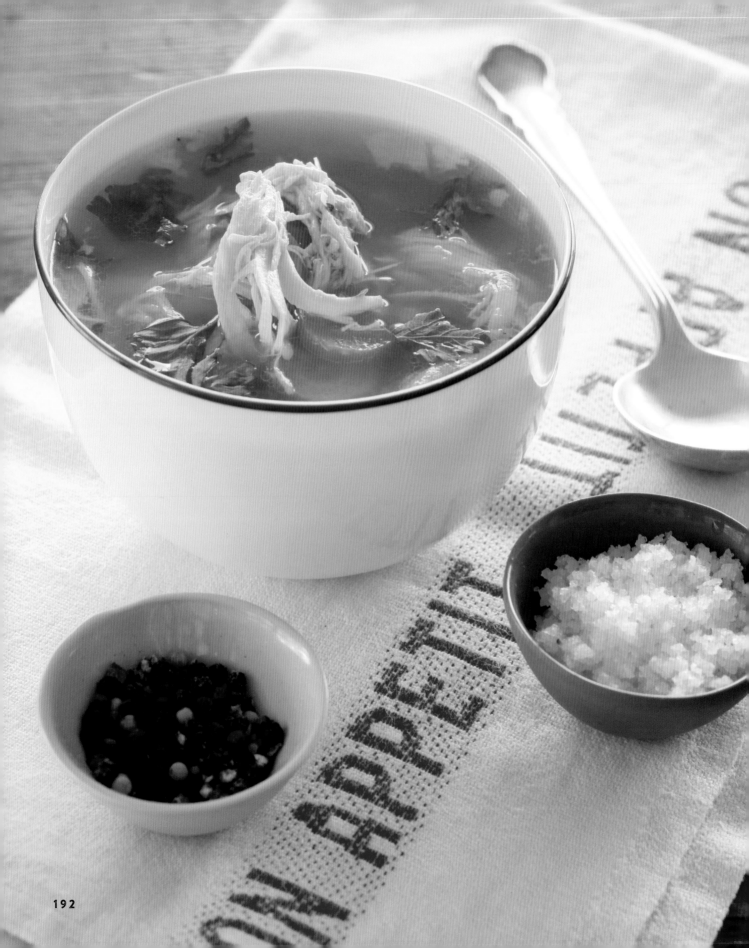

Chicken & Spring Vegetable Soup

There is nothing heartier and more nourishing than homemade chicken soup, because as they say, it really is good for the soul. I like to keep a stash in the freezer for those nights I am short on time to prepare dinner. This way you can simply heat it up in a large saucepan and add any extra fresh vegetables you desire

Method

To make the chicken stock, (see recipe on page 190). Place the stock into a large saucepan and add the chicken meat and vegetables, and season to taste with salt and pepper.

Cover and simmer for 10 minutes or until vegetables are just soft.

Garnish with freshly chopped parsley and serve.

Ingredients

2 -3 litres of chicken stock (see page 190)

Meat from 1 poached chicken

2 carrots, peeled and sliced

1-2 cups of baby kale leaves

1 cup of fresh or frozen peas

1 cup green beans, cut into 4cm pieces

2 celery stalks, finely sliced

Himalayan or Celtic Sea Salt and freshly ground black pepper, to taste

Chopped flat-leaf parsley, to serve

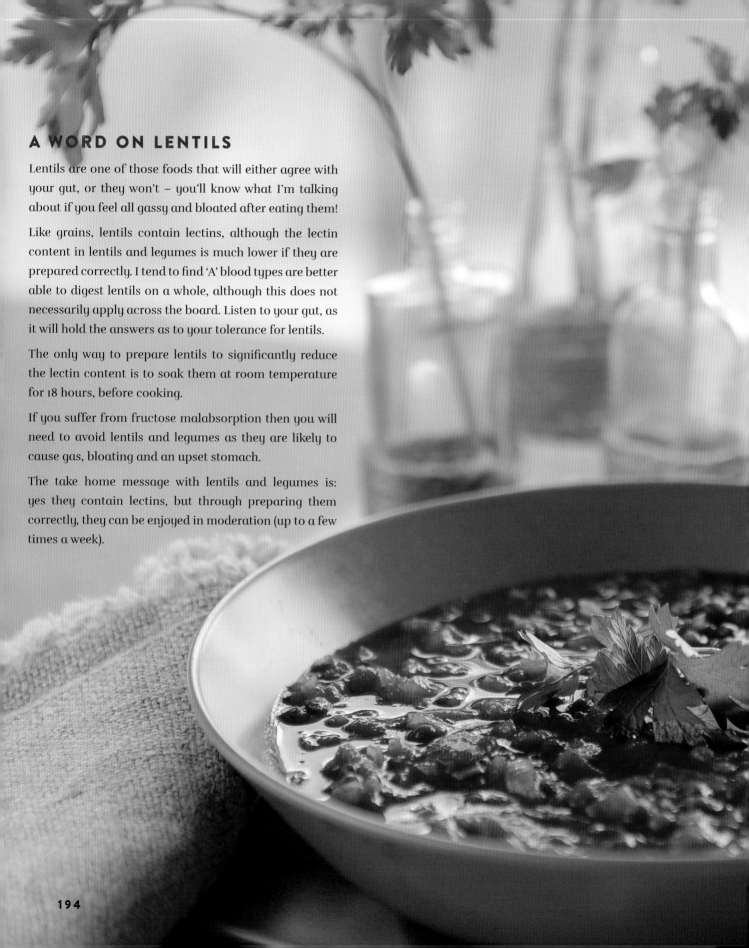

A WORD ON LENTILS

Lentils are one of those foods that will either agree with your gut, or they won't – you'll know what I'm talking about if you feel all gassy and bloated after eating them!

Like grains, lentils contain lectins, although the lectin content in lentils and legumes is much lower if they are prepared correctly. I tend to find 'A' blood types are better able to digest lentils on a whole, although this does not necessarily apply across the board. Listen to your gut, as it will hold the answers as to your tolerance for lentils.

The only way to prepare lentils to significantly reduce the lectin content is to soak them at room temperature for 18 hours, before cooking.

If you suffer from fructose malabsorption then you will need to avoid lentils and legumes as they are likely to cause gas, bloating and an upset stomach.

The take home message with lentils and legumes is: yes they contain lectins, but through preparing them correctly, they can be enjoyed in moderation (up to a few times a week).

Lentil Soup

Prepare this recipe the day before to allow lentils time to soak.

Method

Place the lentils into a large bowl and cover with cold water. Soak for 18 hours, then tip into a strainer and rinse under cold running water until the water runs clear.

Heat a little oil in a large saucepan over medium-low heat and sauté the onions, garlic and ginger for 5 minutes, until soft. Add a pinch of salt. Add the cumin and cayenne pepper and stir for another minute or so, until fragrant.

Add the tomatoes, around three-quarters of the lemon juice, lentils and vegetable stock. Stir to combine then cover and bring to the boil. Reduce the heat and simmer for about 30 minutes, or until the lentils are soft. Add remaining lemon juice.

Serve hot or cold, sprinkled with chopped fresh coriander or flat-leaf parsley, if you like and salt and pepper to taste.

GF DF LS D VV

Ingredients

1 cup red or brown lentils

Virgin coconut oil or macadamia oil

1 large onion, diced

5 garlic cloves, crushed

Pinch Himalayan or Celtic Sea Salt

1 tbsp grated fresh ginger

1 tbsp ground cumin

1/4 tsp cayenne pepper

4 large ripe tomatoes, chopped

1 lemon, juiced

4 cups chicken stock or vegetable stock (see recipes page 190 & 187). May use packaged stock as long as it is organic and yeast free

Himalayan or Celtic Sea Salt and freshly ground black pepper, to taste

Creamy Coconut Zucchini Soup

Ingredients

2 tbsp ghee / virgin coconut or macadamia oil for frying

1 onion, roughly chopped

4 garlic cloves, roughly chopped

6-8 large zucchini, roughly chopped

Himalayan or Celtic Sea Salt and freshly ground black pepper, to taste

1 litre chicken or vegetable stock (see recipes page 190 & 187)

400ml coconut milk or cream

Handful slivered toasted almonds, to serve

Zucchini's make a regular appearance in my recipes, not only because they're so versatile and delicious, but also because they are particularly high in fibre and nutrients like vitamin C and manganese. I love adding them to soups and salads, both raw and cooked, and they taste delicious baked or sautéed. The healthy fat from the coconut milk in this soup will leave you feeling more satisfied, making this recipe a healthy choice for lunch or dinner, served hot or cold.

Method

Heat the ghee or oil in a large saucepan or large deep frying pan over medium heat. Add the onion and sauté for about 3 minutes, until they become transparent. Add the garlic and cook for another minute, being careful not to burn.

Add the zucchini and season generously with salt and pepper. Cook, stirring occasionally for 10 minutes, or until zucchini is lightly golden brown.

Stir in the stock and bring to the boil, then reduce the heat to low and simmer for 15 minutes or until zucchini is very soft. Remove from the heat and stir in the coconut milk. Cool slightly and transfer to a blender, or use a stick blender and blend until smooth.

Return to the pan if you want to reheat. Serve with a sprinkle of ground cinnamon and/or toasted slivered almonds.

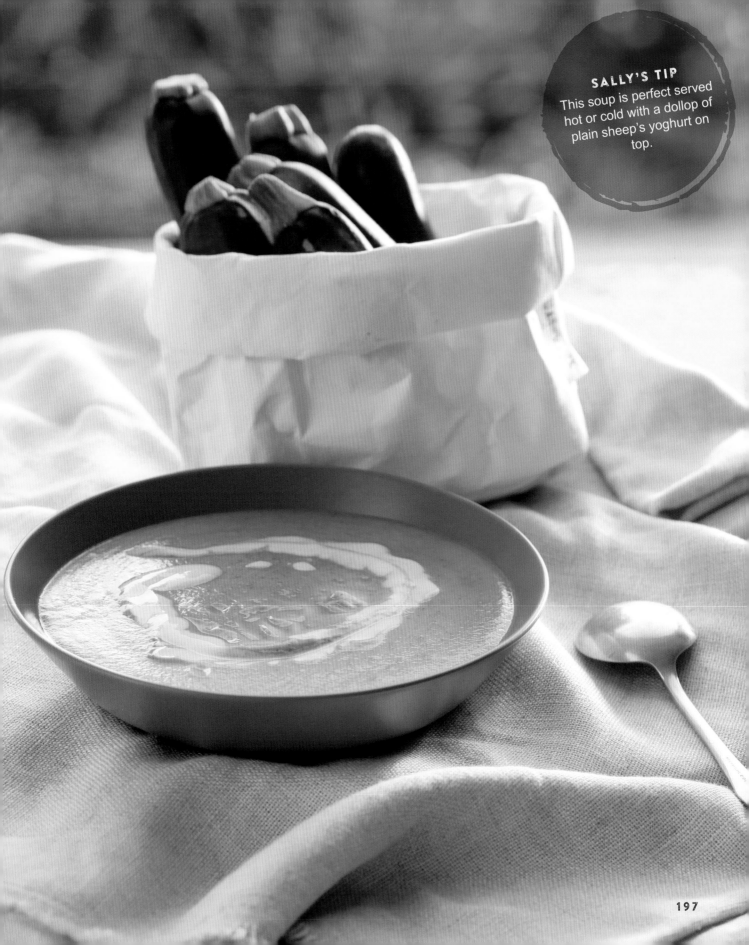

SALLY'S TIP
This soup is perfect served hot or cold with a dollop of plain sheep's yoghurt on top.

Creamy Cauliflower & Leek Soup

If you love potato and leek soup but would rather avoid the high amounts of starch in the potato, then let cauliflower come to the rescue! You can pretty well substitute any dish that contains potato or rice with cauliflower, thanks to its versatility and delicious creamy texture. Cauliflower and leeks are also rich in sulphur, which helps the body to detoxify heavy metals and works as a natural anti-inflammatory, but remember if you are sensitive to sulfur, then its best to avoid these foods.

Ingredients

2 tbsp ghee, coconut or macadamia oil

1 leek, sliced

1 large cauliflower, cut into small florets

2 cups water

1 teaspoon Himalayan or Celtic Sea Salt
cracked black pepper, to taste

4 cups homemade vegetable or chicken stock (see recipes page 187 or 190)

1 - 2 tbsp truffle or parsley oil, to serve (see page 191)

Method

Heat the ghee or oil in a large deep sided frying pan or saucepan, over medium heat. Saute the leek for about 3 minutes, until soft. Add the cauliflower florets, water and salt. Season with salt and pepper.

Cover and bring to the boil, then reduce the heat to low and simmer for 5 minutes, or until the cauliflower is just tender (be careful not to overcook).

Allow to cool slightly, then transfer to a blender and add the stock. Pureé until smooth. Serve warm, with a drizzle of truffle or parsley oil.

Keep any leftovers refrigerated in an airtight container for up to 3 days or freeze for up to 3 months.

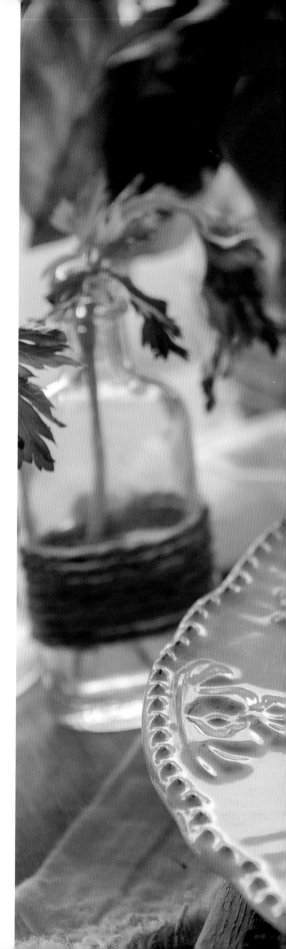

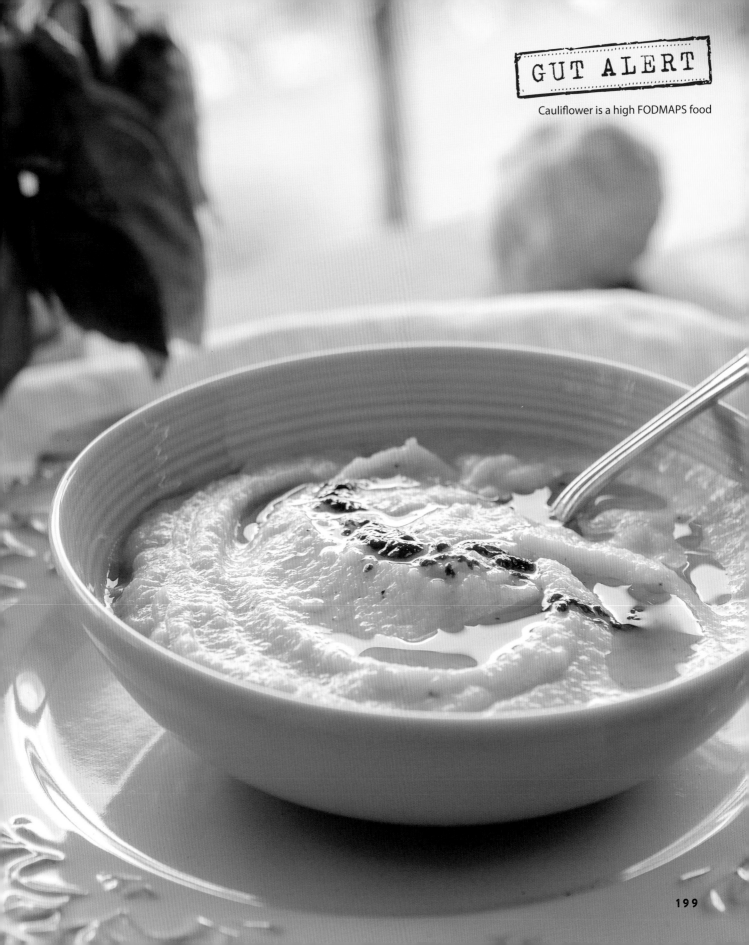

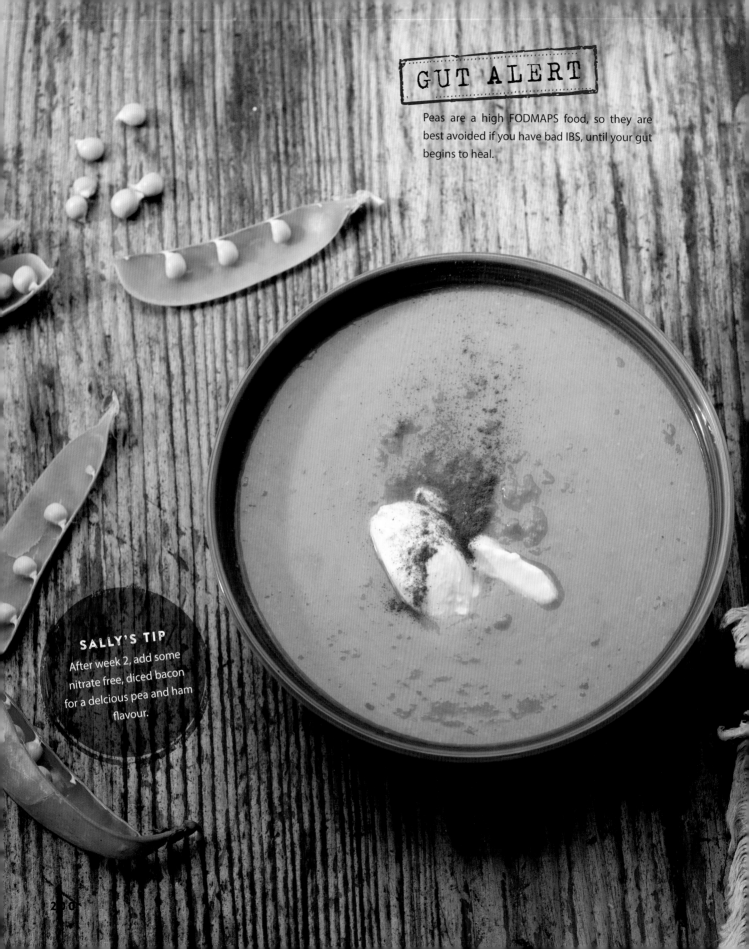

Peas are a high FODMAPS food, so they are best avoided if you have bad IBS, until your gut begins to heal.

SALLY'S TIP

After week 2, add some nitrate free, diced bacon for a delcious pea and ham flavour.

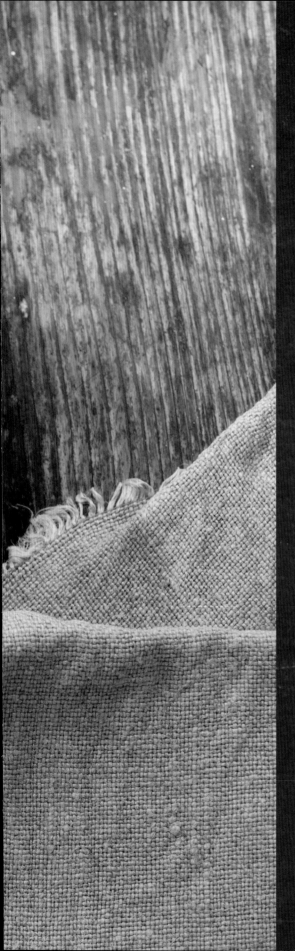

Fresh Pea & Mint Soup

Ingredients

Ghee, macadamia or coconut oil for frying

1 onion, peeled and diced

5 garlic cloves, peeled and crushed

2 tbsp fresh ginger

4 cups fresh or frozen peas

6 cups or 1 litre of vegetable or chicken stock (see recipes page 187 & 190)

Himalayan or Celtic Sea Salt and freshly ground black pepper, to taste

1 handful fresh mint leaves

Juice of 1/2 lemon

Method

Heat ghee or oil in a large saucepan or deep-sided fry pan over medium-high heat. Add onion, garlic and ginger and sauté for 1 minute. Add peas and stock and season with salt and pepper. Cover and bring to the boil.

Cool slightly and transfer to a blender, or use a stick blender in the pan. Add a handful of fresh mint leaves and pureé until smooth. Stir in lemon juice and serve with a dollop of plain sheep's yoghurt. if desired.

Keep any leftovers refrigerated in an airtight container for up to 3 days or freeze for up to 3 months.

GF DF LS P D VV

Lamb Shank & Veggie Soup

Ingredients

2-3 kg lamb shanks

Ghee or coconut oil for frying

1 brown onion, peeled and halved

Himalayan or Celtic Sea Salt, to taste (you will need a generous serve)

1 tsp whole black pepper corns

1 handful of thyme sprigs

3-4 fresh rosemary sprigs

4 garlic cloves, peeled

1 tsp ground allspice

1 cinnamon quill

3 bay leaves

1 medium sweet potato, peeled and diced

1 large carrot, peeled and sliced

2-3 celery stalks, finely chopped

2-3 silverbeet leaves, stalks removed, finely chopped or 1 cup baby kale leaves

This dish is a perfect winter warmer and the healthiest comfort food you can eat! This may sound a little caveman-like, but a little trick I recommend is to suck the marrow from the hollow of the cooked shank bones, not only because it tastes absolutely delicious, but it's also a rich source of essential nutrients. You can also freeze your left over bones to make bone broth with. If you don't already have one, I recommend investing in a slow cooker or crock pot as it will quickly become your best friend in the kitchen for whipping up delicous healthy casseroles and soups.

Method

Add the oil or ghee to a large fry pan on medium heat. Add the onions and sauteé for 1-2 minutes. Add the garlic and continue to stir for a minute, being careful not to burn. Add the shanks one by one and season with salt and pepper and cook on low to medium heat on each side for around 1 minute, or until they turn a light golden brown.

Transfer the shanks to a large stockpot and add the remaining ingredients. Cover with water and set the crock pot on low and cook with the lid on for 4 -6 hours. The meat should be so tender that it easily pulls from the bone.

Allow to cool then place the pot in the fridge until the fat rises to the top and hardens. Using a spoon, skim the fat from the top and discard.

Reheat the broth gently until liquid, then pour through a large colander into a large bowl. Remove the meat from the shank bones and place into the bowl with the broth.

Transfer the lamb and broth to the crockpot or a large saucepan and add all the vegetables. Bring to the boil, then reduce to low. Simmer for around 10 - 15mins, or until the vegetables are soft.

Serve topped with a spoonful of plain sheep's yoghurt and a sprinkle of ground cinnamon and some chopped flat-leaf parsley.

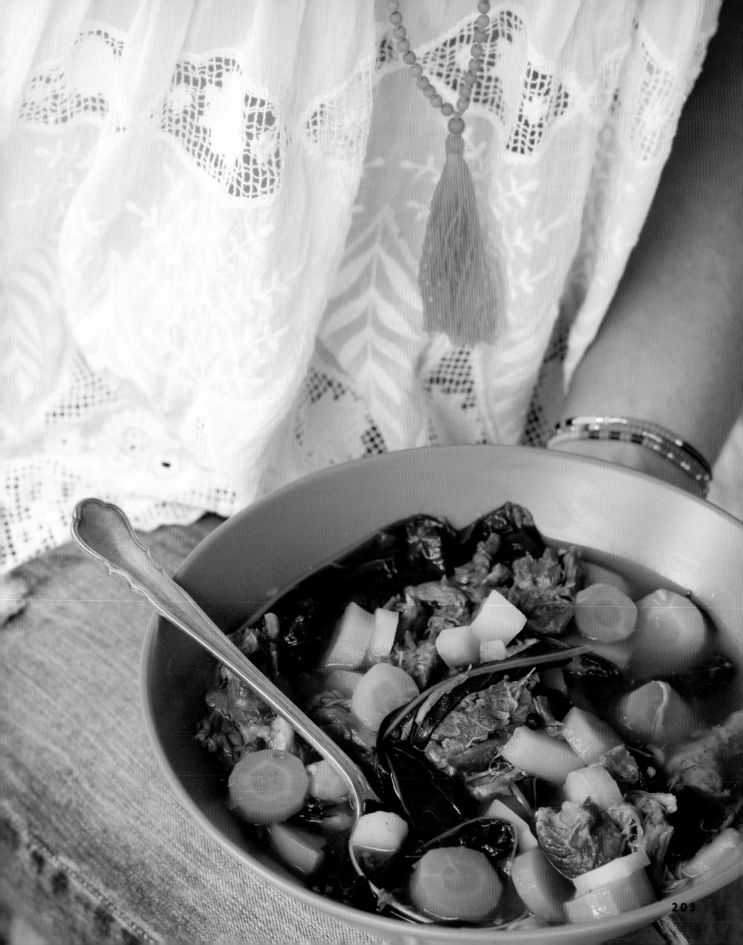

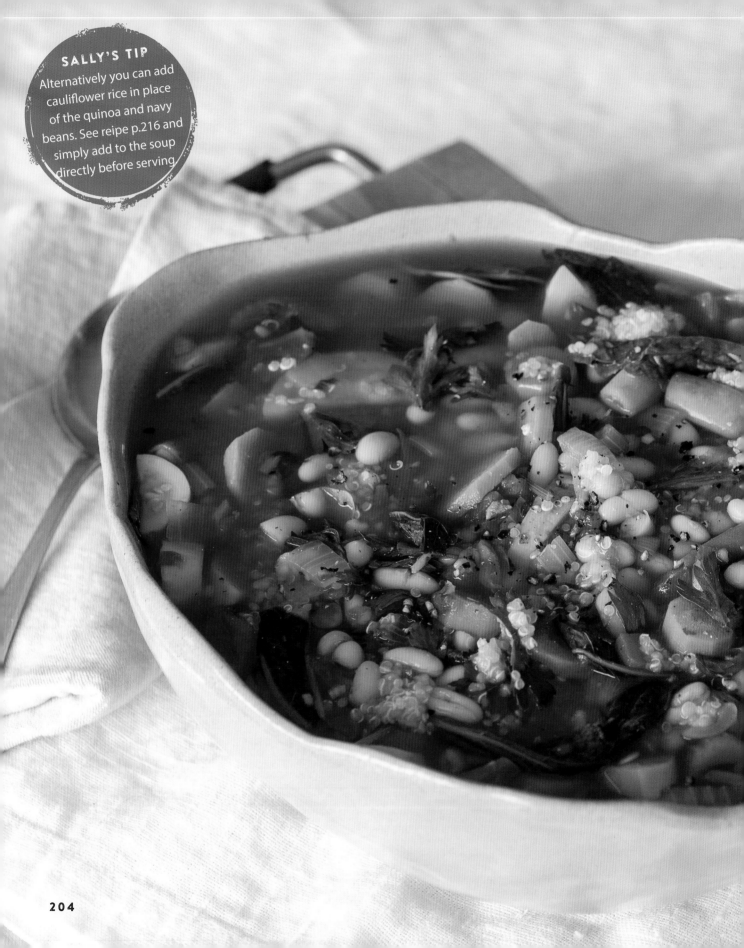

SALLY'S TIP

Alternatively you can add cauliflower rice in place of the quinoa and navy beans. See reipe p.216 and simply add to the soup directly before serving.

204

Quinoa Minestrone Soup

This is my twist on traditional minestrone soup, without the pasta!
Quinoa comes to the rescue and provides a perfect gluten-free substitute.
If you really want to make a hearty soup then you can include the haricot
(navy) beans, otherwise feel free to leave them out if you find they mess
with your gut or you want less starch. Minestrone soup is delicious at
any time of year, served hot or cold.

Method

Heat the ghee or oil in a large saucepan over medium heat, then add the onion, celery and carrot. Cook for about 5 minutes or until softened.

Stir in the garlic and chilli flakes if using and cook for about 1 minute or until garlic begins to change colour, being carefull not to burn

Add the zucchini, beans and turmeric, and season with salt and pepper. Cook, stirring, for about 3 minutes. Add the tomatoes and water and bring to the boil.

Reduce the heat to low-medium and simmer uncovered for 20-30 minutes. Add the rinsed quinoa, cover and cook for 15 minutes.

Uncover and add the kale and the canned beans. Add more water if needed and bring to a gentle boil. Cook for another 5 minutes or until the kale is just tender.

Serve topped with a dollop of sheep's yoghurt and garnish with fresh basil.

Ingredients

2 tbsp ghee or coconut oil

1 red or brown onion, diced

2 celery stalks, diced

3 carrots, sliced

2 garlic cloves, finely chopped

Pinch of chilli flakes (optional)

1 zucchini, halved and sliced (I use yellow but use green if you like)

2 cups chopped green beans

1 tsp ground turmeric (or to taste)

Himalayan or Celtic Sea Salt and freshly ground black pepper, to taste

3 large fresh tomatoes, diced

3 cups filtered water

1 cup quinoa, rinsed

2 cups chopped kale

400g can navy beans, rinsed and drained (optional)

1 bunch flat-leaf parsley, roughly chopped

1 tbsp of plain sheep's yoghurt (optional)

1 tbsp fresh basil, chopped

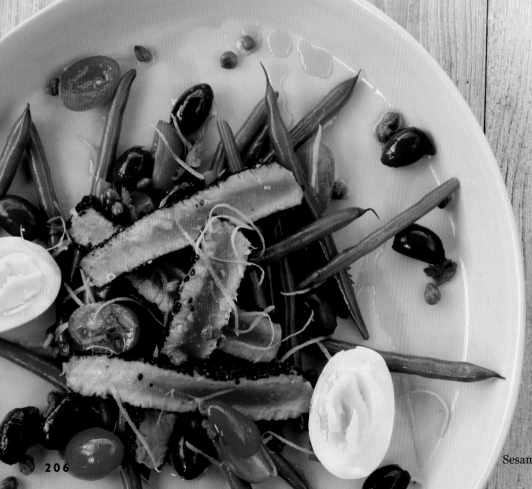

Lunch & Dinner

Sesame Crusted Tuna Nicoise pg.210

Lunch time

If you are making the right food choices at lunch you should feel energised and productive through to around 4 or 5pm, at which time you might be feeling a little peckish and want to grab one of my healthy snack options to tide you over until dinner (see page 170). Try to avoid eating starchy carbs such as rice, quinoa or root vegetables after 4pm if you are trying to lose weight.

THE GOLDEN RULES FOR LUNCH ARE

- **'EAT LIKE A PRINCE'** - make lunch your second largest meal of the day (after breakfast, of course). Definitely don't skip it.

- **LUNCH IS A TIME TO BREAK UP YOUR BUSY DAY,** so avoid eating at your desk, or in the car and take the opportunity to get outside and enjoy the fresh air and soak up some vitamin D from the sun.

- **AVOID BREAD AND STARCHY CARBS.** Most people associate lunch with a sandwich, rice or pasta based dish, which does not constitute as a healthy lunch option. To avoid wheat and glutinous grains, go for a salad, or make a breadless sandwich and include a healthy source of protein and fats to help fill you up.

- **CHOOSE SLOW BURNING, LOW SUGAR CARBS,** like green leafy vegetables, salad greens, quinoa or legumes (if they agree with you).

- **DON'T FORGET YOUR PORTION SIZES:**

Salad greens or vegetables - between 1 – 2 cups

Quinoa or legumes - around 1/2 - 3/4 cup.

Fish - hand size portion

Eggs - 2 per serving

Red meat or organic chicken – around a palm size

- **FATS, CHOOSE FROM** avocado, good oils such as extra virgin olive, coconut or macadamia oil, and / or a little goat or sheep's cheese – around a tablespoon and a ¼ - ½ an avocado.

- **BEWARE OF THE DREADED FOOD COURT!** If you are getting your lunch from a sandwich bar or food hall, remember these places are typically a haven for fast food and hidden sugars and gluten, not to mention artificial additives, and lack any dense nutrition. Consider cooking extra dinner the night before and bring your healthy leftovers to work the next day. If you experience the afternoon slump or tend to bloat like a fish, then take a close look at what you are eating for lunch, as these are classic tell-tale signs of food intolerances.

Dinner time

Dinner should be your smallest meal for the day, because this is the time when your digestive system is winding down and getting ready for rest, but for most people dinner is their largest meal and when they tend to consume foods that are the most difficult to digest – like red meat! Perhaps you are eating too much at dinner time because you are hungry from not eating enough during the day, or maybe you skipped a meal and end up playing 'catch up', with your appetite in the evening. By simply eating earlier and eating less come dinner time, you alleviate the stress on your digestive system which will help you to naturally lose fat, sleep better and improve your digestive function overall.

Here are my top tips for enjoying a healthy dinner and improving your overall gut health.

- **GET YOUR TIMING RIGHT.** For maximum weight loss eat before 6pm or at least 3 hours before bed. If you are regularly eating after 7.30pm stick to light, easily-digestible meals like soups, salads and fish.

- **MAKE DINNER A WINNER.** Avoid high starch carbs like rice, pasta and potato, as this will help you to lose weight. Stick to small servings of quinoa, sweet potato and pumpkin at dinner time.

- **KEEP YOUR PROTEIN CLEAN,** lean and easily digestible. Slow cook red and white meat as much as possible and ensure your red meat is 100% grassfed and only eat chemical free or organic chicken..

- **AVOID DRINKING LIQUIDS** 20 minutes either side of all meals. If you must drink water, limit it to small infrequent sips and avoid adding ice.

- **LOAD UP ON LEAFY GREEN VEGETABLES** or salad greens and include a portion of healthy fat, from avocado, fresh extra virgin olive or macadamia oil, or a little goat or sheeps' cheese or yoghurt to leave you feeling satiated

- **PORTION SIZE -** stick to smaller portions at dinner, except for green leafy vegetables, salads and soups. Aim for a palm size portion or smaller for red and white meat and a hand size portion for fish.

- **COOK UP ENOUGH DINNER TO ENJOY FOR LUNCH THE NEXT DAY.** This will help to ensure you stick to eating healthy food and save on time.

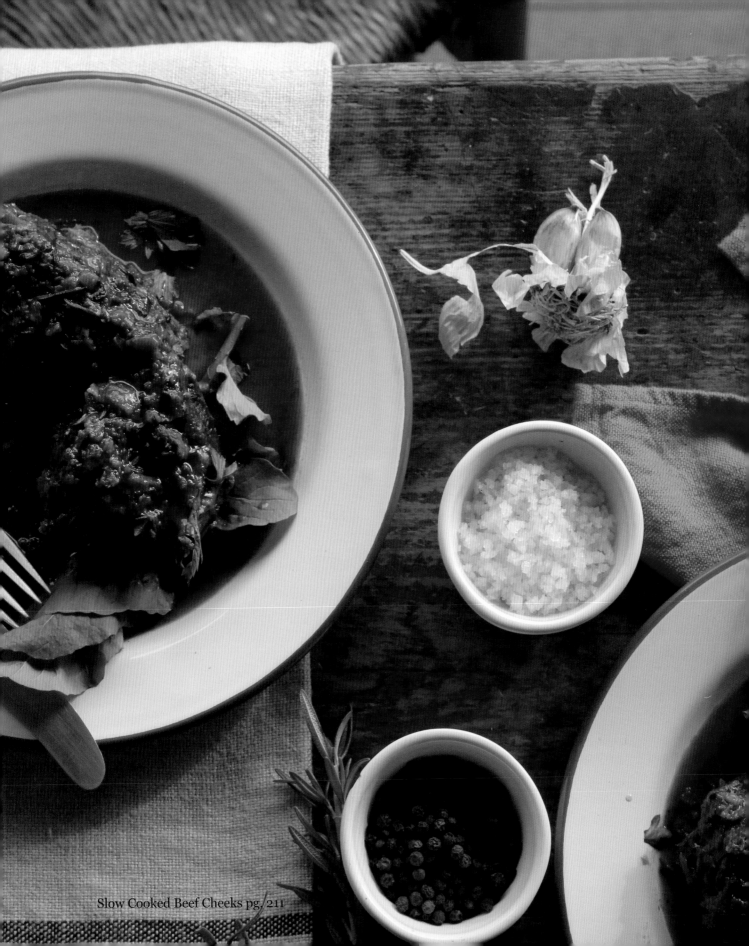

Slow Cooked Beef Cheeks pg. 211

SERVES 1 (SERVING SIZE 2 CUPS)

Sesame Crusted Tuna Nicoise

Ingredients

Approximately 150 gram / 6oz fillet of fresh tuna per person (use sustainably caught canned tuna if not using fresh)

2 tbsp sesame seeds

1 hard boiled egg, cut in half

Handful of blanched green beans, ends removed

6- 8 cherry or grape tomatoes, halved per person

1/4 avocado, sliced (optional)

2 tbsp. of flat leaf parsley, roughly chopped

1/4 cup pitted black Kalamata olives

Juice of 1/2 half a fresh lemon

2 –3 tbsp. extra virgin olive or macadamia oil

Himalayan or Celtic Sea Salt and cracked pepper to taste

Ghee, virgin coconut or macadamia oil for cooking

Method

Coat the tuna fillet in sesame seeds

Place sesame seeds on a plate and coat the tuna in them on all sides. Preheat oil in a pan on medium to high heat, then add the sesame crusted tuna fillet and cook on each side for a few minutes. I prefer to cook my fresh tuna medium rare – so that it is not cooked all the way through. Remove from the pan and set aside on a plate.

Arrange the blanched green beans, cherry tomatoes, parsley, black olives and hard boiled egg halves on a medium sized serving dish. Thinly slice the tuna fillet and arrange on the plate. Drizzle with fresh oil or macadamia and lemon juice and season with salt and pepper to taste

TUNA

Tuna is one of those fish that you need to restrict your consumption of due to contamination from heavy metals such as mercury. It's safe enough to eat once to twice a week, but if you are pregnant I actually recommend avoiding it altogether. But on the plus side, tuna is high in Omega 3 essential fatty acids, which makes it great for combatting inflammation and healthy brain function.

Slow Cooked Beef Cheeks

These beef cheeks are a deliciously nourishing slow cooked dish that can be enjoyed any time of the year. It is an ideal way to enjoy beef because the slow cooking tenderizes the meat, making it easier for your body to digest. It's so simple to prepare - you can cook it in the oven or a slow cooker.

Ingredients

4 100% grass fed beef cheeks (depending on the size I usually allow 1-2 beef cheeks per person)

Rice flour or gluten-free plain flour to dust the beef cheeks in.

Himalayan or Celtic Sea Salt and freshly ground black pepper, to taste - season generously

2 tbsp ghee, coconut or macadamia oil, for frying

2 brown onions, chopped

8 garlic cloves, peeled

4 bay leaves

Handful rosemary sprigs, chopped

Handful sage leaves, chopped

2 thyme sprigs, stalks removed

2 1/2 cups stock (beef, chicken or vegetable)

1 cup fresh flat-leaf parsley, roughly chopped

Method

Preheat the oven to 150°C /300°F. Add around 2 tablespons of rice flour to a plate and coat each beef cheek lightly with flour and season generously with salt and pepper.

Heat oil in a large flameproof casserole dish over medium heat. Cook the beef cheeks in two batches for about 2-3 minutes each side, until well browned. Set aside. Add the onion and cook for 3-4 minutes, until soft. Add the garlic and herbs and cook for a further minute. Return the beef cheeks to the dish.

Pour the stock over and cover with a lid. Place into the oven and cook for 3-4 hours, basting with the stock twice during cooking time. Beef cheeks are ready when the meat is very tender and flakes easily when tested with a fork.

Serve with freshly steamed green vegetables such as green beans and snow peas, or broccoli and a side of Cauliflower rice (see page 216) if desired.

Add a squeeze of fresh lemon juice before serving if desired.

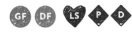

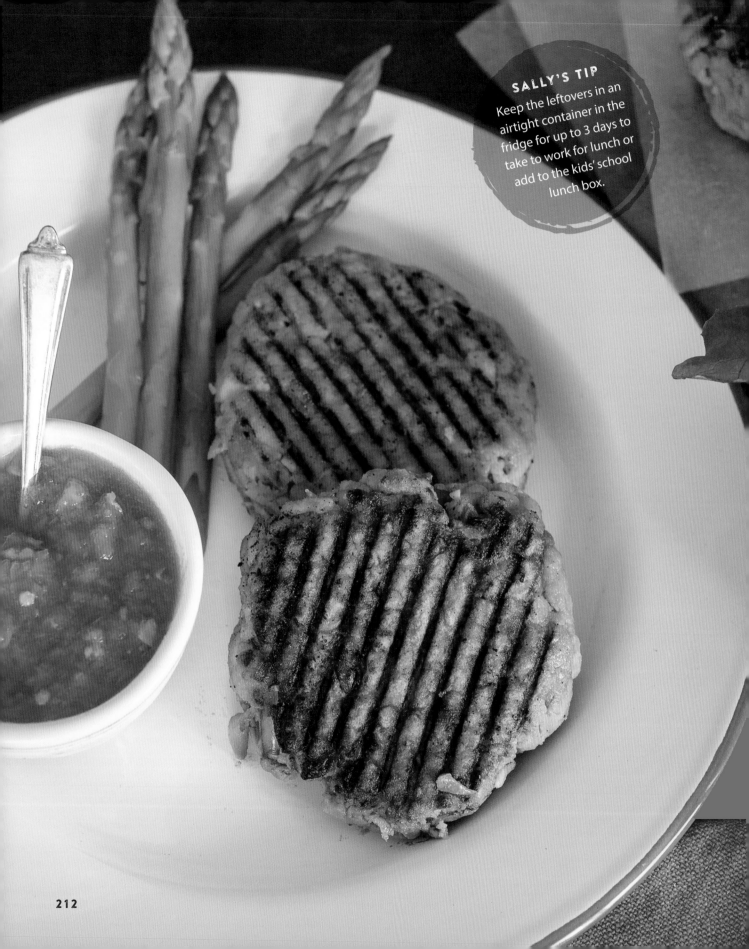

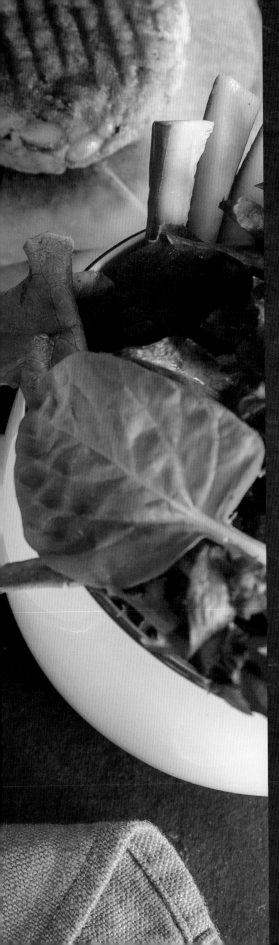

Healthy Beef Rissoles

Beef rissoles or patties, make for a simple yet delicious meal anytime of the week and are a great way to sneak a few extra veggies into the kids. Be sure to always choose 100% grass-fed beef mince to avoid any nasty hormones. and antibiotics

Ingredients

500g 100% grass fed beef mince

1/2 small brown onion, finely diced

1 garlic clove, crushed or chopped

1 small carrot, peeled and grated

1 small zucchini, grated

1 tbsp fresh thyme leaves

1 tbsp roughly chopped fresh flat-leaf parsley

2 tbsp pine nuts (optional)

1 egg, lightly beaten

Himalayan or Celtic Sea Salt and cracked pepper, to taste

Ghee, virgin coconut oil or macadamia oil for cooking

Method

Place the beef mince, onion, garlic, carrot, zucchini, herbs, pine nuts and egg into a mixing bowl and season with salt and pepper. Use your hands to mix until well combined. Scoop out a heaped tablespoon of the mixture and shape into a round patty, around 1.5 inches thick.

Preheat a BBQ or griddle pan over medium-high heat. Brush rissoles with oil and cook for 6-8 minutes, turning once, until golden brown on both sides and cooked through. Remove from the heat and rest for 3 minutes.

Serve with a large green salad and avocado, or with steamed veggies and a dollop of my home-made tomato sauce (see page 276).

GF DF LS   P   D

SERVES 2 (SERVING SIZE A HAND SIZE SLICE)

Salmon, Avocado & Kale Frittata

Frittata is like a low-carb, gluten-free version of quiche and it's a really easy and versatile option for any meal. I often make it when I have veggies or herbs in my fridge that need using up. You could also make individual serving sizes by baking in a large muffin tin - perfect for taking to work for lunch, or to pop in the school lunch box. Feel free to vary the ingredients with whatever vegies you have on hand.

Ingredients

1 tbsp ghee, virgin coconut or macadamia oil

1 spring onion, finely chopped

1 medium roma tomato, cut in quarters

1 cup chopped kale leaves, roughly chopped

4 large eggs, lightly beaten

1 small can of pink or red salmon, drained and flaked. Alternatively use nitrate free smoked salmon or trout.

1/2 avocado, thinly sliced (optional)

2 tbsp roughly chopped coriander, dill or flat-leaf parsley

Himalayan or Celtic Sea Salt and freshly ground black pepper to season

Method

Preheat the oven to 180°C / 350°F. Heat the oil in a small ovenproof frying pan over medium heat and add the spring onion, tomato and kale. Stir for 2 minutes, or until the kale is just wilted. Add the salmon to the pan.

Pour the eggs over the vegetables and salmon, and top with the herbs and avocado, if using. Season generously with salt and pepper.

Transfer pan to the oven. Bake for 10 minutes, or until lightly golden brown and cooked through.

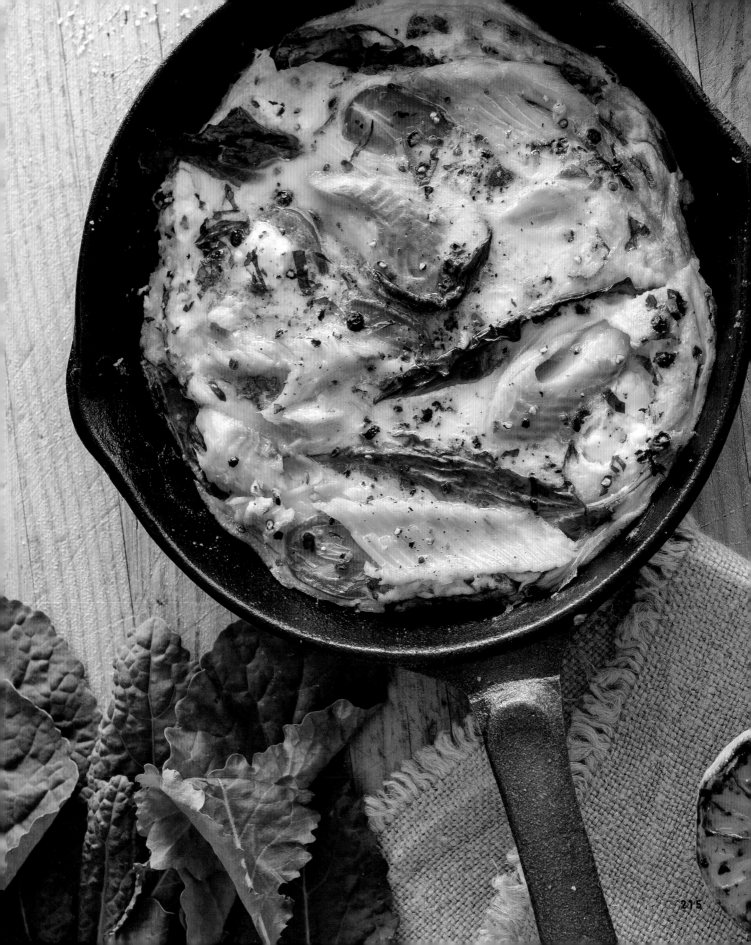

Cauliflower Rice

If you love your rice and mashed potato, but don't love the extra pounds they can add to your hips and thighs, then cauliflower rice might be your new best friend – it's the perfect low carb alternative to high starch grains like rice, or mashed potato. You can mash it to the consistency of rice, or a creamy puree to use as a base under fish, lamb or steak. I promise you will barely taste the difference and the kids will love it too!

Ingredients

1 head of cauliflower, outer leaves and stalks removed

1 tbsp of pure butter

1/4 cup olive or macadamia oil

1 clove garlic, chopped (optional)

1/2 tsp nutmeg and cinnamon (optional)

Celtic Sea Salt and cracked black pepper to taste

Method

Add 1 cup of filtered water to a large saucepan and bring to the boil with the lid on. Cut cauliflower into medium-sized florets

Once the water is boiling, add the cauliflower to the saucepan or to a steam basket and replace lid. Steam until the cauliflower is soft enough for a fork to easily pass through, but be careful not to over cook it or the cauliflower will turn to mush.

Once the cauliflower is cooked, drain all the water from the saucepan and add the butter and oil and season generously with salt and pepper. Use a potato masher to mash to the consistency of rice or if you prefer a cauliflower mash, continue until its soft and creamy. Add extra butter if the cauliflower is too dry. Alternatively you can place the cauliflower into a food processor and pulse a few times until you reach the desired texture.

Sprinkle with a little nutmeg and cinnamon if desired.

SUPER CAULIFRAGALISTIC

Cauliflower is a member of the cruciferous family of vegetables, which contain a powerful anti inflammatory compound called indole-3-carbinol, which has been found to inhibit cancer growth in rats and mice, primarily in breast, colon, bladder, stomach, lung and liver tumors. Just one serving of cauliflower contains 77 percent of your recommended daily vitamin C intake, as well as being a rich source of B vitamins and minerals like magnesium, manganese and potassium. This super dooper vegetable is also high in fibre and antioxidants like Sulforaphane which prevents bacterial overgrowth of Helicobacter pylori bacteria in your gut. But if you suffer from an underactive thyroid, be careful not to overdo your intake of cruciferous vegetables by rotating them around.

GF DF LS P D VV

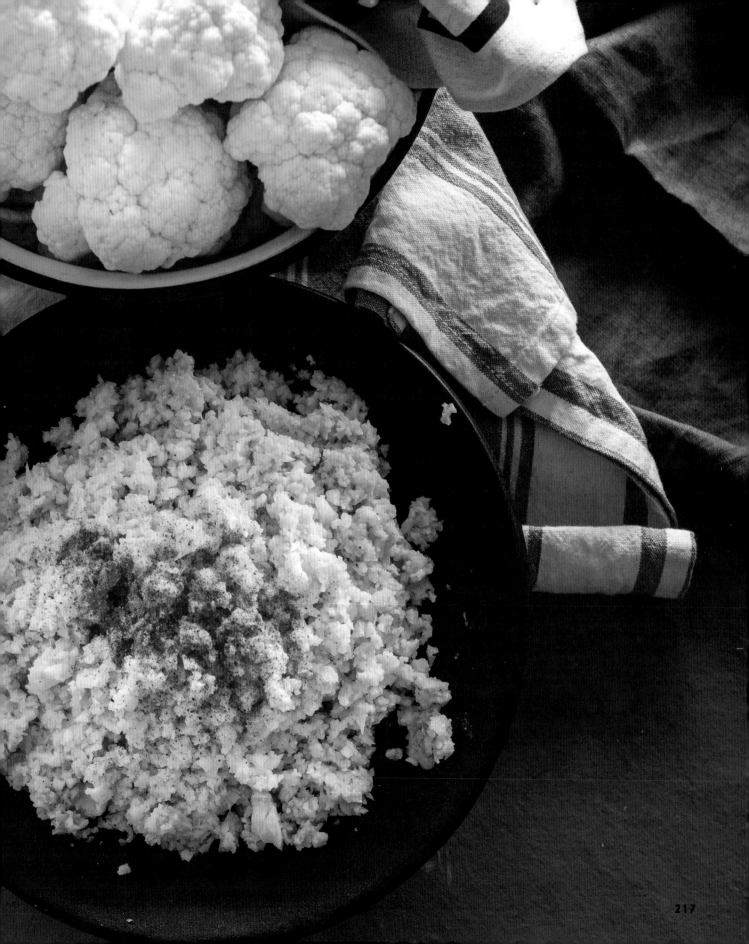

Grilled Chicken with Green Goddess Dressing

Ingredients

4-6 chicken thigh fillets, excess fat trimmed

4-6 garlic cloves, crushed

2 tbsp finely grated fresh ginger

2 tbsp ghee or macadamia oil

Himalayan or Celtic Sea Salt and freshly ground black pepper to taste

1/4 cup virgin coconut oil or macadamia oil

Green Goddess Dressing, to serve (see page 279)

Chicken is a healthy source of animal protein, as long as you buy organic or antibiotic free, that has not been fed GMO soy or corn. I prefer to use chicken thighs over the breast cut, as they are more tender and sweeter in flavour. I recommend consuming the majority of your dense animal proteins like chicken and red meat slow cooked, but when time does not permit or you are entertaining friends, using the grill or BBQ creates a delicious flavour. Try to avoid regularly cooking on an open flame, because this will cause oxidation of specific compounds, especially in red meat, that have been found to be carcinogenic. Instead cook on the BBQ hot plate or use a cast iron chargrill/griddle pan.

Method

Combine the chicken, garlic, ginger and ghee or oil in a large mixing bowl and season with salt and pepper. If you have time, cover with cling wrap or a plate and refrigerate for 1-2 hours to allow the flavours to infuse.

Preheat a BBQ hot plate or a griddle pan over medium-high heat. Cook for 3-4 minutes on each side, until chicken is golden brown and cooked through, but being careful not to overcook or it will become tough..

Serve with Green Goddess Dressing and a fresh green salad, or steamed vegetables. If you want to bulk this meal up a little more, add a serving of cauliflower rice or puree (see page 216) and slow oven roasted tomatoes (see pages 247).

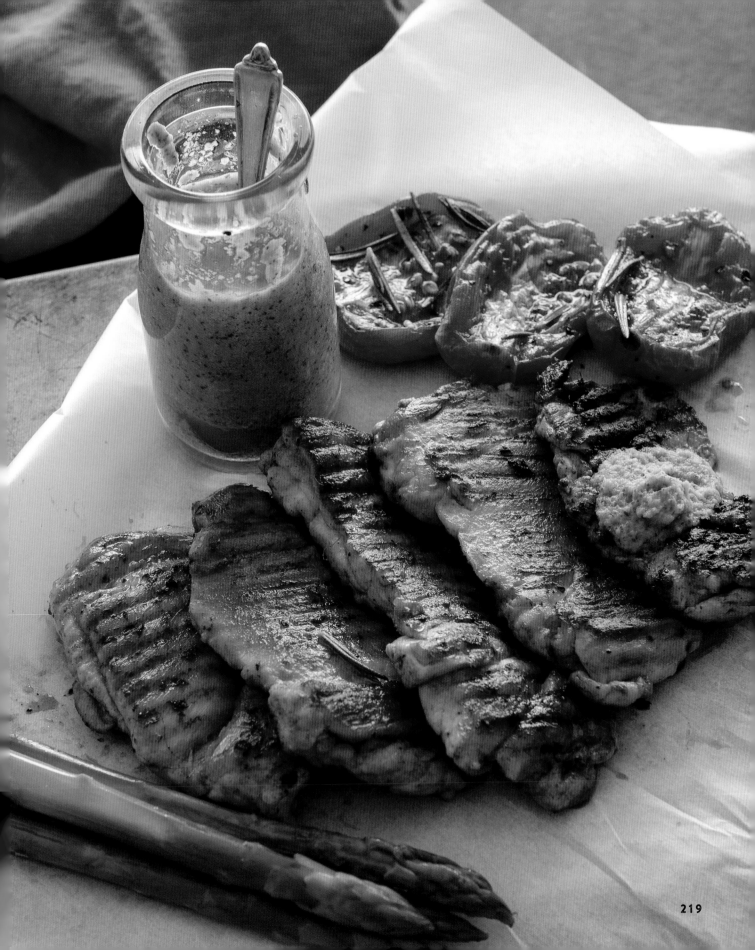

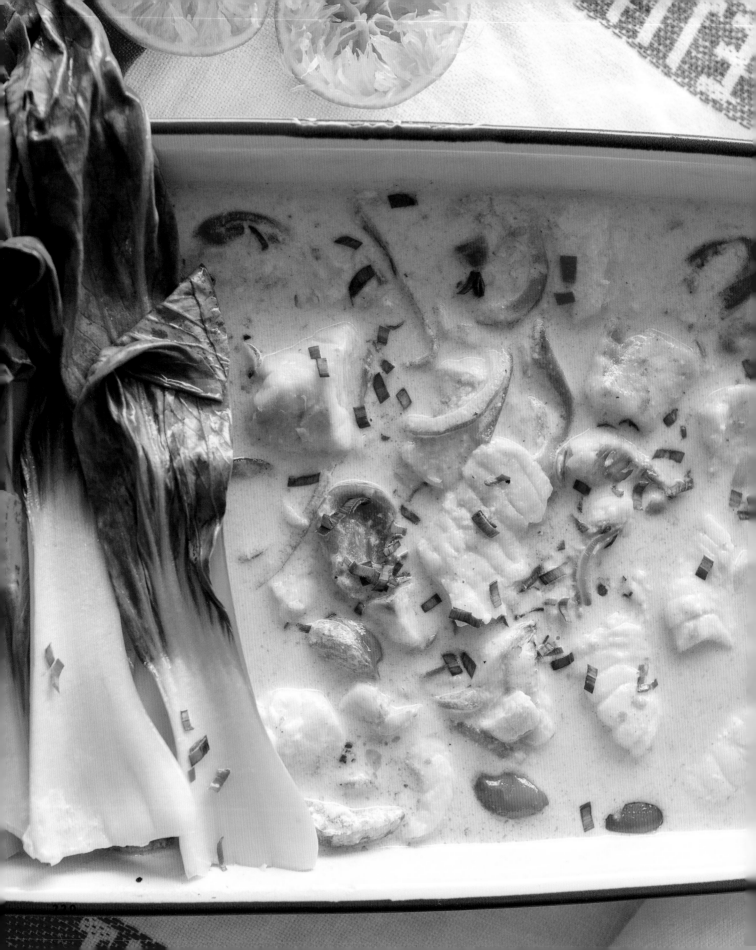

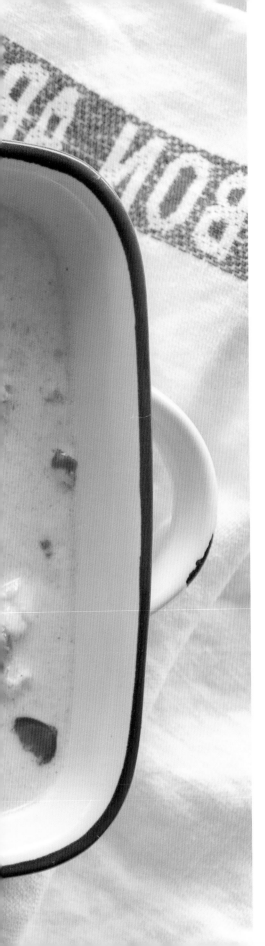

Thai Coconut Fish Curry

This is a healthy and delicious alternative to take-away Thai food (which is often laden with palm sugar and bottled sauces) and it's super-quick and easy to prepare. Further good news: the fat in coconut milk is not fattening, but rather filling! This recipe is a great way to get children to eat fish thanks to the delicious coconut sauce, but you may have to leave out or tone down the chilli and spices depending on the sophistication of your kids' taste buds.

Method

Cut fish fillets into 5cm pieces. Heat the coconut oil in a wok or deep frying pan over medium-high heat. Add the onion, ginger, garlic, lemon grass, kaffir lime leaves (if using) and chilli. Stir-fry for 3 minutes or until soft.

Add the tomatoes and cook for another 3 minutes, stirring frequently to break up. Add the cumin, salt and pepper. Stir to combine and cook for two minutes. Stir in the coconut milk and stevia and bring to a simmer.

Add the fish and cook for 3-5 minutes, depending on the thickness of the fish, until cooked through (it will be opaque).

Add the chives, coriander and a squeeze of lime, and serve with steamed bok choy or other green vegetables, like asparagus or green beans.

Ingredients

500 - 700 g / 18- 24 ounces boneless, skinless white fish fillets (I like to use perch, flathead white cod

1 tbsp virgin coconut oil

1/2 red onion, finely sliced

1 tsp finely grated fresh ginger

2 garlic cloves, crushed

2 stalks of lemon grass, finely sliced

2 fresh kaffir lime leaves (optional)

1 red chilli, seeds removed, finely sliced

250g cherry tomatoes, halved

1 tsp ground cumin

1/2 tsp Himalayan or Celtic Sea Salt

Freshly ground black pepper, to taste

1 1/2 cups coconut milk

5-6 drops of liquid stevia

1 tbsp finely chopped fresh chives

1/2 cup fresh coriander leaves, roughly chopped

1 lime, quartered

Steamed bok choy, to serve

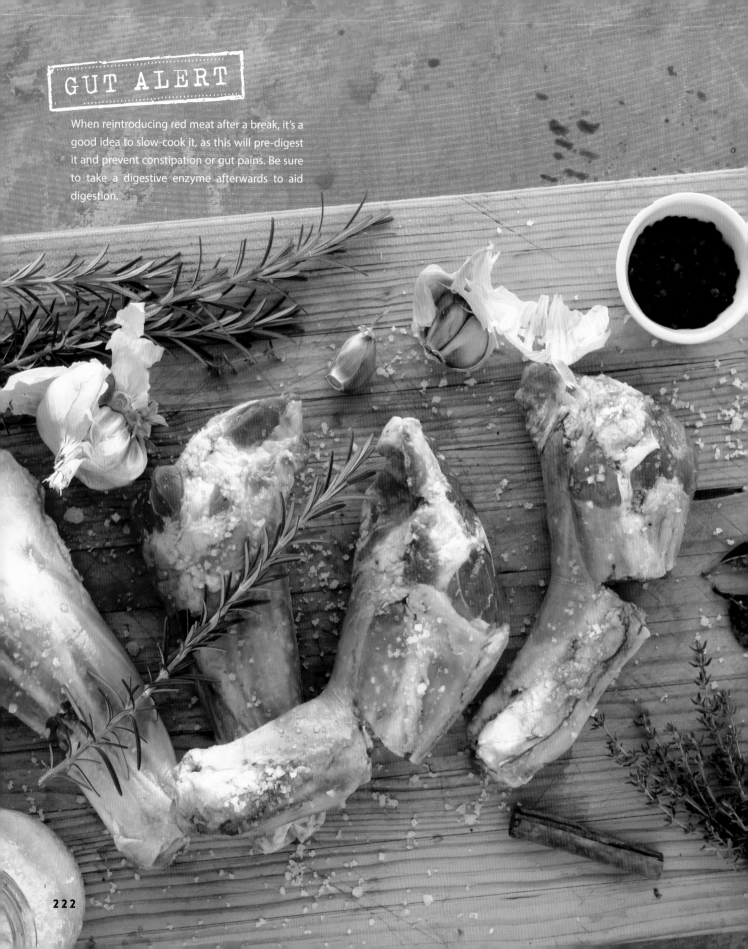

When reintroducing red meat after a break, it's a good idea to slow-cook it, as this will pre-digest it and prevent constipation or gut pains. Be sure to take a digestive enzyme afterwards to aid digestion.

Slow Cooked Lamb Shanks

Slow cooked lamb shank is hands-down my favourite meat dish. Your gut will love it too, because the slow cooking method tenderizes the meat, making it super easy to digest compared to baked or grilled meat. If you don't already have one, I recommend investing in an electric slow cooker or crockpot with a timer, to help you create everything from soups to slow cooked chicken and meat casseroles.

Method

You can also cook this dish in the oven, simply preheat it 150°C/350°F.

Heat the ghee or oil in a large, deep sided fry pan or casserole dish, over medium heat. Add the onion and sauteé for 3-4 minutes, until soft. Add the garlic and cook for another minute. Add the shanks and turn to coat in the ghee or oil. Cook for 3-5 minutes on each side, or until the shanks are slightly brown (you may need to do this in batches, depending on the number of shanks you are cooking and the size of your fry pan or casserole dish).

Transfer the shanks and cooked onion to your crockpot if using, and add the stock, all remaining ingredients and season generously with salt and pepper. Cover and set on 'low' and allow to cook for 4 - 6 hours. If cooking in the oven, transfer the shanks and all remaining ingredients to an oven proof cassserole dish and replace the lid. Place in the oven for 4- 6 hours, until meat is very tender and separates easily from the bone. Baste the shanks with pan juices twice during cooking.

Serve with freshly steamed green vegetables or salad and a little cauliflower rice (see page 216) to soak up the delicious juices. Add a squeeze of fresh lemon juice to serve if desired.

GF DF LS P D

SALLY'S TIPS

If not making your own stock, choose a brand free from added sugar, yeast and artificial additives.

Cool then freeze any leftover portions for convenient meals.

Ingredients

2 tbsp ghee or coconut oil

1 brown onion, finely diced

4 garlic cloves, crushed

4-6 lamb shanks

1 litre vegetable or chicken stock

4-6 small fresh vine-ripened or Roma tomatoes

1/2-3/4 cup Kalamata olives, pitted

1 dessert spoon of rice malt syrup (optional)

1 cup fresh flat-leaf parsley, roughly chopped

2 tbsp fresh oregano

2 tbsp fresh tarragon

4 sprigs fresh rosemary

2 bay leaves

1 cinnamon quill or 1 tsp ground cinnamon

1 tsp freshly grated or ground nutmeg

Himalayan or Celtic Sea Salt and freshly ground black pepper-season generously

Fish Cakes with Green Goddess Dressing

These fantastic fishcakes are super-easy to make and are rich in Omega-3 fatty acids and protein. I recommend limiting your tuna and salmon intake to no more than twice a week, because large oily fish like tuna and wild salmon can be contaminated with high levels of mercury from the ocean – depending where they are caught. I recommend choosing a brand of tinned fish that uses only sustainable 'pole and line' fishing methods. These can easily be found in the supermarket.

Ingredients

1 large can (415g /or 3 x 6 oz) of salmon, drain excess liquid

500g sweet potato or butternut pumpkin / squash, peeled and sliced into chunks

1 small bunch of fresh dill , stems removed, roughly chopped

2 spring onions, finely chopped finely grated rind and juice of 1 lemon

Himalayan or Celtic Sea Salt and freshly ground black pepper, to taste

1 egg, lightly beaten

1/4 cup pine nuts, toasted (optional)

Ghee / virgin coconut or macadamia oil, for frying

Green goddess dressing, to serve (see page 279)

Method

Steam the sweet potato or pumpkin in water until soft, drain excess water and mash with a little salt and pepper.

Add to a large mixing bowl along with the salmon, dill, onions, lemon rind and juice, pine nuts and egg. Season with salt and pepper and use your hands to mix until all ingredients are combined.

Take 2 tablespoons of mixture and shape into round patties - around 1.5-2 inches thick. Heat a little ghee or oil in a frying pan over medium heat and cook for 4-5 minutes on each side, until golden brown.

Serve with your choice of steamed greens, or leafy green salad with avocado. Add a dollop of plain sheep's yoghurt, with fresh lemon juice instead of the dressing, if you desire.

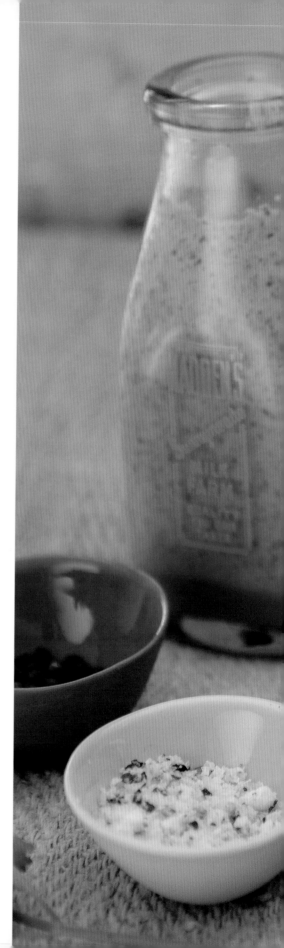

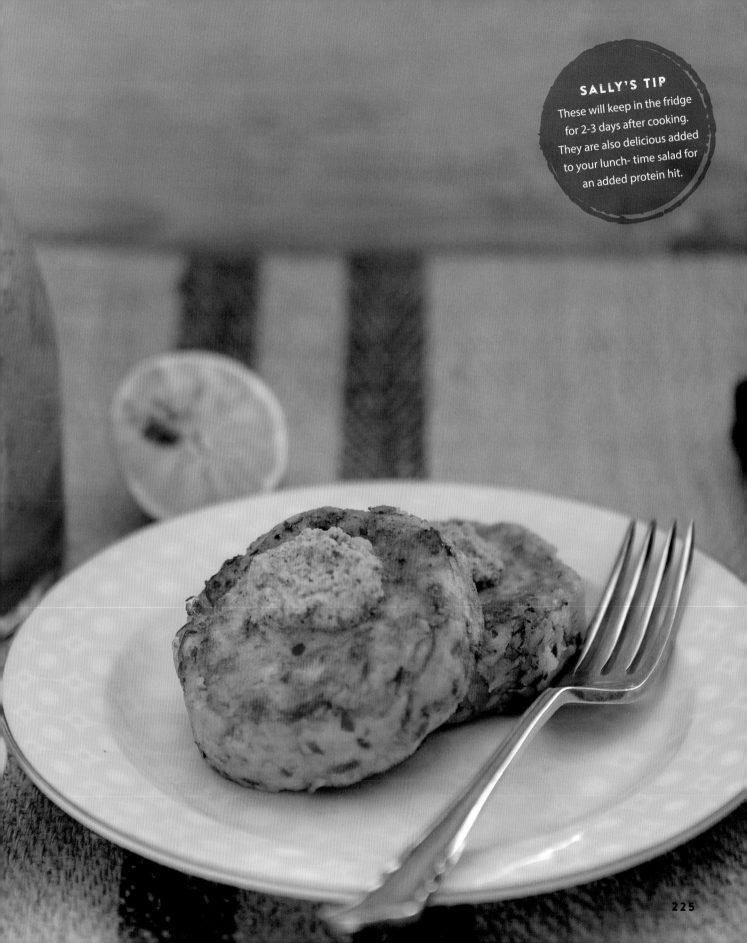

Pan Fried Flathead With Aioli

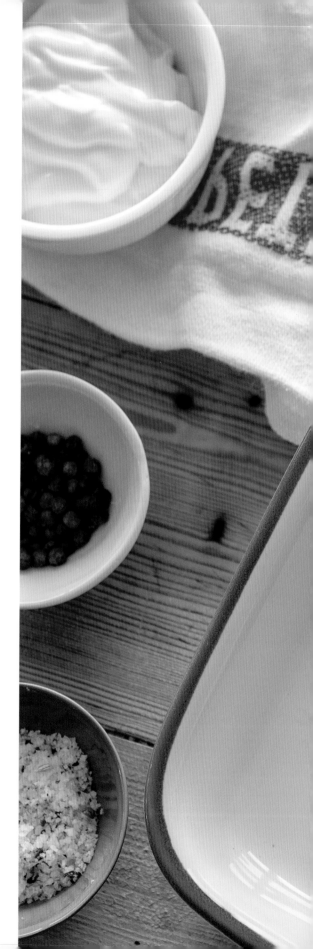

If you're like most people, you could probably do with a little more fish in your diet and I find even the fussiest fish eater can be won over with flat head, thanks to its really delicate and mild flavour, so I challenge you to try this simple fish recipe if you're struggling to eat fish, or don't know how to cook it. Fish is an excellent source of easy to digest protein, as well as being rich in essential fatty acids.

Method

Add the rice flour to a plate and mix through the salt and pepper and herbs.

Dust each flathead fillet in the rice flour mix until the whole fillet is finely covered, shaking off any excess.

Heat the oil and butter in a medium to large fry pan on medium heat and before adding the flathead fillets.

Cook each fillet on each side for approximately 2 - 3 minutes or until fish is cooked through.

Serve immediately with a dollop of whole egg aioli and a wedge of fresh lemon.

Season with extra salt and pepper if desired and a green salad or a big bowl of steamed greens.

Ingredients

180 - 200gm fillet of freshflat head – per person

1/4 cup of rice flour (optional)

2 tbsp finely chopped flat leaf parsley or coriander

1 teaspoon of pure butter and virgin coconut or macadamia oil for frying

Wedge of fresh lemon

Himalayan or Celtic Sea Salt and pepper to taste

CHOOSING THE BEST FISH

The healthiest fish are small white-fleshed varieties, because they tend to be less contaminated with heavy-metals than large oily fish. Always go for wild-caught varieties over farmed fish like barramundi and salmon. Be conscious of where your fish and seafood comes from as some oceans are more polluted than others.

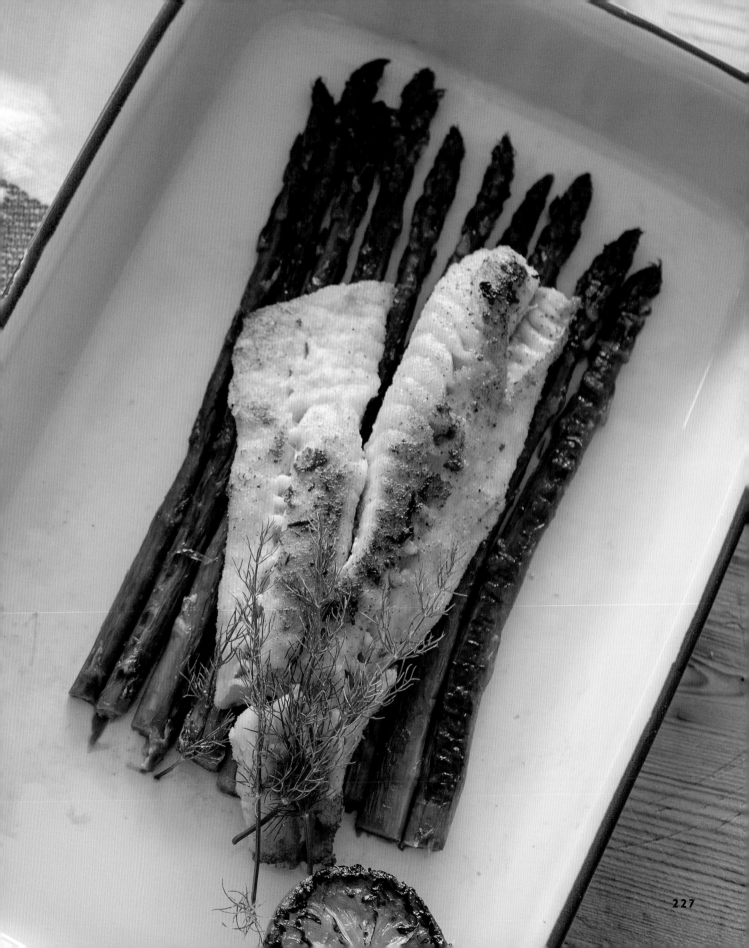

Prawn Zucchini Linguine

Ingredients

4 – 6 cooked prawns / shrimp per person (heads and outer shell removed)

3/4 cup zucchini noodles per person

1/3 - 1/2 cup extra virgin olive oil (depending on number of serves)

Juice of 1-2 limes, or to taste

1 small red chilli – seeds removed and finely sliced

Lightly blanched asparagus, julienned (optional)

1/4 -1/2 cup coriander/cilantro leaves

1/4 - 1/2 cup mint leaves loosely chopped

1/2 cup macadamia nuts, chopped and toasted (alternatively use pine nuts)

Himalayan or Celtic Sea Salt and freshly ground black pepper, to taste

If you love the combination of shrimp with pasta, then this recipe will serve as a delicious gluten and grain free alternative on those hot summer nights you feel like treating yourself, or entertaining friends while on the LYG Program. I've used pre-cooked prawns, but feel free to use green and grill them on the BBQ or griddle pan with a little crushed garlic and oil. As shrimp are a crustacean, they tend to be higher in heavy metals compared to other sources of seafood, so I recommend occasional consumption and avoid farmed prawns, or those imported form Asia. Shrimp or 'prawns' as we call them in Australia, are a delicious source of protein.

Method

To make your zucchini linguine or noodles, see recipe on page 241.

Meanwhile, add the zucchini noodles to a large mixing bowl along with all other ingredients and toss through to coat generously with the olive oil and lime dressing.

Serve on a large serving dish and garnish with extra mint and coriander/cilantro leaves and roast macadamia nuts.

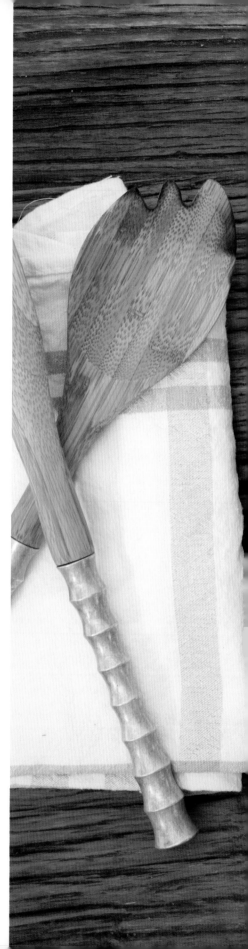

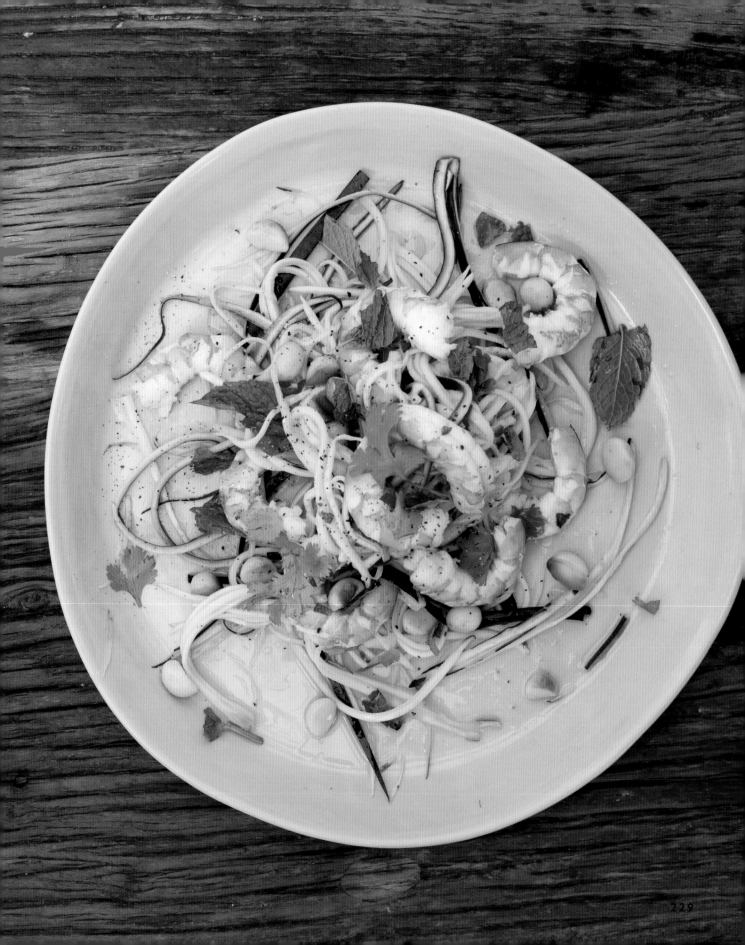

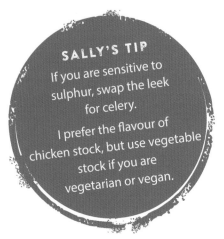

SALLY'S TIP

If you are sensitive to sulphur, swap the leek for celery.

I prefer the flavour of chicken stock, but use vegetable stock if you are vegetarian or vegan.

SERVES 4 (SERVING SIZE 1 1/2 CUPS)

Butternut Pumpkin & Adzuki Bean Casserole

Traditionally a 'winter warmer', the flavours in this dish actually make it a delicious meal to enjoy anytime of the year when you're looking for a vegetarian or vegan option. Whilst not strictly Paleo because of the adzuki beans, if your gut tolerates a few serves of legumes here and there, there's no reason to exclude them completely. Nutritionally this recipe is beautifully grounding, perfect for those with an overly stimulated nervous system.

Ingredients

1 tbsp ghee, virgin coconut oil

1 leek, finely sliced

1/2 brown onion, diced

1-2 cups butternut pumpkin/ squash peeled and cut into 2.5cm/1 inch cubes

1/2 tsp ground nutmeg

1/2 tsp ground cinnamon

1/2 tsp ground ginger

2 tsp rice malt syrup

2 tbsp slivered almonds

1 cup organic chicken or vegetable stock

400g can organic adzuki beans, rinsed and drained

2 bunches of fresh asparagus, woody ends trimmed

1/2 cup fresh coriander/ cilantro leaves

Method

Heat oil in a large frying pan over medium heat. Add the leek and onion and sauté for 3-5 minutes, until soft. Add the pumpkin, cinnamon, nutmeg, ginger, rice malt syrup and almonds. Cook, stirring frequently, until the pumpkin begins to brown.

Add the stock and adzuki beans and simmer, covered, for 10-15 minutes, until pumpkin is soft. Add the asparagus for the remaining 1-2 minutes, then transfer to a serving dish and top with fresh coriander leaves.

Make up extra to store in the fridge for lunch or dinner the next day, and serve warm or cold.

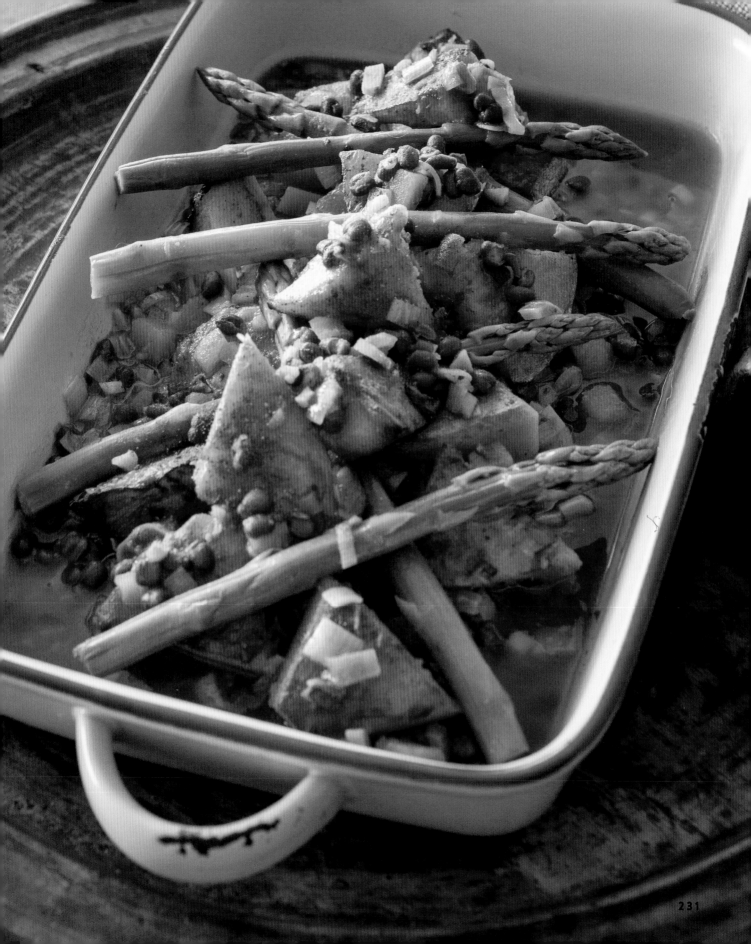

Chicken Cacciatore

Everyone seems to have their own spin on this classic Italian dish but no matter what your personal twist, it's a guaranteed crowd pleaser! Best of all it's so simple to make and the perfect dish when you either have a lot of mouths to feed or to keep on hand for extra meals during the week..

Ingredients

¼ cup ghee or coconut oil

2 kg (4.5 lb.) whole organic chicken, cut into 8 pieces, or use the equivalent amount of chicken pieces – eg: drumstick, Maryland / thighs

Himalayan or Celtic Sea Salt and freshly ground black pepper

Rice flour for dusting

1 small red or brown onion, thinly sliced

4-5 cloves garlic, 3 cloves crushed and the others whole

½ cup black olives, pitted

6 anchovy fillets (optional)

6-8 bay leaves

2–3 sprigs fresh rosemary

2–3 sprigs fresh thyme

4–6 large whole ripe tomatoes (I prefer Roma or vine ripened)

¼ cup capers, drained (optional)

1/2 litre (17oz) organic chicken stock.

Finely chopped fresh flat-leaf parsley to serve

Method

Dust the chicken pieces in a little white rice flour and season with salt and freshly ground black pepper and put aside.

Preheat the oven to 180ºC/350ºF and heat the oil or ghee on medium to high in a deep heavy based 12-inch fry pan or casserole dish. Add the onion and sauté for 1-2 minutes until soft. Reduce the heat slightly and add the crushed garlic and anchovies if using and continue to sauté for a couple more minutes.

Shake off any excess flour from the chicken pieces and add to the fry pan and brown slightly on each side - around 5 -10 minutes.

Add the olives and capers if using, fresh tomatoes and continue to sauté for around 5 minutes. Add the chicken stock, rosemary sprigs, remaining garlic cloves and bay leaves and season with a little extra salt and pepper if necessary. Cover with a lid and bring to the boil then place in the preheated oven to bake for 1 1/2 hours.

When ready to serve, remove the bay leaves and sprigs of rosemary and thyme and transfer the chicken to a serving platter and top with freshly chopped parsley. Serve with the sauce spooned over the top and a large green salad or steamed veges.

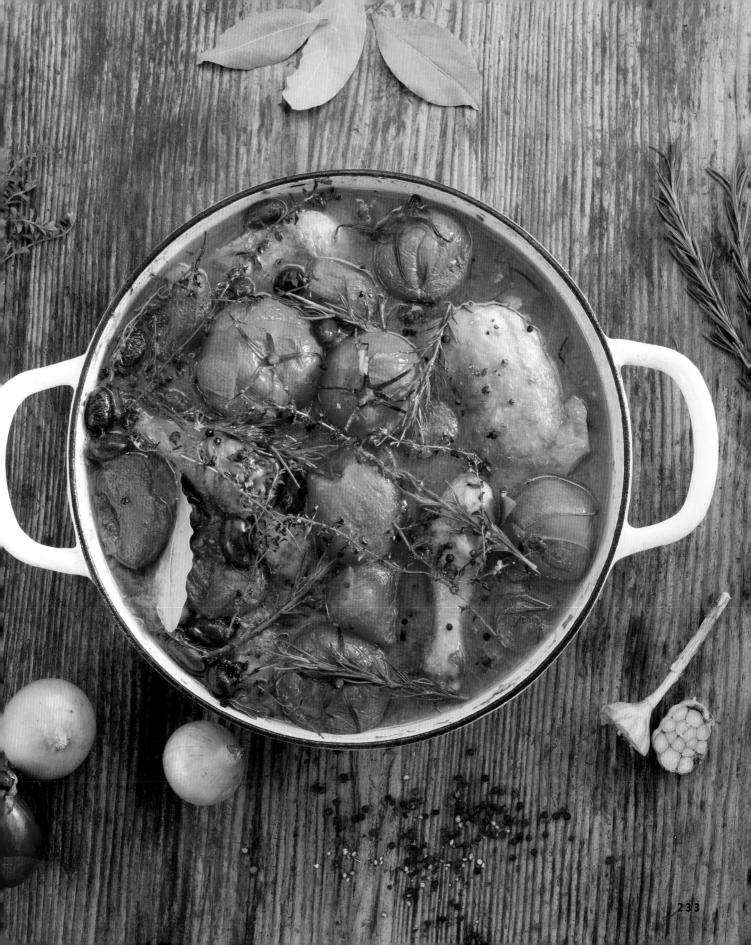

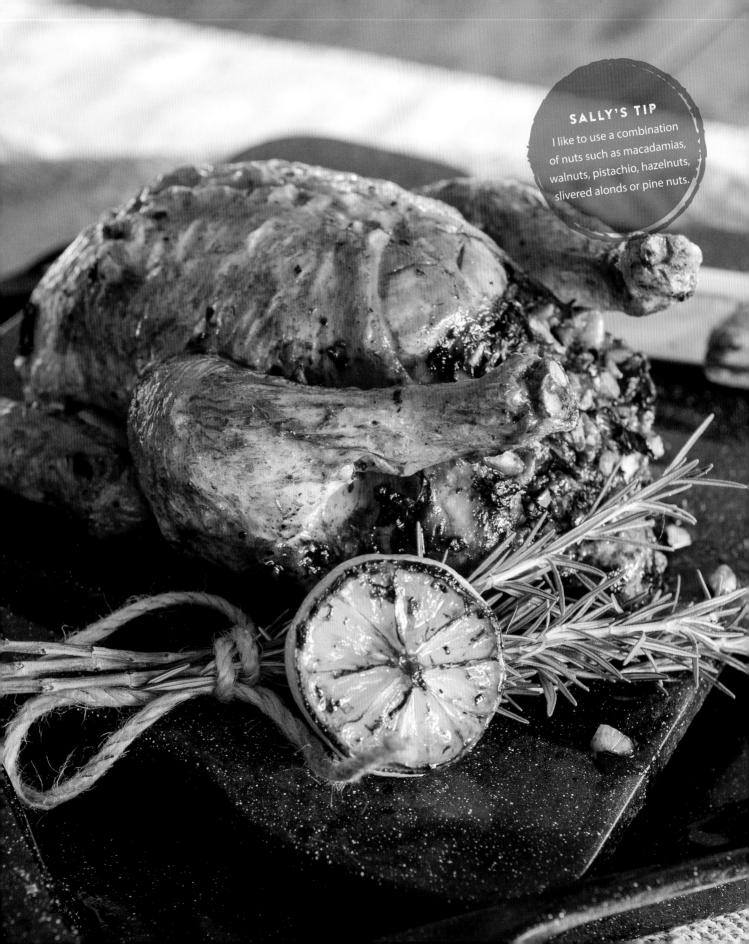

SALLY'S TIP

I like to use a combination of nuts such as macadamias, walnuts, pistachio, hazelnuts, slivered alonds or pine nuts.

Roast Chicken With Fig, Herb & Nut Stuffing

I created this recipe especially for those who, like me, love eating stuffing with their roast chicken, but don't love the gut pain caused by eating gluten. I've swapped the breadcrumbs for crushed nuts and combined them with fresh figs and herbs and the result... well, this stuffing is good enough to eat on its own! So give it a whirl after Stage I and enjoy with family and friends. Remember to always buy organic or antibiotic-free chicken.

Method

Preheat oven to 180°C/350°F. Combine the herbs, fennel, fig, feta, oil, 1 teaspoon of the lemon rind and all of the juice in a mixing bowl. Season generously with salt and pepper.

Use a mortar and pestle or food processor to coarsely grind the nuts and add to the mixing bowl with other ingredients. Use your hands to combine well.

Spoon the stuffing into the chicken cavity.

Lightly grease a roasting pan with ghee oil and place the chicken into the pan. Baste the chicken skin with ghee or oil until well coated and season with salt and pepper and the remaining lemon rind.

Bake for approximately one hour (depending on the size of your chicken and force of your oven) or until the skin is golden brown and the chicken juices run clear. Be careful not to overcook the chicken or it will become tough.

Rest the chicken for ten minutes, then carve into serving size pieces. Serve with freshly steamed green vegetables or green salad with avocado and a side of the stuffing.

Ingredients

1 whole chicken - organic or at least antibiotic free

Ghee, macadamia or virgin coconut oil

Stuffing

1 cup fresh mixed herbs, roughly chopped. eg: flat-leaf parsley, mint and thyme

1/3 cup fennel fronds, chopped

2 fresh figs, chopped - if figs are not in season, you can use dried figs

1-2 tbsp goat's feta

1/3 cup extra virgin olive oil or macadamia oil

1 tbsp finely grated lemon rind

Juice of 1 lemon

1/2 tsp Himalayan or Celtic Sea Salt and freshly ground black pepper, to taste

3/4 cup mixed raw nuts

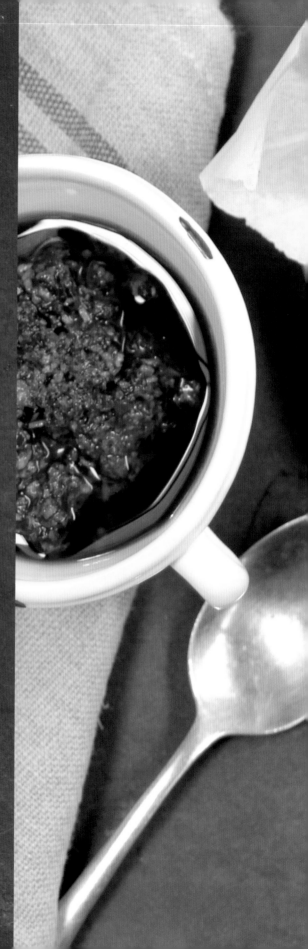

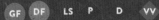

GUT ALERT

Root vegetables and zucchini are high in soluble fibre, making them easier to digest than vegetables with insoluble fibre. If you suffer from IBS, then you may want to stick to this vegetable combo until your gut and digestion heals.

SERVES 4 (SERVING SIZE 1/4-1 1/2 CUPS)

Mixed Baked Vegetables

Ingredients

2 small red onions, quartered

2 baby fennel bulbs, trimmed and halved lengthways

2 zucchini, quartered lengthways

2 beetroot, peeled and quartered

1 medium butternut pumpkin / squash, peeled and cut into even-sized chunks

3-4 sprigs of fresh rosemary

4-6 whole cloves of garlic

1 tbsp ghee, virgin coconut oil or macadamia oil

Himalayan or Celtic Sea Salt and cracked pepper

Dairy-free pesto (see page x), to serve (optional)

Method

Preheat oven to 180°C/350°F. Place the vegetables onto a pre-greased baking tray and drizzle with oil or coat with the ghee. Season with salt and pepper and add the rosemary sprigs and whole garlic cloves. Place in the oven and cook for 25–30 minutes or until tender and slightly golden brown. Serve warm or cold, and drizzle with a little dairy-free pesto (see page 277) if desired.

GF DF LS P D VV

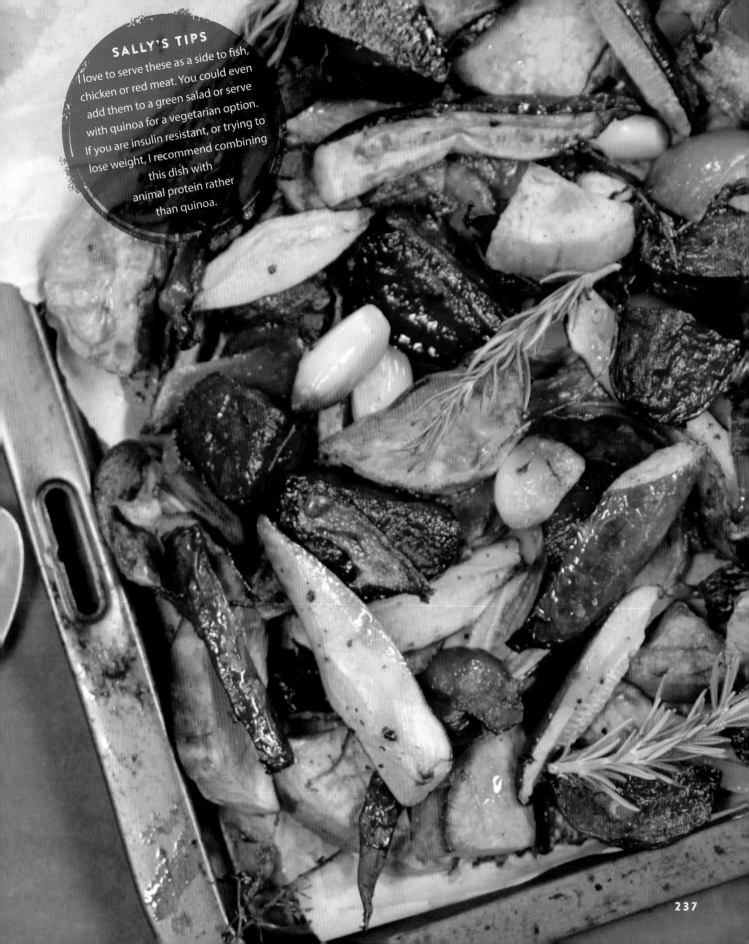

Zucchini Noodles with Home-made bolognaise

I like to keep a stash of bolognaise on hand in the freezer for those nights when you're tight on time, or if unexpected guests drop in. It's easy to prepare and this recipe is so full of flavour that you will never want to buy bottled bolognaise sauce again. I've replaced traditional pasta in this recipe with zucchini noodles, which make a great grain and gluten-free alternative. This recipe is also a hit with the kids and is a great way to sneak a few extra vegetables into them.

Ingredients

1 tbsp ghee, macadamia or virgin coconut oil

1 brown onion, diced

3-4 garlic cloves, crushed

500g 100% grassfed beef or lamb mince

2 carrots, peeled and grated

2 sticks celery, thinly chopped (optional)

1/2 cup pepita seeds

800g fresh, ripe tomatoes, chopped

2 dessert spoons fresh rosemary, leaves removed from stems and roughly chopped (use dried rosemary as an alternative)

2 dessert spoons dried oregano

Handful fresh basil, roughly chopped, plus extra to serve

Juice of 1/2 lemon

Himalayan or Celtic Sea Salt and freshly ground black pepper to taste

Zucchini noodles, to serve (see page 241)

Method

Heat the ghee or oil in a large deep frying pan over medium heat. Add the onion and sauteé for a few minutes, before adding the garlic. Continue to sauteé for 1-2 minutes, until soft, being careful not to burn.

Add the mince and cook for 5 minutes or until brown, using a fork to break up the lumps as it cooks. Season with salt and pepper and herbs.

Add the carrot, celery and pepita seeds and cook for a further 5 minutes. Stir through the tomato, cover and allow to simmer over low heat for 45 minutes, or until the liquid reduces and sauce thickens (remove the lid for the last 10 minutes if the sauce needs to thicken further).

Check the flavour and season with any additional herbs, salt or pepper, if required and add a squeeze of fresh lemon juice.

Garnish with fresh basil leaves and/or chopped parsley. Serve on top of with zucchini noodles (see recipe page 241). If you are really missing your grated parmesan cheese, substitute with pecorino which is made from sheep's milk if tolerated.

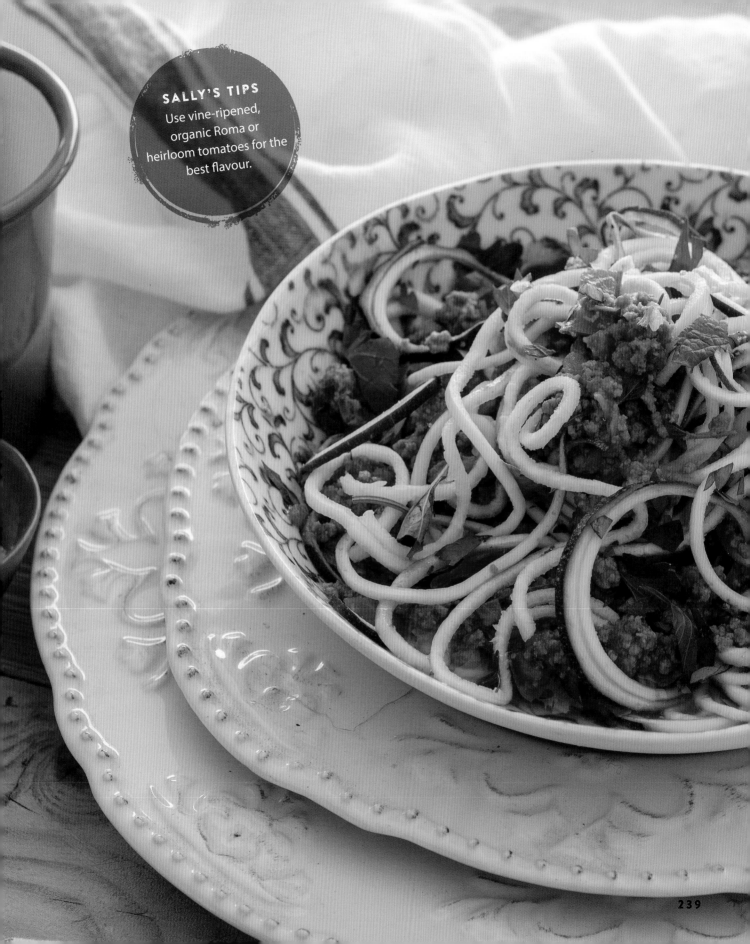

SALLY'S TIPS
Use vine-ripened, organic Roma or heirloom tomatoes for the best flavour.

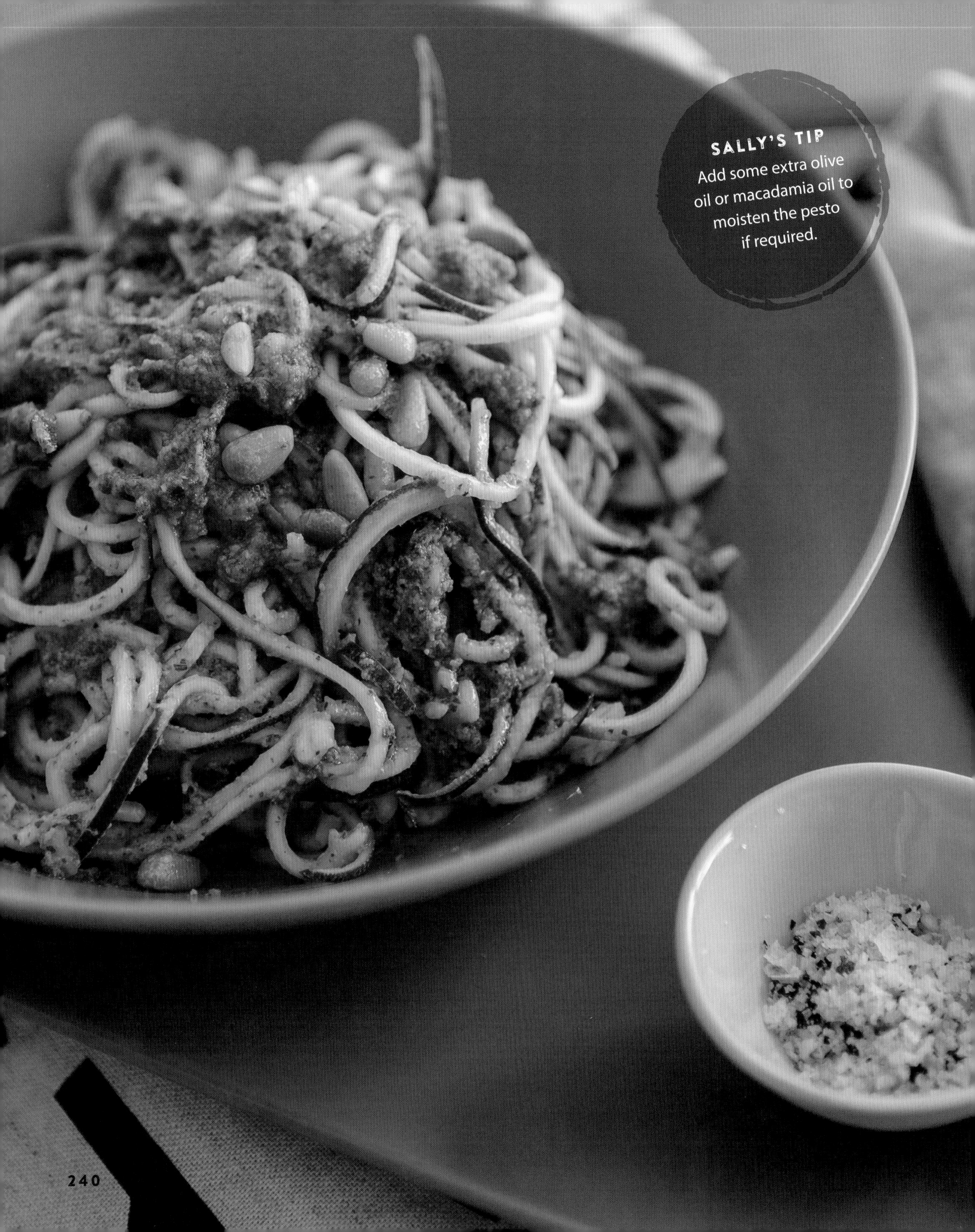

SALLY'S TIP
Add some extra olive oil or macadamia oil to moisten the pesto if required.

Zucchini Pesto Noodles

This makes a delicious vegetarian option to enjoy when you are eating meat-free on the program and, because it's made on a base of zucchini noodles, it won't leave you feeling bloated, or end up on your hips like wheat or even gluten free pasta can! Enjoy the noodles raw or slightly blanched, whatever works best for your gut.

Method

To make the zucchini noodles

Remove ends from the zucchini and place into the opening of the vegetable spiraliser to make your zucchini noodles. If you don't have a zucchini spiraliser, you can use a julienne vegetable peeler to cut the zucchini lengthways into long strips and separate the strands of zucchini with your hands to resemble spaghetti. You can then serve them raw (I prefer this) or sauté lightly in a little olive oil for 1 minute.

Transfer the zucchini noodles to a large mixing bowl along with toasted pine nuts and combine well with the pesto sauce. Add to a serving dish and drizzle with a little fresh lemon juice and season with salt and pepper to taste.

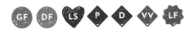

Ingredients

For the zucchini noodles

2 - 4 large zucchini's

Extra virgin olive oil (optional)

Pinch of Celtic Sea Salt and freshly ground black pepper (optional)

For the pesto

2-3 tbsp dairy-free pesto (see recipe page 277)

2-3 tbsp pine nuts, lightly toasted

1 lemon wedge, (optional)

Himalayan or Celtic Sea Salt and freshly ground black pepper, to taste

Poached Chicken

Poaching is a really healthy way to cook chicken. Preparing some in advance to keep on hand in the fridge makes light work of knocking up quick and easy meals when you're short on time. It's also a great way to add protein to your meals, so you will feel fuller and more satisfied. Be sure to use organic chicken.

Method

Place all the ingredients into a large stockpot or flameproof casserole dish and cover with water. Bring to the boil, then cover and reduce heat to low a simmer and cook for a further 40-50 minutes, until meat is very tender and no longer pink.

Carefully remove the chicken from the stock. Place into a large bowl and allow to cool slightly, then pull apart and shred, or slice the meat thinly. Store in an air tight container in the refrigerator for up to 3 days.

Ingredients

2 kg chicken breasts

1 handful fresh flat-leaf parsley

4 bay leaves

Good pinch Himalayan or Celtic Sea Salt

1-2 tsp black peppercorns

1/2 fennel bulb, chopped

2 spring onions (use tops only for Low FODMAPS)

1 large carrot, peeled and cut in quarters

1–2 celery stalks, halved

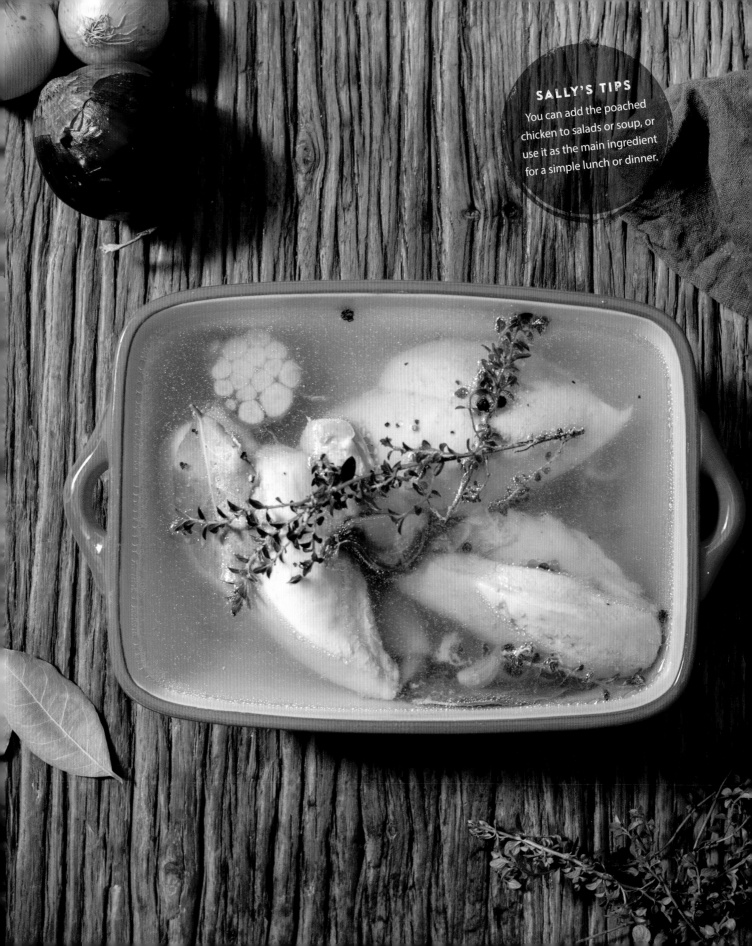

SALLY'S TIPS
You can add the poached chicken to salads or soup, or use it as the main ingredient for a simple lunch or dinner.

Chicken & Quinoa Patties

Ingredients

200g / 7oz chicken mince

1 cup cooked quinoa (see page 254)

1 egg, lightly beaten

1 zucchini, grated

1/2 cup fresh flat-leaf parsley or coriander/cilantro, roughly chopped

1/2 red onion, finely diced

1 tbsp pepitas (pumpkin seeds)

1 tbsp coriander seeds, ground

1 tbsp black sesame seeds

1/4 tsp ground turmeric

Celtic or Himalayan Sea Salt and freshly ground black pepper to taste

1/4 cup rice flour or almond meal

1tbsp ghee, coconut oil or macadamia oil for frying

This is one of my 'go-to' recipes if I'm rushing around and need to grab healthy food fast. These delicious rissoles are packed with protein and have oodles of flavour thanks to plenty of fresh herbs and spices. I've added cooked quinoa for a little slow burning carbohydrate to keep you feeling fuller for longer, but feel free to exclude it if you prefer.

Method

Place the chicken mince and all the other ingredients (except the rice flour and oil) into a large mixing bowl. Use your hands to mix until well combined. Scoop a heaped tablespoon of the mixture into your hands and shape into a small patty about 1 inch thick.

Add the rice flour or almond meal to a plate and roll each patty in it until well coated.

Heat the ghee or oil in a frying pan on medium heat, then add one patty and cook for 3 minutes on each side, or until a light golden brown and cooked through. Transfer to a paper towel to drain excess oil. Taste to see if you need to add any more seasoning, such as salt and pepper and/or ground spices. Repeat the same method for each patty.

Serve with a dollop of plain sheep's yogurt or my Yoghurt and Herb Tahini Dressing (see page 280), and serve with a big green salad and avocado or steamed veggies.

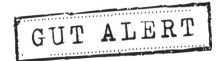

Substitute the red onion for spring onions - using the green tops only, to make this Low FODMAPS

Simple Roast Pumpkin

Roast pumpkin, or butternut squash as it's known in America, makes a delicious side to any meal, although because they are a starchy vegetable like sweet potato, I recommend limiting your intake so as to avoid feeding your gut flora too much starch. You may need to experiment with your guts tolerance of starchy vegetables initially, especially if you suffer from bad IBS and or Candida overgrowth. If you find they don't leave you feeling gassy or bloated then a moderate intake is A oK!

Method

Preheat oven to 210°C/410° F

Line a large baking dish or tray with baking/parchment paper

Arrange the pumpkin on the tray and coat with the ghee/coconut or macadamia oil. Sprinkle with cinnamon if using and salt and pepper. If you are using rosemary in place of the cinnamon, arrange the fresh sprigs on top of the pumpkin

Bake for 30 minutes. Turn the pumpkin pieces and cook for another 30 minutes or until pumpkin is tender and slightly golden brown.

Ingredients

1 kg piece of pumpkin, peeled and cut into slices or cut into 4cm pieces

2 tbsp ghee, coconut or macadamia oil

1 tsp ground cinnamon or sprinkle with fresh rosemary sprigs

Himalayan or Celtic Sea Salt to taste

Cracked black pepper to taste

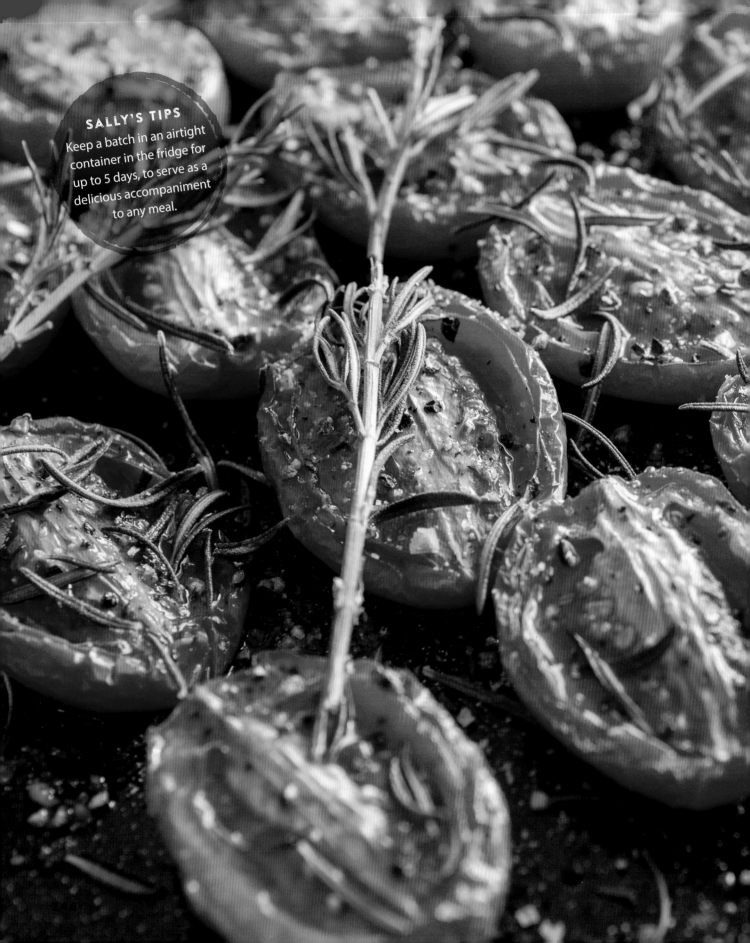

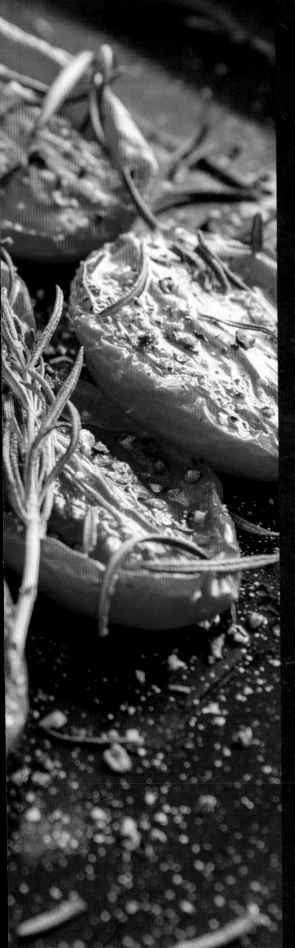

Slow-Roasted Tomatoes

There is nothing quite like the delicious sweet flavour of slow roasted tomatoes, oozing olive oil and the aroma of fresh herbs. Slow roasted tomatoes are probably one of my favourite accompaniments to any meal and the good news is that recent research has found cooking tomatoes increases the levels of the powerful antioxidant - lycopene. Serve these with poached eggs and avocado for breakfast, toss through a salad, or serve as a side with lamb, chicken or beef for dinner.

Ingredients

12 vine-ripened or Roma tomatoes, cut in half horizontally

2 tbsp extra virgin olive oil or macadamia oil

Himalayan or Celtic Sea Salt and freshly ground black pepper, to taste

1 tsp dried or 1 tbsp freshly chopped herbs, such as rosemary, basil, thyme

Method

Preheat the oven to 120°C/250°F. Lightly grease an oven tray with a little oil. Arrange tomatoes on tray, cut side up. Drizzle with oil. Season with salt and pepper and sprinkle herbs over the tomatoes.

Roast for 2 hours. If you have the time, reduce the oven temperature to 80°C/175°F and cook for another 2 hrs to further caramelise.

Dukkah Crusted Lamb Cutlets

Lamb is a healthy source of lean animal protein. The dukkah is full of natural herbs and spices, adding a delicious flavor to the lamb

Ingredients

2 lamb cutlets per person (depending on the size)

1 tbsp dukkah (see page 285)

Ghee, coconut or macadamia oil, for grilling if required

Method

Preheat a griddle pan or BBQ grill plate to medium-high heat. Sprinkle both sides of the cutlets with the dukkah.

If cooking on the BBQ, heat 1 tbsp of oil on the grill. Cook the cutlets for 2-3 minutes each side or until lamb is cooked how you like it.

Serve with Mediterranean salad or Roasted Brussel Sprouts with Pine Nuts (see recipe page 269)

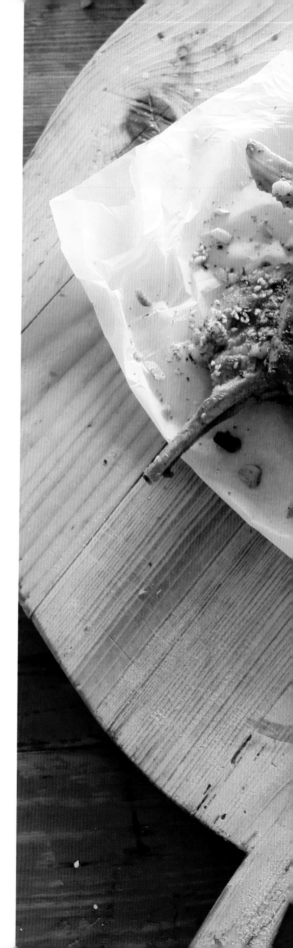

GUT ALERT

Although I recommend you eat the majority of your red meat slow cooked because it is easier to digest, eating it grilled or barbecued occasionally is fine. If you experience any bloating or gas afterwards, I recommend taking a digestive enzyme or a little apple cider vinegar in water, and stick to eating slow cooked meat for a while.

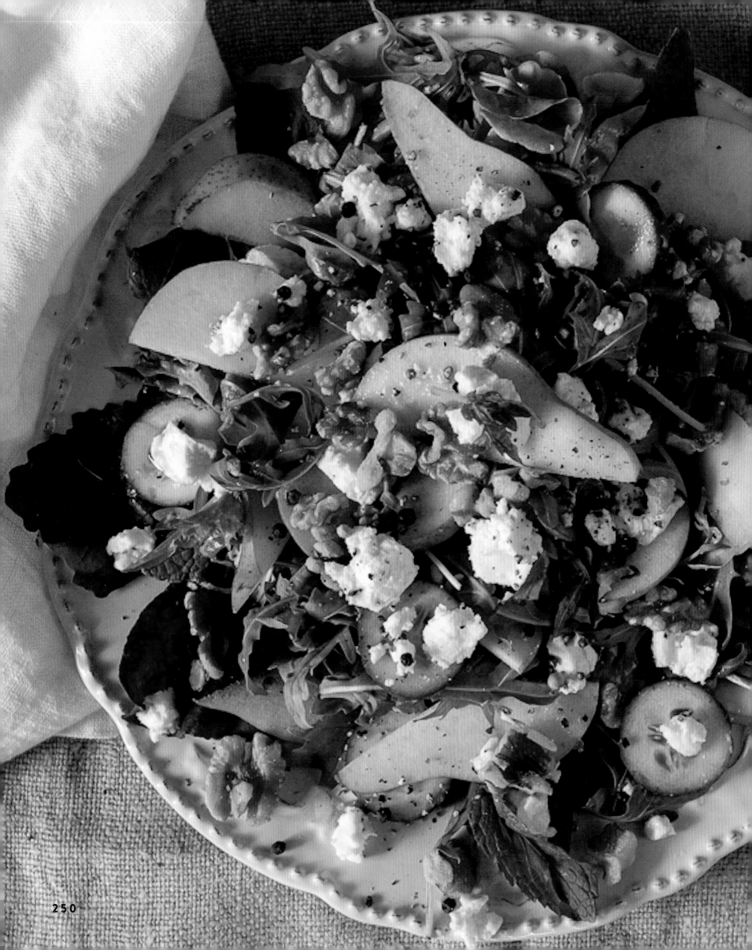

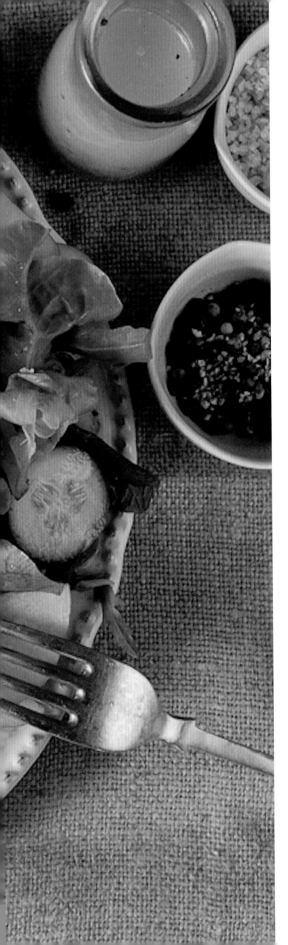

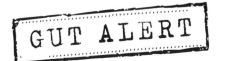

GUT ALERT

I don't usually recommend mixing fruit with other foods because it can cause bloating and gas from fermentation, and exacerbate symptoms associated with IBS. But unless you suffer from fructose malabsorbtion syndrome (see page 38) or really bad IBS, then it should be tolerated by your gut, as long as it's an occasional indulgence.

SERVES 2 (SERVING SIZE 2 CUPS)

Pear, Walnut & Goat's Feta Salad

I like to add a little goat's feta to salads, as a low allergy alternative to cheese made from cow's milk. This salad is a delicious accompaniment to chicken or lamb or can be enjoyed on its own as a light meal. Walnuts are known to be great for brain health, so this salad is a chance to get your grey matter firing!

Ingredients

1-2 large handfuls of rocket and mixed lettuce leaves

1 Lebanese cucumber, thinly sliced

1 pear, cored and thinly sliced

2 tbsp soft goat's feta, crumbled (my favourite is Meredith Valley)

1/2 cup walnuts, toasted

Himalayan or Celtic Sea Salt and freshly ground black pepper, to taste

Method

Arrange the rocket and lettuce on a large platter or individual plates, and top with the cucumber, pear, feta and walnuts. Season with salt and pepper.

Dress with Sally's simple salad dressing (see page 282).

Cauliflower & Pistachio Tabouli

Cauliflower makes a delicious grain free alternative to the cracked wheat in traditional tabouli recipes. It's also grain-free - a great combo for keeping your gut happy and your hips and thighs trim! Enjoy this salad as a side with any animal protein, like fish, chicken or red meat, or as a vegetarian option during Stage I of the program.

Ingredients

2 cups cauliflower rice (see page 216)

3 stalks of shallots or scallions, ends removed and finely sliced

1 bunch fresh flat-leaf parsley, leaves picked and finely chopped

1/2 bunch fresh mint, leaves removed and finely chopped

1 Lebanese cucumber, finely diced

250g organic cherry tomatoes, halved

1/2 - 3/4 cup shelled pistachio nuts

1/2 tsp ground cumin

Juice of 1 lemon

1/4 cup extra virgin olive oil

Himalayan or Celtic Sea Salt and freshly ground black pepper, to taste

Method

Combine all the ingredients in a large mixing bowl. Cover and refrigerate for 1-2 hours before serving to allow the flavours to infuse.

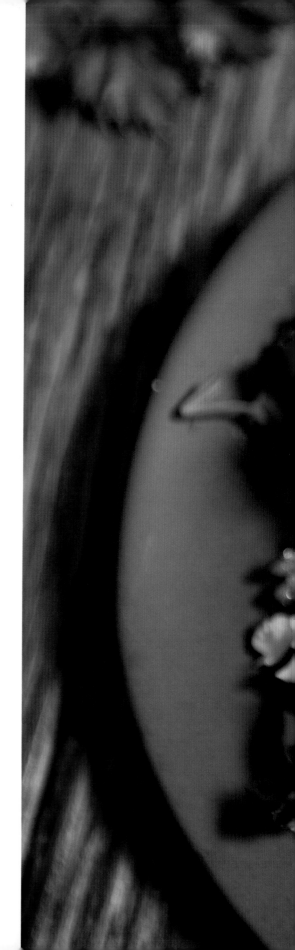

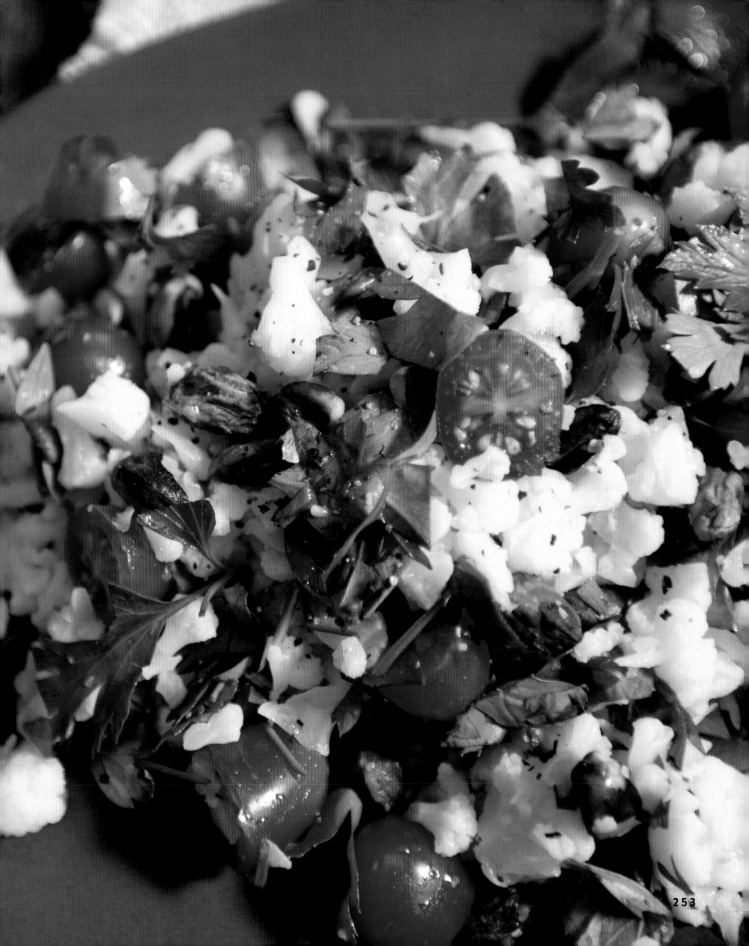

Simple Quinoa

Quinoa is really simple to prepare and you cook it the same way you would rice. I like to cook up a batch every week or so and store in the fridge to add to salads. It comes in three varieties, red, white and black, the most common being white. You can pretty well add any flavours to it that take your fancy. I've kept this recipe really simple and delicious, but feel free to serve it plain with just a little olive oil, salt and pepper, especially if you are adding it to my chicken quinoa patties or vegetable minestrone.

Ingredients

1 cup quinoa

2 cups water

Pinch of Celtic Sea or Himalayan rock salt

1/4 cup extra virgin olive or macadamia oil

Optional

Finely grated rind of 1 lemon

Juice of 1/2-1 lemon (you could a little freshly squeezed orange juice as well)

1/2 cup slivered almonds or pine nuts, toasted

1/2 cup fresh flat-leaf parsley, roughly chopped

Method

I like to pre-soak my quinoa in water overnight to reduce the phytic acid levels and make it more digestible, but if you are short on time, just ensure you rinse the quinoa well in a fine sieve under cold running water,before draining.

Add the quinoa to a large saucepan with the water and salt and replace lid. Place on the stove and set heat to high and bring to the boil.

Reduce heat to low and simmer, covered, until the water has been absorbed into the quinoa. If quinoa is not quite soft enough, add a little more water and continue cooking until absorbed. Quinoa should be soft and fluffy when ready.

Transfer the quinoa to a large mixing bowl and add the remaining ingredients if desired. Use a wooden spoon to mix through.

Store in an airtight container in the fridge for up to 4 days.

GF DF LS P D VV LF

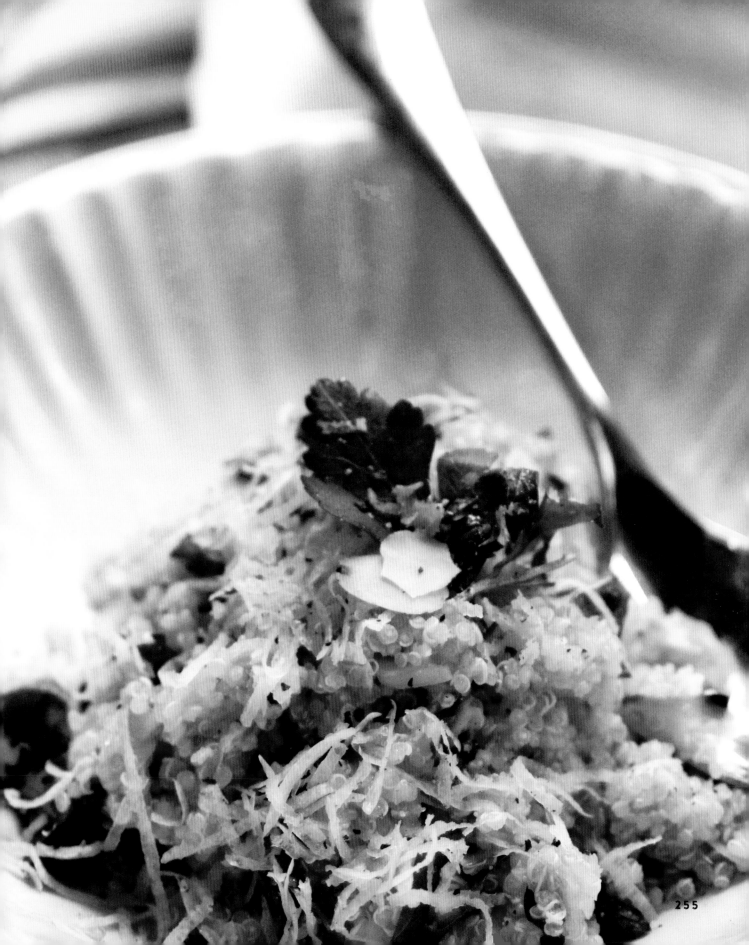

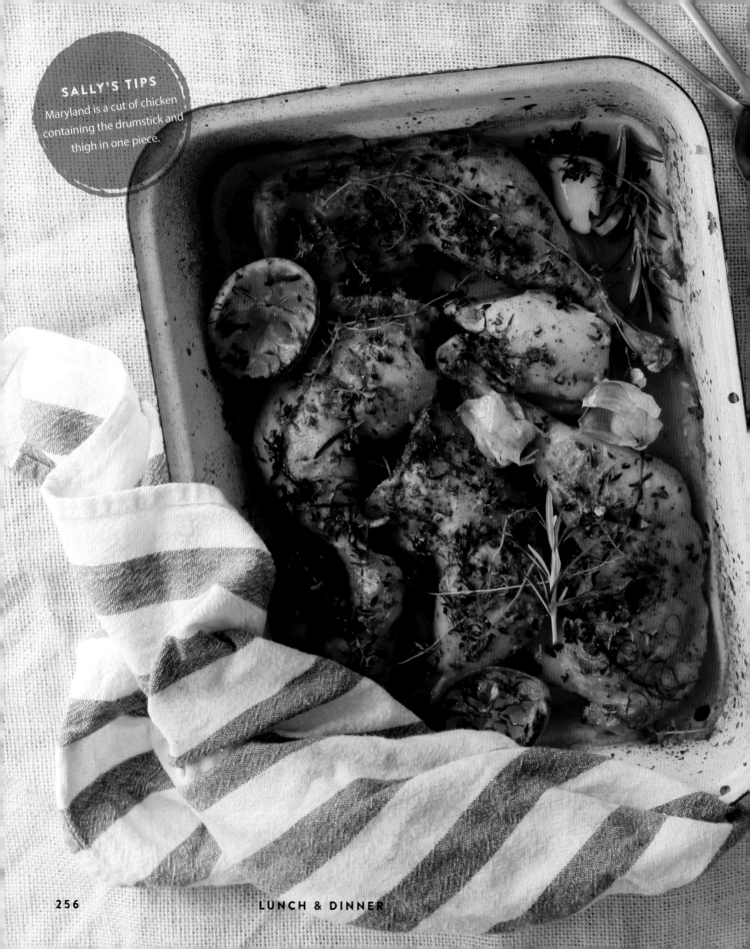

SALLY'S TIPS

Maryland is a cut of chicken containing the drumstick and thigh in one piece.

LUNCH & DINNER

Lemon & Herb Garlic Chicken

I owe this delicious recipe to my mum and it's one of my all-time favourites It is so simple and quick to prepare and the flavours are beautifully fresh and light. It's also the perfect recipe to whip up when you don't have a lot of time, but have a lot of mouths to feed and the best part is it's pretty well foolproof! Be sure to use organic or antibiotic free chicken to avoid any chemical nasties - and also because the flavour is so much better.

Method

Preheat the oven to 180°C/350°F. Arrange the chicken pieces in a large baking dish and coat the chicken pieces generously with the ghee or oil. Arrange the garlic evenly between the chicken pieces. Squeeze the lemon juice over the chicken and top with the zested lemon rind and plenty of fresh herbs. Season generously with salt and pepper.

Place into the preheated oven and cook for 45 minutes to an hour, or until the chicken pieces are golden brown on top and cooked through.

Divide between plates and drizzle with cooking juices. Serve with a green salad or steamed greens.

GF DF LS P D

GUT ALERT

Leave out the garlic to make it Low FODMAPS.

Ingredients

4 chicken Marylands and 3-4 drumsticks

1/2 cup ghee. coconut or macadamia oil

12 garlic cloves, peeled

Juice of 1 lemon and rind of 2

3 large sprigs of fresh rosemary

4 sprigs of fresh thyme

Himalayan or Celtic Sea or Salt and freshly ground black pepper to taste

Zucchini and Pea Fritters with Tzatziki

Ingredients

4 zucchini, grated

2 tsp Himalayan or Celtic Sea Salt

1 cup fresh or thawed frozen peas

4 spring onions, finely sliced

2 tbsp chopped fresh dill

2 tbsp chopped fresh flat-leaf parsley

2 tbsp chopped fresh mint

2 eggs, lightly beaten

180g goat's feta, crumbled

1/2 cup rice flour or coconut flour

1/2 tsp gluten-free baking powder

1/2 teaspoon each Himalayan or Celtic Sea Salt and freshly ground black pepper

2 tbsp virgin coconut oil or macadamia oil for cooking

Tzatziki (see page 182), to serve

Lemon wedges, to serve

Method

Place the grated zucchini in a colander lined with cheesecloth or a nut milk bag. If you don't have either of these, you can place the zucchini directly in the colander. Sprinkle with salt and toss to combine, then set aside for 20 minutes.

In the meantime, shell and cook the peas if using fresh.

Gather up the ends of the cheesecloth or nut milk bag and wring out the liquid. If you're not using either of these, you can squeeze the water out of the zucchini with your hands in batches. It is important to squeeze out as much water as possible so that the fritters won't be soggy.

Place the zucchini into a large mixing bowl and add the peas, spring onions, herbs and eggs. Mix with a fork to combine.

Add the feta, flour, baking powder, salt and pepper and mix with a fork to combine all ingredients well.

Heat 1 tablespoon of oil in a non-stick or cast iron frying pan, over medium heat. Drop around 2 tablespoons of the mixture into the pan for each fritter, being careful not to overcrowd the pan, and flatten each fritter slightly with a spatula. The more you flatten them, the crispier the fritters will be. Cook for 3-4 minutes on each side, or until golden brown.

Remove the fritters from the pan and place on paper towel. Add the remaining oil into the pan and repeat the process with the remaining mixture.

Serve fritters warm topped with tzatziki, and a squeeze of fresh lemon juice.

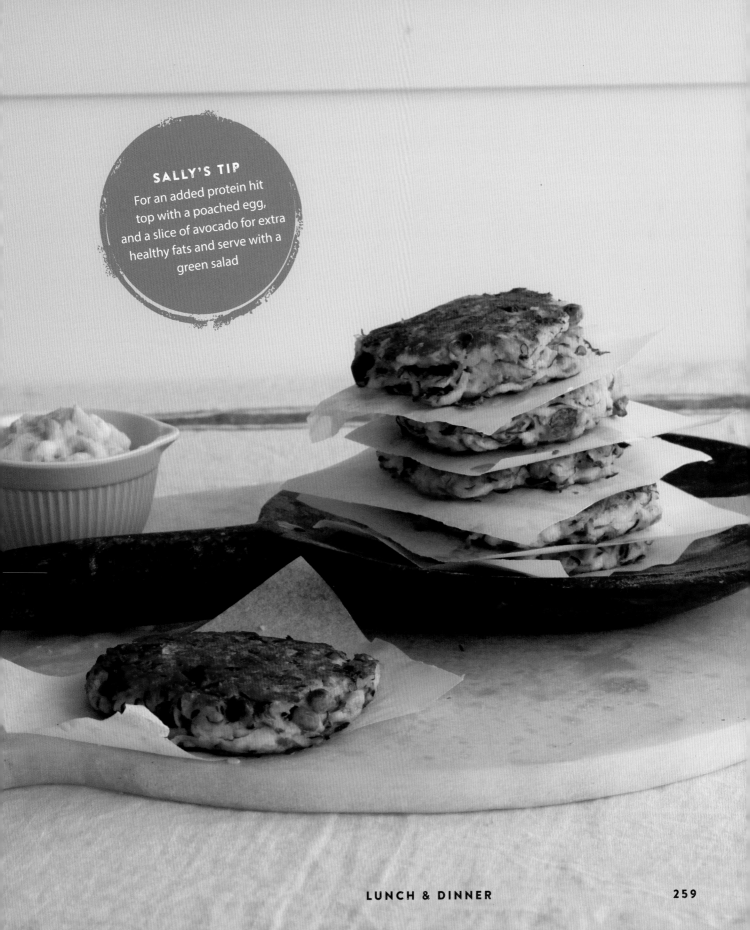

SALLY'S TIP
For an added protein hit top with a poached egg, and a slice of avocado for extra healthy fats and serve with a green salad

Shepherd's Pie

Ingredients

1 ½ tbsp ghee, coconut or macadamia oil

1 brown onion, diced

1 carrot, grated

1 zucchini, grated

2-3 garlic cloves, crushed

1 kg 100% grass fed beef or lamb mince

1 cup beef or chicken stock

2 ripe tomatoes, roughly chopped

1/4 cup flat-leaf parsley, roughly chopped

2 tbsp fresh rosemary

1 tbsp fresh thyme leaves

Himalayan or Celtic Sea Salt and freshly ground black pepper, to taste

1 quantity Cauliflower rice (see page 216)

Paprika to dust, optional

If you're a fan of conventional Shepherd's Pie, then this is a great low-carb alternative – perfect if you are watching your weight or eating Paleo. It's a breeze to prepare and freezes well, making it the perfect meal to keep on hand for those nights you don't feel like cooking, or when unexpected guests pop in. The kids will also love it!

Method

Preheat the oven to 200°C/390°F. Heat the coconut oil in a large frying pan over medium-high heat. Add the onion, carrot and zucchini. Reduce heat to medium-low heat and cook, covered, for 5 minutes or until the vegetables are soft but not browned. Add the garlic and cook, stirring, for 1 minute.

Add the mince to the pan and cook for 5 minutes or until well browned, breaking up lumps with a wooden spoon as it cooks.

Stir in the stock, tomatoes and herbs. Bring to a simmer and cook, uncovered, until the liquid has reduced and the mixture has thickened slightly. Season to taste. Spread the mince mixture evenly into the base of a medium-sized casserole dish.

Spoon the cauliflower rice on top and place in the oven. Cook on the middle rack of the oven for 25-30 minutes, until the top begins to brown. Allow to stand for 5-10 minutes before serving.

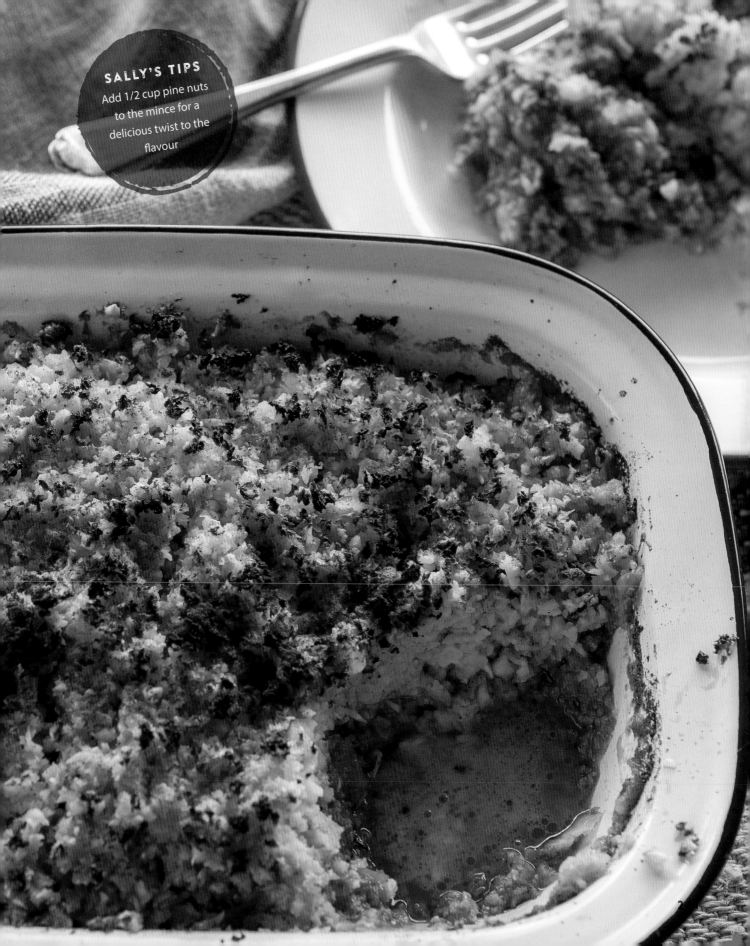

SALLY'S TIPS

Add 1/2 cup pine nuts to the mince for a delicious twist to the flavour

Haloumi & Avocado Wraps

This is my version of a breadless sandwich, made with my favourite cheese, haloumi, which is traditionally made from unpasteurized sheep or goat's milk. Nowadays haloumi made from cow's cheese is more popular, although you will find sheep's haloumi in some super markets. Pan fried haloumi also makes a super filling snack, thanks to being a rich source of saturated fat.

Method

Heat the coconut oil in a frying pan and cook the haloumi over medium-low heat for 1-2 minutes each side or until just golden brown. Remove from the pan and drain on paper towel.

Arrange the lettuce or Witlof leaves on a plate and top with the haloumi and avocado.

Drizzle with a little olive oil or macadamia oil, fresh lemon juice and add a dollop of pesto.

Garnish with fresh herbs and snow pea sprouts or alfalfa.

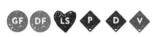

Ingredients

1 tbsp virgin coconut oil

150g/2oz sheep's haloumi, cut into 2- 2.5cm thick slices

Cos lettuce or Witlof, washed and dried

1/2 large or 1 small avocado, thinly sliced

Ghee, coconut or macadamia oil for frying

1/2 lemon, to squeeze

Freshly ground black pepper to taste

Dairy Free pesto (see page 277)

Fresh herbs and snow pea sprouts or alfalfa, to garnish

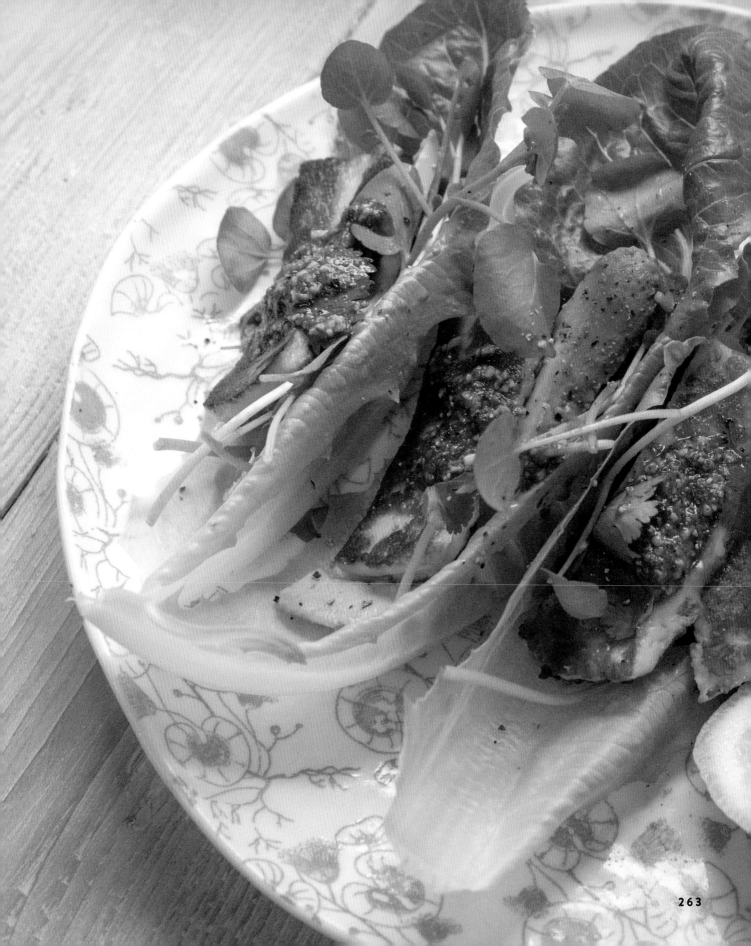

Cauliflower Rice Vegetable Stir-fry

This has to be another one of my favourite recipes, as far as the flavours, nutritional value and convenience go. It's also a real crowd pleaser, especially with kids, and the best part is they will have no idea just how many veggies they're having! If you want to add a different source of protein, simply replace the chicken with fish, prawns or 100% grass-fed meat, or even a beaten egg and some free range, nitrate free bacon, to make it fried rice style. There's no need to cook with any bottled sauces with this stir-fry, and it's also low in starch, thanks to the cauliflower rice.

Ingredients

2 tsp sesame oil

2 tsp ghee or coconut oil

2 organic chicken thigh fillets, chopped (optional)

1/2 red or brown onion, diced

3 spring onions, finely chopped

2 garlic cloves, crushed

2 tsp finely grated fresh ginger (or use 1 tsp ground

2 tsp finely grated fresh turmeric (or use 1/4 tsp of ground)

1 large carrot, peeled and cut julienne style

1 cup chopped kale leaves, or baby English spinach

1 cup small broccoli florets

6 asparagus spears, woody ends trimmed, finely sliced

4 yellow squash, chopped

10 snow peas, sliced

2 tbsp pepitas

2 tsp sesame seeds

1 tsp ground cinnamon

Ground nutmeg, to taste

1 serving of Cauliflower Rice (see page 216)

2 tbsp fresh coriander / cilantro leaves or flat-leaf parsley, leaves removed from the stems

Method

Heat the oil in a large frying pan or wok on medium- high heat, then add the chicken or meat if using and stir-fry until golden brown and cooked through. Transfer to a plate and set aside.

Add the onion, spring onions, garlic, ginger and turmeric and stir-fry until onion becomes transparent.

Add all the vegetables along with the pepitas and sesame seeds. Stir-fry for 3-5 minutes or until vegetables are just soft, but still a little bit crunchy.

Add the chicken and Cauliflower Rice, and sprinkle with cinnamon and nutmeg. Toss with a wooden spoon until well combined and heated through.

Serve topped with fresh coriander leaves or flat-leaf parsley.

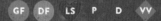

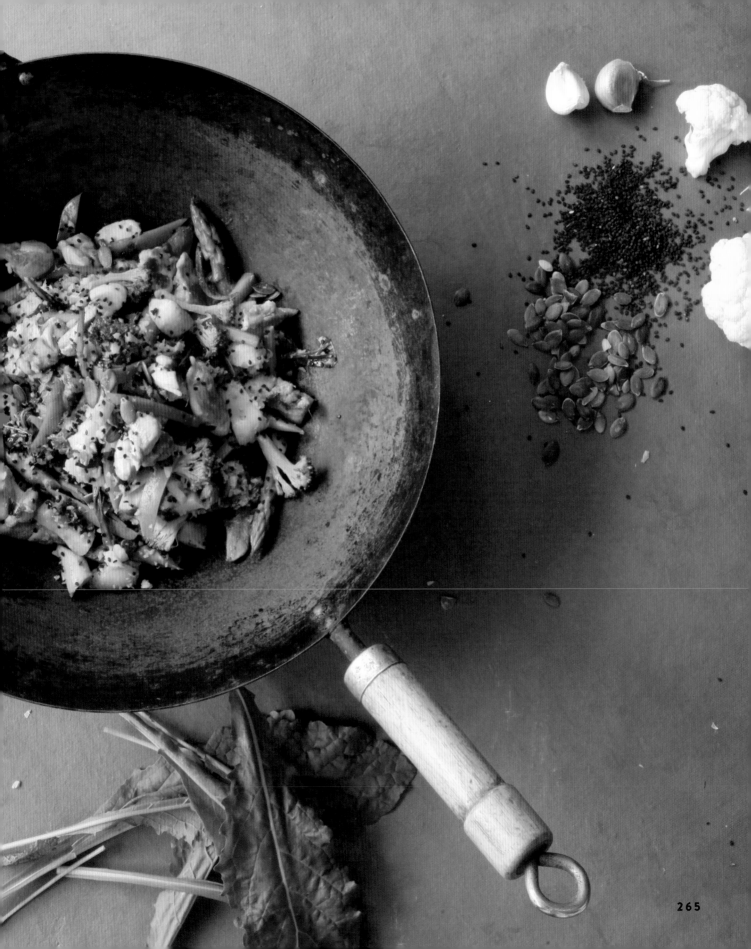

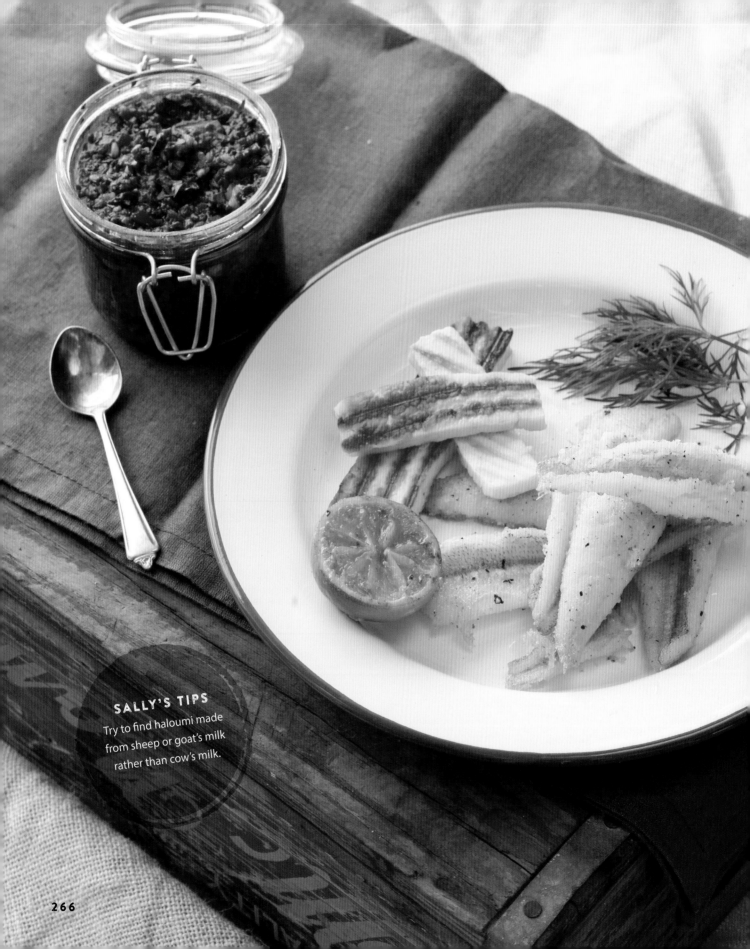

Pan-fried Whiting with Haloumi & Olive Tapenade

Method

Place flour onto a large dinner plate and season generously with salt and pepper. Mix to evenly combine.

Dust the whiting fillets lightly in rice flour to cover evenly. Heat a little ghee or oil in a frying pan over medium-high heat. Shake off excess flour and cook for 1-2 minutes each side, or until crispy and cooked through.

Warm a small amount of oil and buitter in a separate small frying pan and cook the haloumi over medium-low heat for 1-2 minutes each side or until lightly golden.

Transfer the fish and haloumi to plates and top with a little olive tapenade. Sprinkle with herbs and drizzle with a little extra virgin olive or macadamia oil. Season with pepper and serve with lemon to squeeze over.

I recommend serving this dish with a green salad and sliced avocado.

Ingredients

1/4 cup rice flour or coconut flour (optional)

Himalayan or Celtic Sea Salt and freshly ground black pepper

150g/5 oz sheep's haloumi, cut into 1cm thick slices (optional)

300- 400g/10-14 oz fresh whiting fillets or another white fish like cod.

Coconut or macadamia oil, for cooking

1 tsp of pure butter for cooking

1 tbsp freshly-made olive tapenade (see page 279)

Dill sprigs or roughly chopped fresh flat-leaf parsley, to serve

Extra virgin olive oil or macadamia oil, to serve

1/2 lemon (lightly chargrilled if you like), to serve

Yummy Zucchini

It would be hard to pick a favourite vegetable but if I had to I'd vote for zucchini. It's so versatile and full of flavour, and eaten raw or cooked it's super healthy. You can prepare this dish in minutes and it's a fresh and zesty accompaniment to your chosen protein.

Ingredients

1 tsp butter

1 tbsp macadamia oil

1 large zucchini, grated

Juice of 1/2 lemon

Pinch of Himalayan or Celtic Sea Salt and freshly ground black pepper, to taste

Method

Combine the butter and oil in a frying pan and melt over medium heat. Add the zucchini and lemon juice, and season with salt and pepper. Cook, stirring, for a minute or two, until just softened. Serve immediately.

GF **DF** **LS** **P** **D** **VV** **LF**

ZUCCHINI

Zucchini are particularly high in insoluble fibre, so your gut will also love this vegetable for getting things moving!

SALLY'S TIPS

Serve as an accompaniment to any dish. Alternatively, add to cooked quinoa with other salad veggies for a healthy vegetarian salad.

Pan Fried Brussel Sprouts with Pine Nuts

If you're like me and had a major aversion to the humble Brussel sprout as a child, then this recipe is sure to convert you being a Brussel sprout lover! Pan fried Brussel sprouts are a delicious accompaniment to any meal and also make a handy snack, hot or cold.

Ingredients

10 or more Brussels sprouts (or as many as you want)

Ghee, macadamia or coconut oil

Squeeze of fresh lemon juice a

2 -3 cloves of garlic, crushed

2 tbsp pine nuts (optional)

Himalayan or Celtic Sea Salt and freshly ground black pepper, to taste

Method

Trim the ends slightly from each Brussel sprout. Preheat the oil or ghee on medium to high heat in the pan. Add the sprouts and sauteé for 2 minutes. Add a splash of lemon juice to the pan and the garlic. Continue sauteéing for a further 4 minutes and add the pine nuts towards the end to toast. The sprouts are ready when they start to crisp up slightly on the outside.

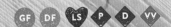

THE HUMBLE BRUSSEL SPROUT

These little green nuggets are a nutrient powerhouse, bursting with vitamins and minerals, including B6, K1 and C. When it comes to fibre they really pack a punch - great for helping to lower cholesterol and blood pressure. They are also rich in antioxidants. A word or warning however, if you suffer from IBS you should test your sensitivity to cruciferous vegetables to see if you experience any discomfort after eating them. Being so dense in fibre they can irritate your gut.

SERVES 4 (SERVING SIZE 1-2 CUPS)

Pomegranate & Fennel Salad

I like to serve this nourishing and delicious salad, along with grilled white fish or poached chicken, when I'm entertaining.

Ingredients

1 bunch asparagus, woody ends trimmed (or 1 cup snow peas)

Virgin coconut oil or macadamia oil

Couple of large handfuls mixed lettuce and rocket

1/2 cup fresh mint leaves, roughly chopped

1 fennel bulb, thinly sliced, leafy tops reserved

1/2-3/4 cup toasted macadamias or walnuts

120g soft goat's feta, crumbled (optional)

2 pomegranates, halved, seeds removed

Sally's Simple Salad dressing see page 282)

Method

Preheat a BBQ grill or chargrill pan to medium-high heat. Drizzle asparagus with a little oil and cook for 3-4 minutes, turning occasionally, until just tender but still slightly crisp. Remove and set aside on paper towel to cool. (Alternatively lightly steam or blanch the snow peas and rinse under cold water to cool.)

Arrange the lettuce, rocket and mint on a serving platter and sprinkle the fennel, nuts, feta, pomegranate seeds and asparagus (or snow peas) over.

Garnish with fennel tops and dress with Sally's Simple Salad dressing when ready to serve.

POMEGRANATE

Pomegranate is renowned for being rich in antioxidants, which can prevent LDL (bad cholesterol) from oxidizing, helping to reduce the build of plaque in the arteries, whilst increasing levels of HDL (good cholesterol). Research has indicated that the compounds in pomegranate may reduce the risk of breast and prostate cancer and even slow down its growth. Be aware though that pomegranate juice bought in stores usually has sugar added – as always, check the label!

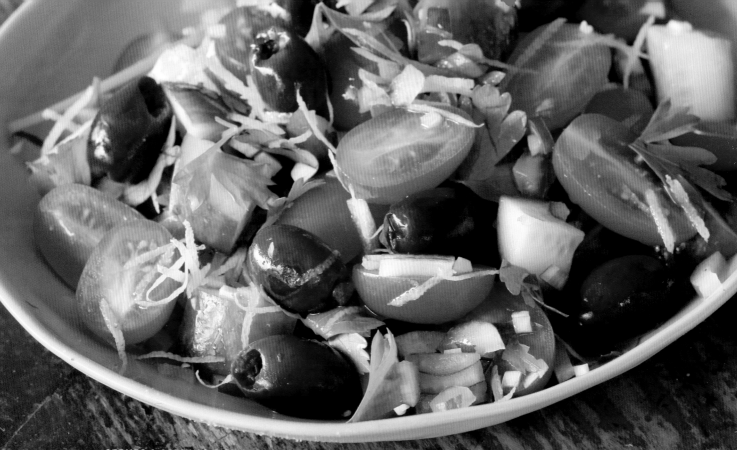

Mediterranean Salad

This salad makes a delcious fresh and zesty side to any dish, in particular lamb or fish. It's my twist on the traditional Greek salad where I have replaced the cow's feta with goats feta. The best part is you can whip this salad up in a matter of minutes!

Method

Place all the ingredients into a mixing bowl and toss to combine. Transfer to a serving dish and enjoy!

GF DF LS P D VV

Ingredients

6- 8 organic cherry or grape tomatoes, halved

2 Lebanese cucumbers, diced

Finely grated rind of 1 lemon

1/4 of a red onion, finely chopped (optional)

Juice of 1/2-1 lemon

1/2 cup flat-leaf parsley, roughly chopped

1/4 cup pitted kalamata olives

1/4 cup extra virgin olive or macadamia oil

Himalayan or Celtic Sea Salt and freshly ground black pepper, to taste

2 tbsp goat's feta (optional)

I recommend pre-soaking the almonds, seeds and buckwheat kernels (if using), overnight, as this will make them easier to digest and reduce the levels of phytic acid.

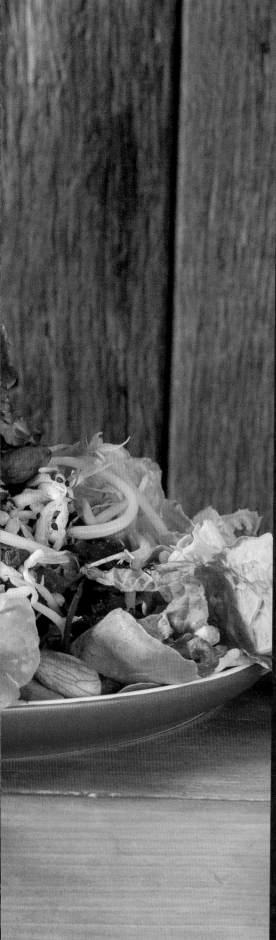

Sally's Super Food Salad

This is one of my 'go-to' salad recipes, because it's packed with an abundance of nutrients and fibre, making it far more satisfying and nutritious than simply eating a salad made on lettuce or rocket. I've used many standard pantry items I recommend you keep on hand, but feel free to add any ingredients you like, as long as they are in keeping with the LYG program.

Ingredients

1 zucchini, grated

1/2 cup fresh beetroot, peeled and grated

1 large handful of baby kale, or baby spinach leaves

1 handful of mixed salad greens

1 handful mung bean sprouts or alfalfa

4 tbsp buckwheat kernels, soaked overnight (optional)

1 handful raw almonds, soaked overnight

1 handful pepitas, soaked overnight

1 handful sunflower seeds, soaked overnight

1 tsp fresh turmeric, finely grated or 1/4 tsp ground tumeric

Dressing

Juice of 1/2 lemon

1/4 cup extra virgin olive oil

1 tsp rice malt syrup (optional)

Himalayan or Celtic Sea Salt and freshly ground black pepper, to taste

Method

Place all the salad ingredients in a mixing bowl and toss to combine.

For the dressing, place the ingredients to a glass jar and seal lid tightly. Shake vigorously until well combined.

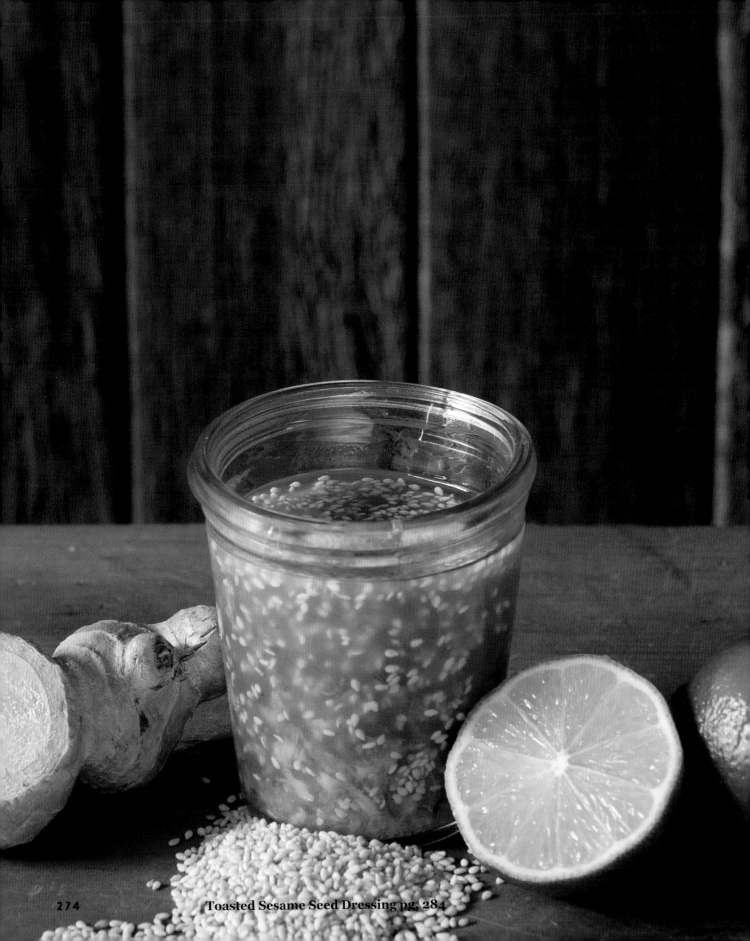

Toasted Sesame Seed Dressing pg. 284

Dressing & Sauces

Dressings and sauces are what often make a meal, but if you have been relying on processed bottled brands, then it's more than likely you have been getting your fair share of hidden sugars, artificial additives and vegetable oils - like canola and soy -which are often genetically modified. My advice is to make your own, this way you know exactly what ingredients you are putting into them. I hope these recipes will show you just how quick and easy it can be, not to mention they taste so much better than processed brands!

Homemade Tomato Sauce

If you love tomato sauce, but don't love all the artificial additives in processed brands, then this recipe is for you! It's a healthy alternative to the dreaded bottled brands which are loaded with sugar and artificial ingredients. After trying this recipe, I guarantee you will leave that bottled sauce in the supermarket aisle behind for good!

Ingredients

2 tbsp macadamia oil

3 large garlic cloves, crushed

8 large vine-ripened tomatoes (use Roma if you prefer)

1 tbsp Italian or mixed dried herbs (or to taste)

3/4 cup fresh basil, roughly chopped

1/4 cup rice malt syrup

1 tsp Himalayan or Celtic Sea Salt and freshly ground black pepper, to taste

Method

Heat the oil in a deep frying pan over medium-low heat. Add the garlic and cook, stirring for about 30 seconds.

Add the tomatoes salt and pepper and herbs and simmer for 10 - 15 minutes or until very soft and pulpy. Stir in the basil and rice malt syrup and cook for a further 5 minutes.

Set aside to cool, then transfer to a blender and blend to your preferred consistency (I like mine a bit chunky).

Keep in an airtight jar in the fridge for up to 5 days.

   GF DF LS P D VV

Basil Pesto

Pesto is a delicious addition to so many dishes, from roast veggies to chicken, poached eggs or salads. The only challenge is in choosing which herb to make it from ! I have included coriander (cilantro) as an alternative, but you could even try kale or Swiss chard. For a deliciously light and detox-friendly meal, stir some pesto through my raw zucchini noodles on page 241.

Method

Place all the ingredients in a food processor and blend until smooth and creamy – add more olive oil , lemon juice or salt to adjust flavour if desired.

Store in a jar or airtight container in the fridge for up to 1 week.

GF DF LS P D VV

Ingredients

1 bunch of fresh basil leaves or coriander / cilantro

2 - 4 garlic cloves, outter skin removed

2/3 cup extra virgin olive or macadamia oil,

Juice and rind of 1 lemon

1/2 cup raw pine nuts or you could use cashews or walnuts

Himalayan or Celtic Sea Salt and cracked pepper to taste

SALLY'S TIPS

If you are making coriander pesto, replace the lemon juice with the juice of 1-2 limes.

Pesto also freezes really well, just cover with a little extra olive oil.

279

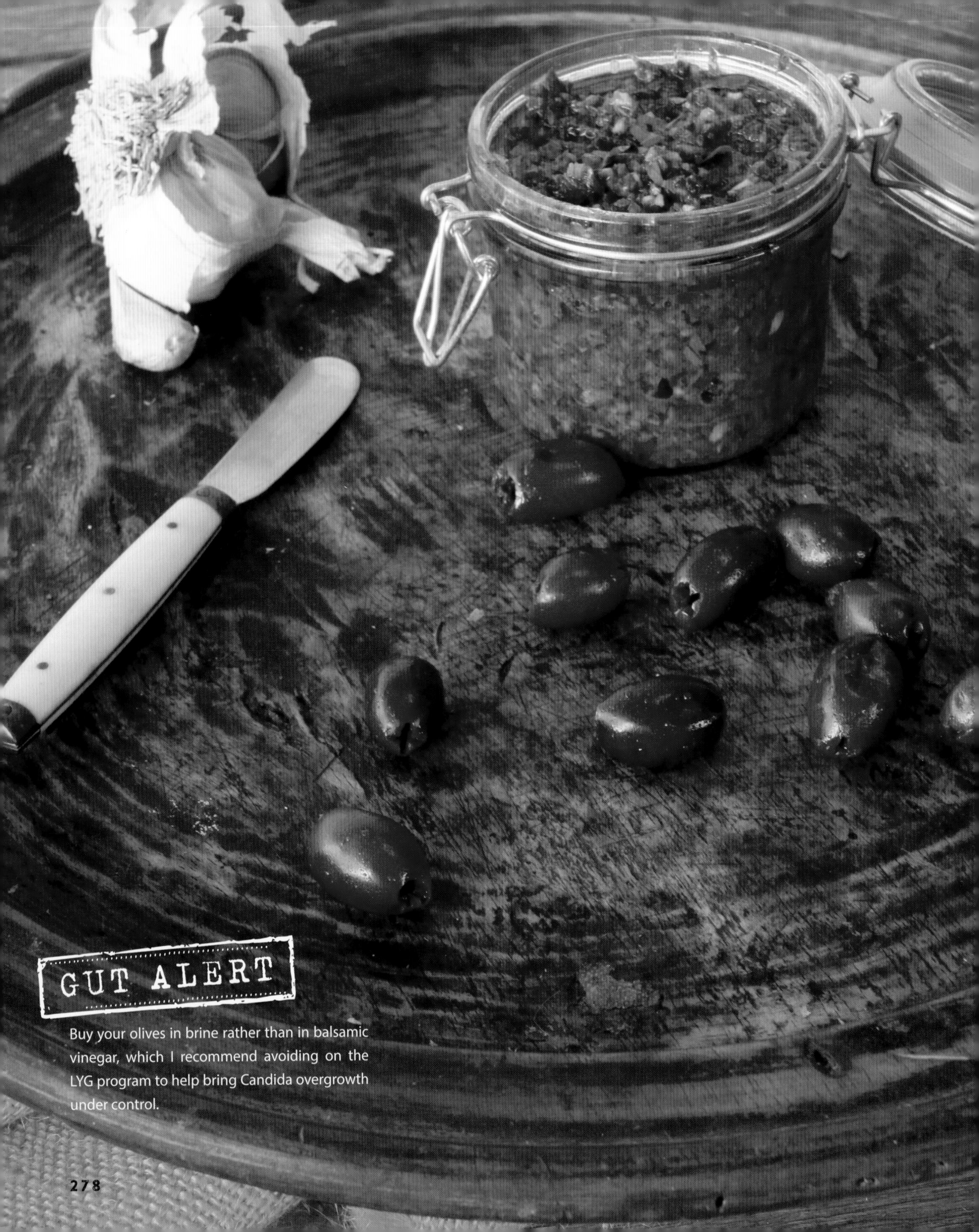

GUT ALERT

Buy your olives in brine rather than in balsamic vinegar, which I recommend avoiding on the LYG program to help bring Candida overgrowth under control.

Black Olive Tapenade

Olives are rich in monounsaturated healthy fats, making them great for heart health and regulating inflammation. Healthy fats are filling and make a delicious addition to any meal leaving you feeling more satiated and reducing those sugar cravings! I love to add olive tapenade to any savoury dish for a little extra flavour, or to serve as an hors d'oeuvre alongside goats feta.

SALLY'S TIPS
Use as a condiment with grilled haloumi or fish. Finely grate the rind from one lemon over the top for a little extra zing.

Method

Place all the ingredients into a food processor and use the pulse button to process to a chunky consistency.

Keep in an airtight container or sealed jar in the fridge for up to 5 days.

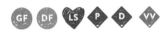

Ingredients

1 cup Kalamata olives, pitted

1/2 red onion, diced

1/2 cup extra virgin olive or macadamia oil

1/2 cup flat-leaf parsley, roughly chopped

Juice of 1/2 lemon

MAKES 1 CUP (SERVING SIZE 2 TBSP)

Green Goddess Sauce

I love to serve this sauce with just about any dish, but it goes particularly well with seafood.

Method

Place all the ingredients into a food processor and mix until smooth and creamy. Add a little filtered water if you would prefer a slightly runnier consistency.

Serve as a dressing over salads, seafood or chicken for added flavour . This sauce can be frozen for up to 2 months.

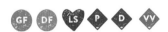

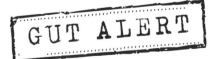

This recipe contains capsicum, which is a nightshade so you may want to avoid it if you are suffering acute symptoms of arthritis or heavy Candida overgrowth, until your gut has healed.

Ingredients

1 green capsicum (sweet pepper)

7cm piece fresh ginger, peeled and sliced

1 large green chilli, seeds removed

1 large bunch coriander (cilantro)

3 tbsp extra virgin olive or macadamia oil

1/2 cup rice malt syrup or xylitol

2-3 garlic cloves, peeled

Herb Tahini & Yoghurt Dressing

Ingredients

1 tbsp plain sheep's yoghurt

1/4 cup extra virgin olive oil

1 tbsp tahini

1/4 cup fresh mint or coriander leaves

1/4 cup flat-leaf parsley

1 tsp rice malt syrup

Juice of 1 lemon

Himalayan or Celtic Sea Salt and freshly ground black pepper, to taste

This is my favourite salad dressing. It's so easy to make and is super healthy, thanks to being loaded with healthy fats. Healthy fats help to reduce inflammation, nourish your skin and hair and balance your hormones. I add this dressing to any salad, or serve over cooked quinoa with roast veggies. For an even creamier texture, add half an avocado.

Method

Place all ingredients except the salt and pepper into a blender (or use a hand held stick blender) and blend until smooth and creamy. Add more olive oil if you prefer a runnier consistency. Season with salt and pepper to taste.

GF DF LS P D V

SALLY'S TIP
This sauce also makes a tasty dip with celery and cucumber sticks.

Anchovy Sauce

Ingredients

3 garlic cloves, peeled

200ml/7oz sheep's yoghurt

8 anchovy fillets in oil

2/3 cup extra virgin olive oil

Juice of 1 lemon

Being a small fish, anchovies are a healthier alternative to larger oily fish. They are far less exposed to contamination from heavy metals like mercury, which is commonly found in ocean-caught salmon, tuna and swordfish. Anchovies have a salty, pungent flavour which some people profess not to like, but I have converted many with this yummy sauce.

Method

Place all the ingredients into a food processor (or use a stick blender) and blend to a creamy consistency.

GF DF LS P D

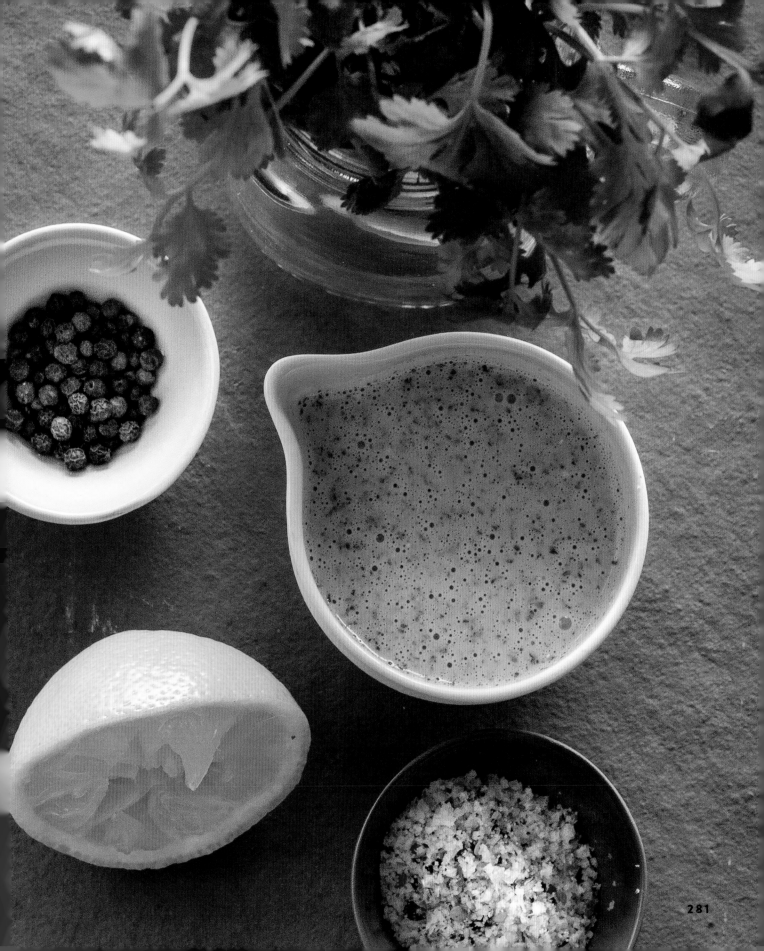

Sally's Simple Salad Dressing

Ingredients

1/4 cup extra virgin olive or macadamia oil

juice of 1/2 lemon

1 tsp wholegrain mustard

1 tsp brown rice malt syrup or 2- 3 drops of stevia

1 garlic clove, crushed (optional)

Himalayan or Celtic Sea Salt and
freshly ground black pepper, to taste

Method

Place the oil, juice, mustard, syrup and garlic into a glass screwtop jar. Seal tightly and shake vigorously to combine. Season to taste.

Store any leftover dressing in the fridge for up to 5 days.

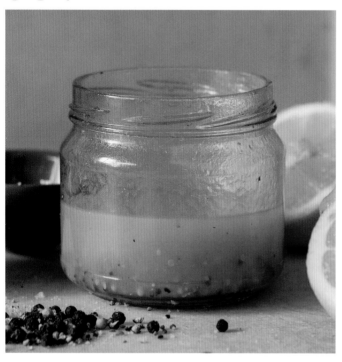

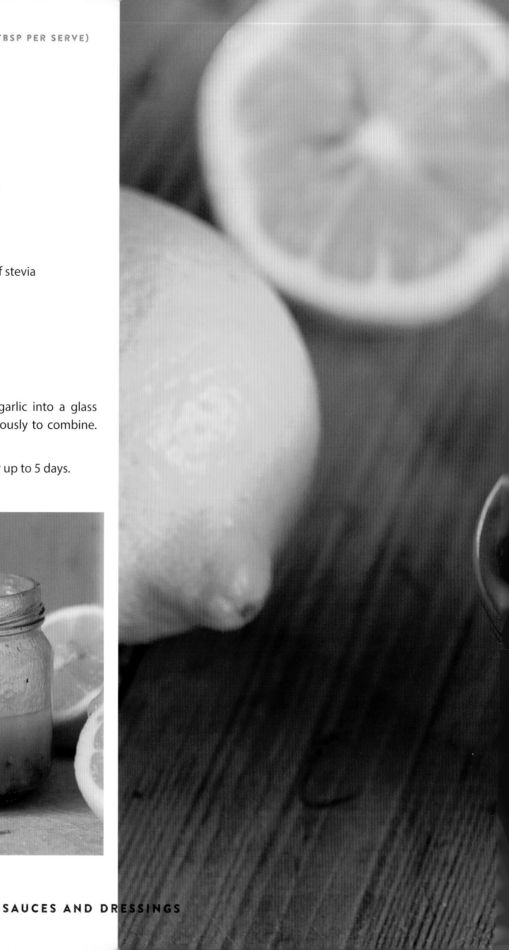

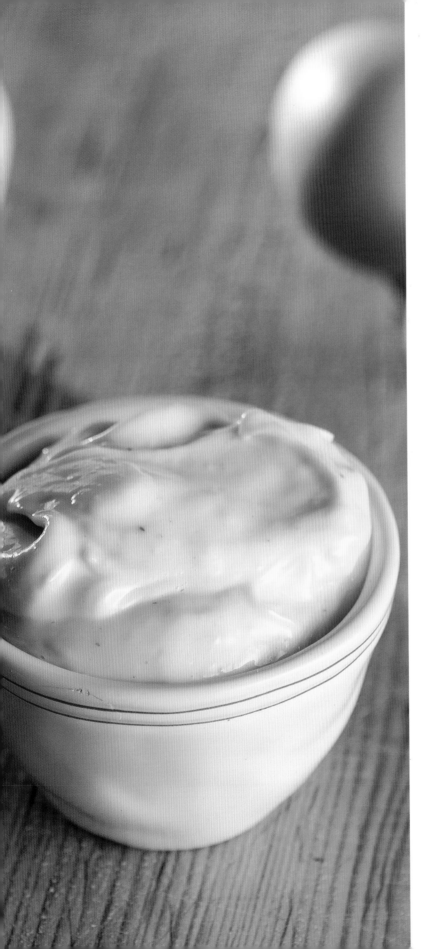

Homemade Mayonnaise

Store-bought mayonnaise is typically loaded with sugar and artificial additives, as well as being made with processed vegetable oils like soy and canola – a BIG no no and often GMO! So making your own mayonnaise guarantees you know exactly what you're eating. To make aioli, simply add some crushed garlic and serve with salads or grilled fish.

Ingredients

2 egg yolks

1 tsp mustard

3/4 cup extra virgin olive oil

Juice of 1 large lemon, or to taste

Pinch each Himalayan or Celtic Sea Salt and white pepper

Method

Combine the egg yolks and mustard in a food processor. With the motor running, add the oil slowly in a thin stream. The mixture will become thick and creamy. Add the lemon juice and process briefly to combine. Season to taste.

Store in an airtight container in the fridge for up to 3 days.

MAKES ABOUT 1 CUP (SERVING SIZE 2 TBLSP)

Toasted Sesame Seed Dressing

The combination of ingredients in this recipe combine to create a deliciously zesty, Asian style flavour – perfect over fish, seafood or salads, but totally free of any artificial additives or hidden sources of gluten, commonly found in many bottled Asian style dressings or sauces.

Ingredients

Finely grated rind of 1 lime

Juice of 2 limes

2 tsp finely grated ginger

1 tsp brown rice malt syrup or xylitol

1 tbsp mirin

3 tsp sesame oil

1/2 cup extra virgin olive oil

2 tbsp sesame seeds, toasted

Himalayan or Celtic Sea Salt, to taste

Method

Place the lime rind, juice, ginger, rice malt syrup, mirin and sesame oil in a bowl. Gradually add the olive oil, whisking constantly until combined. Stir in the sesame seeds and season to taste

Dukkah

Dukkah is a fragrant seasoning made from nuts and spices. You can use it to add delicious natural flavour to anything that takes your fancy - from salads to fish, chicken or lamb!

Method

Place the coriander, fennel and cumin seeds into a heavy based fry pan (with no oil) and stir over medium heat for about 2 minutes, until fragrant.

Use a mortar and pestle to grind the seeds along with the peppercorns until pulverized (you can also use a coffee grinder or small food processor).

Toast the nuts in the frying pan for about 8 minutes on low - medium heat (watch they don't burn). Transfer to a plate and allow to cool. Use a mortar and pestle to grind until finely chopped, but still a little chunky.

In the same frying pan, toast the sesame seeds for about 2 minutes, until lightly golden. Transfer to a plate to cool.

Combine the sesame seeds, nuts, spices and salt. Taste and adjust seasoning if necessary. Store in an airtight glass container in a dark pantry for up to one month.

Ingredients

1 tsp coriander seeds

1 tsp fennel seeds

1 tsp cumin seeds

1 tbsp black peppercorns

1 cup hazelnuts

1/2 cup almonds

1/2 cup macadamia nuts

2 tbsp white sesame seeds

1 tsp Himalayan or Celtic Sea salt

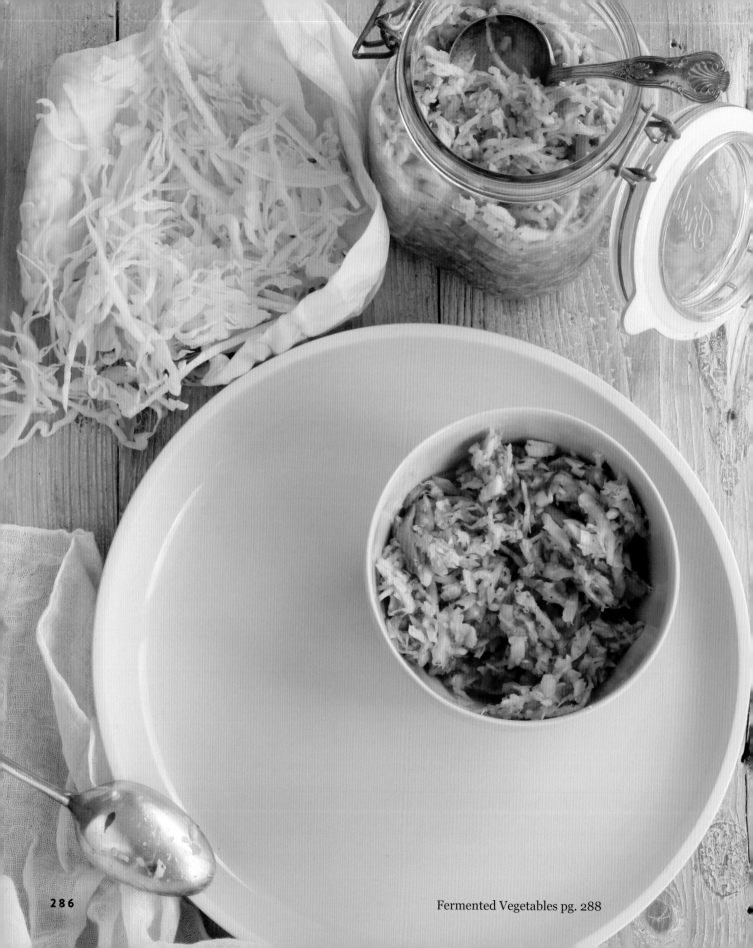

Fermented Vegetables pg. 288

Fermented Foods

I've explained that there are 'good' and 'bad' sources of yeast and bacteria. The good news is that by making your own cultured and fermented foods from recipes like these, you'll not only be saving money, but you'll be feeding your colonies of good gut flora, which will help to keep the growth of Candida at bay. These recipes all contain a healthy source of good bacteria and yeast and have been part of a healthy diet in many traditional cultures for thousands of years. Many people ask me why I don't promote kombucha tea on my LYG program, and the reason is because Kombucha contains wild strains of yeast, which can compromise your ability to over come Candida overgrowth. This is also why I recommend making fermented foods using either a starter culture, or quality probiotic - to protect against the growth of harmful wild yeast and bacteria .

I recommend including a serve of fermented foods from these recipes in your diet each day - just enough to keep your gut happy.

Fermented Vegetables

Ingredients

6 cups of cabbage, a few leaves reserved

4 carrots, peeled and grated

1 tbsp ginger, peeled thinly and sliced

2 green apples, peeled and grated (optional)

1 cup freshly made celery juice (make in your juicer)

2 tsp Himalayan or Celtic Sea Salt

1/4 teaspoon probiotic capsule or vegetable starter culture for every 3 cups of vegetables

1/4 cup of black sesame seeds or caraway seeds (optional)

1-1.5 litre/34 fl oz glass jar

I'll admit: making your own fermented vegetables does require some time and it's a bit of a learning curve, but it's worth the effort considering the health benefits to your gut, not to mention the money you will save in buying them. I promise you will get quicker at making them with practice, so don't give up after your first attempt!

Method

Remove the outer leaf of the cabbage, wash and set aside. Shred remaining cabbage very finely, using a mandolin if possible, or a very sharp large knife.

Measure all the vegetables (including the carrot, ginger, and apples) in cups so you know how much culture to use. Sterilise a large stainless steel or glass bowl in boiling water and dry before adding all the ingredients sprinkle with salt. Dissolve the probiotic culture in a sterilized glass with a little filtered water, add to the vegetables and combine well by massaging the ingredients with your hands. Transfer the mixture, one handful at a time to a large sterilised glass jar and press the mixture down firmly with a wooden spoon to tightly pack and remove any air pockets allow a 2cm gap at the top. Place a cabbage leaf on top of the mixture, tucking it down the sides to keep the vegetables beneath the brine.

Place the lid on the jar, being careful not to screw it on too tightly, or the jar may crack or explode. Store the jar in a relatively warm place (ideally about 23°C/73°F) but away from direct sunlight for several days. During the summer it will take 3-4 days to fully ferment. In winter it will take up to 7-10 days. You may need to wrap the jar in a towel to keep warm enough for fermentation to occur.

Once the veggies have fermented for long enough, store them in the fridge to prevent ongoing fermentation. The fermented veggies will keep for 2-6 months. Over time the vegetables will lose their crispiness.

Remember to be patient with your first attempt as this may not work out as well as when you have had some practice – it took me a couple of goes! Serve as an accompaniment with any meal.

Pickled Vegetables

Pickling was originally done to preserve food, before refrigerators were invented. I love to add pickled vegetables as a condiment to my meals. Not only does it add a delicious flavour, but they also encourage the growth of beneficial bacteria. I don't recommend buying commercially pickled vegetables as these are pasteurized to prevent ongoing fermentation, negating any nutritional benefit.

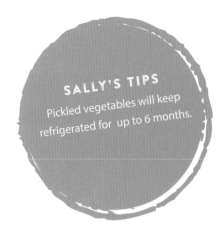

SALLY'S TIPS
Pickled vegetables will keep refrigerated for up to 6 months.

Method

Wash and slice your vegetables finely, or if using cauliflower, cut into small bite size chunks.

Add to a sterile glass jar, along with the spices of your choice.

Bring the vinegar, water and salt to boil in a saucepan then pour over the vegetables.

Replace the lid on the jars and place in the refrigerator for between ten to 20 days.

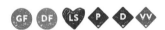

Ingredients

Any vegetable of your choice – I like to use either cucumber, red cabbage, ginger cauliflower, radish or carrots.

1/4 to 1/2 tsp dried spices such as: whole peppercorns, cumin, caraway, coriander or mustard seeds

1 cup of apple cider vinegar

1 cup filtered water

1 tbsp. Himalayan or Celtic Sea Salt

1 tsp. rice malt syrup (optional)

FERMENTED VEGETABLES

I believe the key to successfully fermenting your own veggies is to use a starter culture instead of using salt. This will give you a more consistent result and cut down on the fermentation time, and provide your gut with a broader range of beneficial bacterial strains. Be aware that starter cultures can vary in quality. You could use the whey from sheep's yoghurt as an alternative to using a probiotic capsule. Be sure to use really fresh, organic vegetables. Cabbage should form the bulk of your mixture and feel free to use green or purple, or even add some grated beetroot.

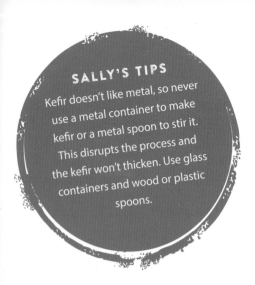

SERVES 1 (SERVING SIZE 100-200ML)

Coconut Milk Kefir

Kefir is essentially drinking yoghurt and makes a fantastic addition to my grain free granola recipe, or as a gut-loving snack! If you're like me and can't tolerate cow's dairy, then kefir made from coconut milk is your next best alternative. It may not be as potent in beneficial bacteria as found in kefir made from raw cow's milk, but it's better than an unhappy gut. Kefir grains can be purchased from your local health food store or online.

Ingredients

1 tablespoon kefir grains or kefir starter

1-2 cups unsweetened coconut milk or you can make it fresh (see recipe on page 138)

Glass jar

Muslin or cheese cloth

Rubber band

Method

Combine the kefir grains or kefir starter (as directed on packet) with the coconut milk in a glass jar. Cover with a cloth secured with a rubber band and let it sit on the kitchen bench (a warm environment is best for fermenting) for 12-24 hours. Give your kefir a few shakes or stirs, after about 12 hours.

Once the coconut milk becomes thick and has a slightly sour flavour, it has turned into kefir. Strain the mixture through a fine plastic strainer to remove the grains (you can re-use the grains later by storing them in a glass jar in the refrigerator). Store the kefir in the fridge and enjoy for breakfast or a gut-loving snack. If your kefir doesn't thicken within 24 hours, it might be that the temperature in your house isn't warm enough

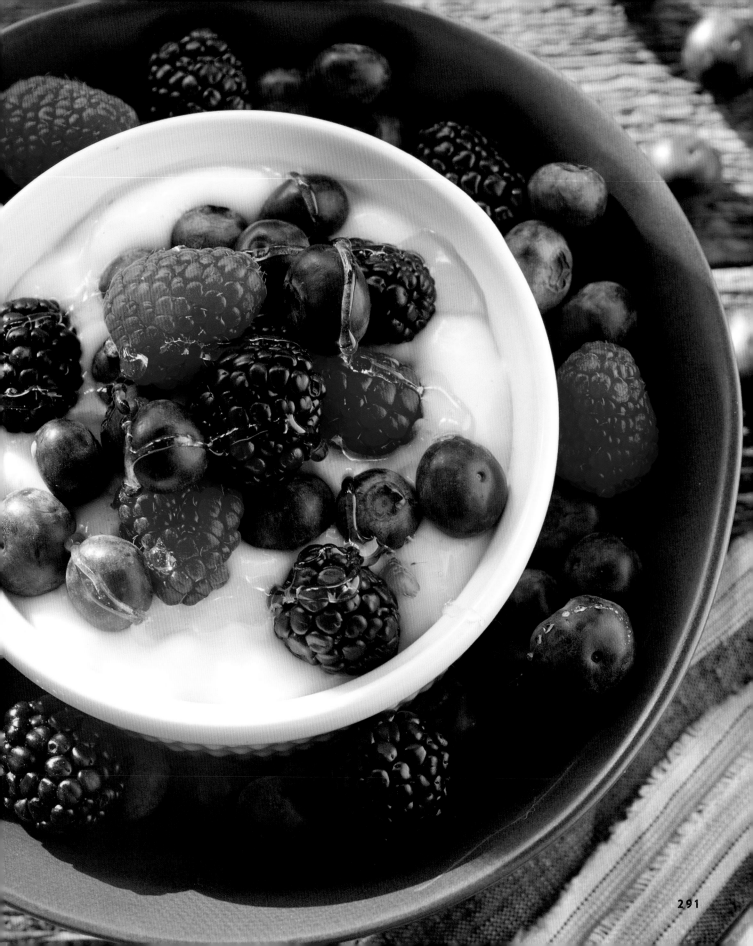

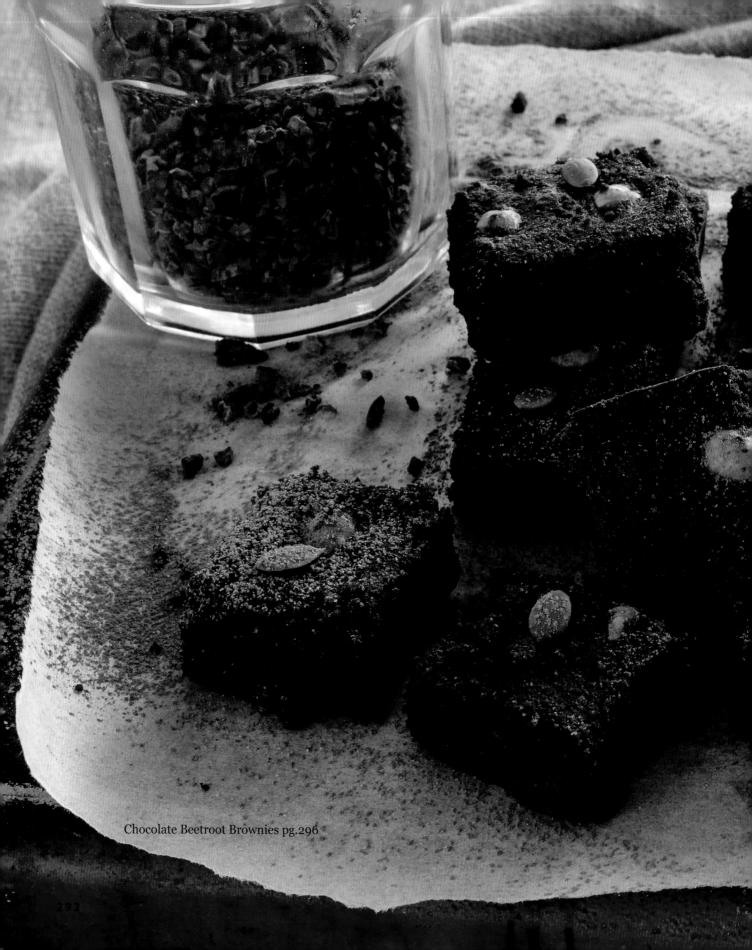

Chocolate Beetroot Brownies pg.296

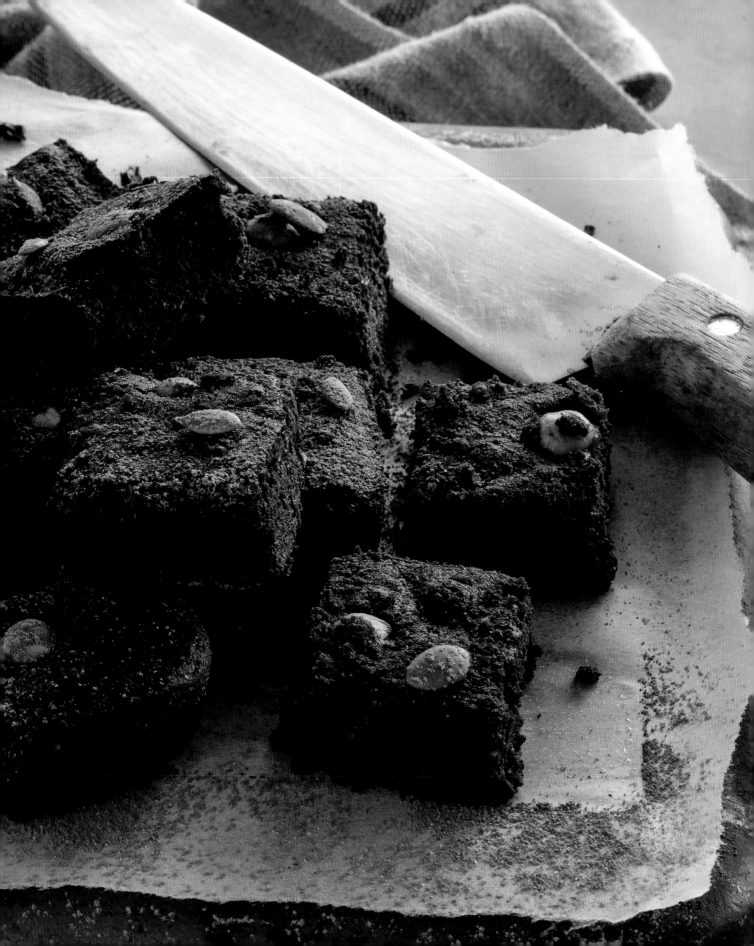

Nothing Naughty Treats

There's no doubt we all love a little sweet treat, but one of the main aims of the LYG Program is to wean you off the sweet stuff because sugar is extremely problematic, not just for maintaining a healthy weight, but also your overall health - especially your immune, brain and gut function! The most challenging part of getting off sugar is finding ways to overcome those all-consuming cravings. Remember sugar is highly addictive, so go easy on yourself as you wean off it and check in with my tips for kicking those cravings, on page 75. But life without a little sweetness would be a tad dull, so the key to healthy sugar consumption lies in the amount and type of sugar you consume. I do not recommend consuming too many of the Nothing Naughty Treats in the initial stages of the program, even though they contain fructose free sweeteners, because the idea is to shift your taste buds towards consuming more veges, healthy fats and clean proteins, in an effort to rebalance your appetite hormones. So if you are going to indulge in any of my Nothing Naughty Treats, keep them as just that – treats! They are not designed for daily snacks, with the exception of the Bellisimo Balls, as these are so low in sugar.

Nothing Naughty Rocky Road

Ingredients

1/3 cup cacao butter

1/3 cup virgin coconut oil

1/4 cup raw cacao powder

2 tbsp brown rice malt syrup

1 tsp vanilla powder or essence

1 tsp ground cinnamon or nutmeg

1 tsp maca powder (optional)

2 cups raw mixed nuts

1 cup shredded coconut or coconut flakes

1/2 cup pepitas

1/4 cup chia seeds

1/2 cup frozen raspberries

This is a great low-sugar indulgence when you're struggling with sugar cravings, because it is naturally rich in magnesium, plant proteins and good fats to help regulate your blood sugar and insulin levels. It's super quick to make and you should have most of the ingredients handy in your pantry.

Method

Lightly grease a bread loaf or slice tin and line with baking / parchment paper. Place the cacao butter and coconut oil in a small saucepan and melt over low heat. Whisk in the cacao powder, rice malt syrup, vanilla, cinnamon and maca powder (if using) until well combined.

Scatter the mixed nuts, coconut, seeds and raspberries over the base of the prepared tin. Pour the cacao mixture over to coat evenly.

Place in the refrigerator (or freezer if you are in a hurry) until set. Lift from the tin and cut into small fingers, about 5cm x 3cm each.

Enjoy with a cup of fresh herbal or chai tea (see recipe page 315)

GF DF LS P D VV

SALLY'S TIPS

Replace the raspberries with dried goji berries if preferred- Store in an airtight container in the fridge.

If you don't have cacao butter, substitute it and the cacao powder with 2 x 100g (3oz) blocks of 85% dark chocolate.

Chocolate Beetroot Brownies

Let's face it, everyone loves a brownie, but most are packed with sugar and gluten. I have developed a recipe that is not only free of all the inflammatory gut-bloating nasties, but also contains superfoods such as raw cacao, coconut oil, pepitas and the goodness of beetroot. So there really is nothing naughty in this treat! Enjoy for an afternoon treat here and there, with a cup of fresh herbal tea.

Ingredients

1/2 cup almond meal

3/4 cup finely grated raw beetroot

1/2 cup virgin coconut or macadamia oil

2 eggs, lightly beaten

1/2 - 3/4 cup rice malt syrup

1 teaspoon liquid stevia or 1/2 cup xylitol

1/2 cup roughly chopped hazelnuts or walnuts (optional)

1/2 cup raw cacao powder

1 tbsp pepitas

1 tsp natural vanilla extract

1/2 tsp ground cinnamon

1/4 tsp gluten-free baking powder

Method

Preheat the oven to 180°C /350°F. Lightly grease a small (28 x 18 cm) slice tin and line with grease proof/parchment paper.

Place all the ingredients into a large mixing bowl and use a spatula or wooden spoon to combine.

Pour into the prepared tin.

Bake for 25 - 30 minutes, or until firm when tested with a gentle touch to the centre. Allow to cool before slicing with a sharp knife into 4cm x 4cm portions.

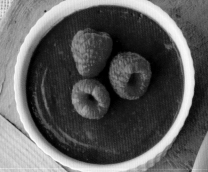

Raw Chocolate Mousse

When I occasionally make dessert I usually go for anything made with dark chocolate, not only because it tastes so good, but because the natural antioxidant compounds it contains have been found to improve heart health, lower blood pressure and reduce LDL ("bad") cholesterol. Be aware that this only applies to chocolate with a high cacao content, not the processed variety with added milk and sugar! I've added avocado to this recipe, not only because it is also one of my favourite foods, but because it adds a creamy texture and healthy fats, but feel free to leave it out if you prefer. The healthy fats in avocado and coconut milk / cream will leave you feeling satisfied and help to reduce sugar cravings.

Method

Place all the ingredients into a food processor (or use electric beaters) and process or beat until thick and creamy. Alternatively you can use a hand whisk.

Spoon into individual ramekins or glasses and place in the fridge for 2-3 hours, until set. Serve topped with berries and toasted coconut or cashews.

Ingredients

1 can of organic coconut cream chilled in the fridge overnight

1/4 cup raw cacao powder, unsweetened

1 tsp vanilla extract

1/4 cup brown rice malt syrup or 5-10 drops of stevia

1/2 tsp ground cinnamon, or to taste

Pinch of Himalayan or Celtic Sea Salt

Fresh berries, toasted coconut flakes (unsweetened) or chopped cashews, to serve (optional)

GF   DF   LS   P   D   LF   VV

Ingredients

6 apples, peeled, cored and cut into thick slices.

2 cinnamon quills

Finely grated rind of 1 lemon

1 cup raspberries (frozen if not in season)

Pinch ground cinnamon (optional)

2 cups mixed raw nuts - eg: almonds (I prefer slivered), hazel nuts, or brazil, macadamias walnuts or pecans

1 tsp ground cinnamon, plus extra to serve (optional)

1 tsp ground nutmeg

1 tsp ground ginger

1/2 - 3/4 cup shredded coconut

1/2 cup virgin coconut oil - add more if mix is too dry

2 tbsp rice malt syrup

1/4 teaspoon vanilla bean paste or 1 tsp natural vanilla extract

Cashew Cream

1 cup organic raw cashews

1-2 tbsp brown rice malt syrup or xylitol (optional)

1 tsp natural vanilla extract or powder

Pinch Himalayan or Celtic Sea Salt

1/4-1/2 cup filtered water, depending on desired consistency

Apple "Grumble" With Cashew Nut Cream

This is one of my signature recipes that I created many years ago for a friend who has severe coeliac disease and was eating all the wrong foods! Apple crumble also happens to be my favourite dessert, but after developing Lupus and Hashimoto's I realised I had to be super strict in avoiding grains and gluten, including oats. But that didn't mean giving up my favourite treats in life, including this dessert – because there's no tummy 'grumble' with this crumble! You'll find this recipe is a real crowd pleaser and kids can't get enough of it, so serve it up when you have a crew for dinner, but want to stick to the LYG Program.

Method

Preheat the oven to 180°C /350°F and lightly grease a baking dish with a little coconut oil.

Place the apple, cinnamon quills and lemon rind into a large saucepan and add 1/2 - 3/4 cup water.

Cover and simmer over medium-low heat for about 5 minutes, until the apple is soft and opaque, but not mushy. Drain excess water.

Transfer the apple to the prepared dish (discard cinnamon quills). Arrange the raspberries over the apple and sprinkle with a little ground cinnamon if desired. Set aside.

To make the topping, combine the nuts and spices in a food processor and process to a crumble-like consistency. Transfer the mixture to a large bowl and add the shredded coconut, coconut oil, rice malt syrup and vanilla bean paste or extract. Use your hands to mix until evenly combined.

Sprinkle the crumble mixture evenly over the apple. Bake for about 20 minutes, or until topping is golden brown.

Serve crumble warm, topped with a spoonful of Cashew Nut Cream or plain sheep or coconut yoghurt and a light dusting of extra cinnamon.

To make the Cashew Cream, place all the ingredients except the water into a food processor. Process on high until smooth and creamy, adding water gradually until you reach the desired consistency. Transfer to a serving jug or glass jar.

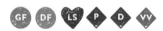

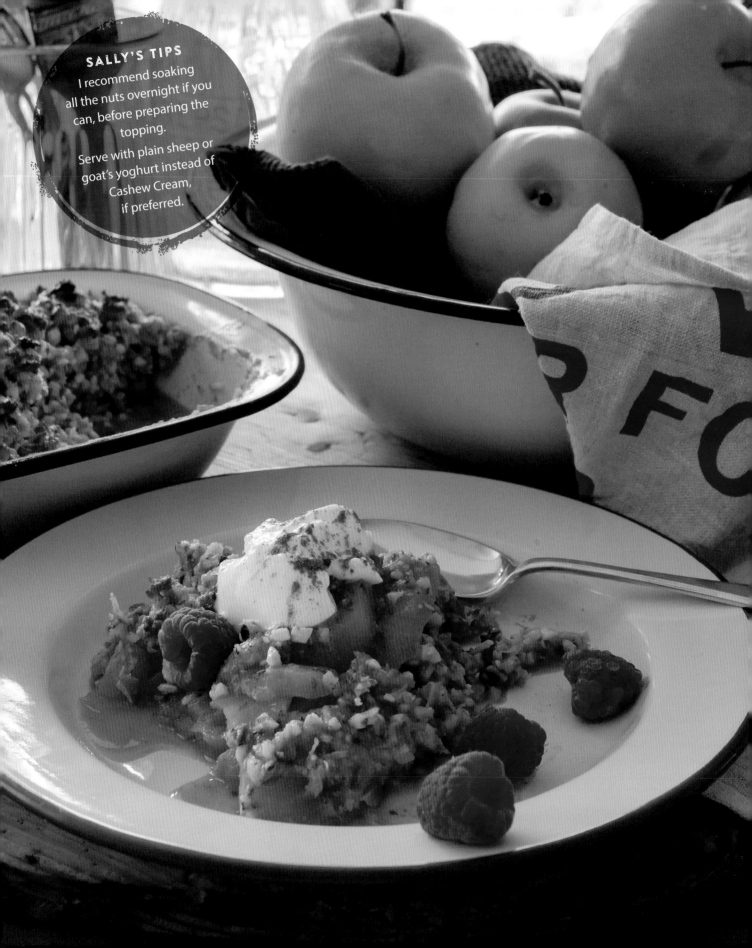

SALLY'S TIPS

I recommend soaking all the nuts overnight if you can, before preparing the topping.

Serve with plain sheep or goat's yoghurt instead of Cashew Cream, if preferred.

Coconut Berry Muffins

Everyone loves a muffin but often they are loaded with sugar and processed fats. I developed this recipe when I was at university, in an attempt to re-create the muffin experience without the adverse impact on my health. Admittedly it took a few goes, but eventually I got there! If you want to make them nut-free for the kids, replace the almond meal with coconut flour. Use any type of berry you prefer, but I recommend avoiding adding high-fructose fruits like bananas or apple. I've included a few macadamias and chunks of 85% dark chocolate which makes these muffins truly decadent, yet still low in sugar.

Ingredients

2/3 cup desiccated coconut

1/2 cup almond meal

2/3 cup coconut flour

2 tsp gluten-free baking powder

1 /2 tsp ground cinnamon

3/4 cup coconut milk or cream

1/2 cup rice malt syrup

3 eggs, beaten

2 tsp natural vanilla extract, vanilla bean powder or paste

1/4 cup virgin coconut oil or macadamia oil

1/2 cup frozen raspberries or blueberries (or a combination of both)

60g 85% dark chocolate, cut into small chunks

3/4 cup macadamias or walnuts, roughly chopped (optional)

Method

Preheat the oven to 160°C/320°F. Lightly grease a 12-pan small (cup capacity) muffin tray, or line with paper cases.

Place all dry ingredients into a mixing bowl and whisk with a fork to combine.

Combine the coconut milk, rice malt syrup, eggs and vanilla in a food processor and process for about 4 minutes, until light and creamy. With the motor running, add the oil gradually. Add the dry mixture and process until combined.

Transfer to a mixing bowl and fold in the raspberries, chocolate and macadamias. Spoon into the prepared pans.

Bake for 35 minutes or until a skewer inserted into the centre of a muffin comes out clean. Cool in the pan before lifting out. Enjoy for afternoon tea with a pot of fresh herbal tea.

Store in an airtight container in the fridge for up to 4 days.

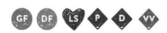

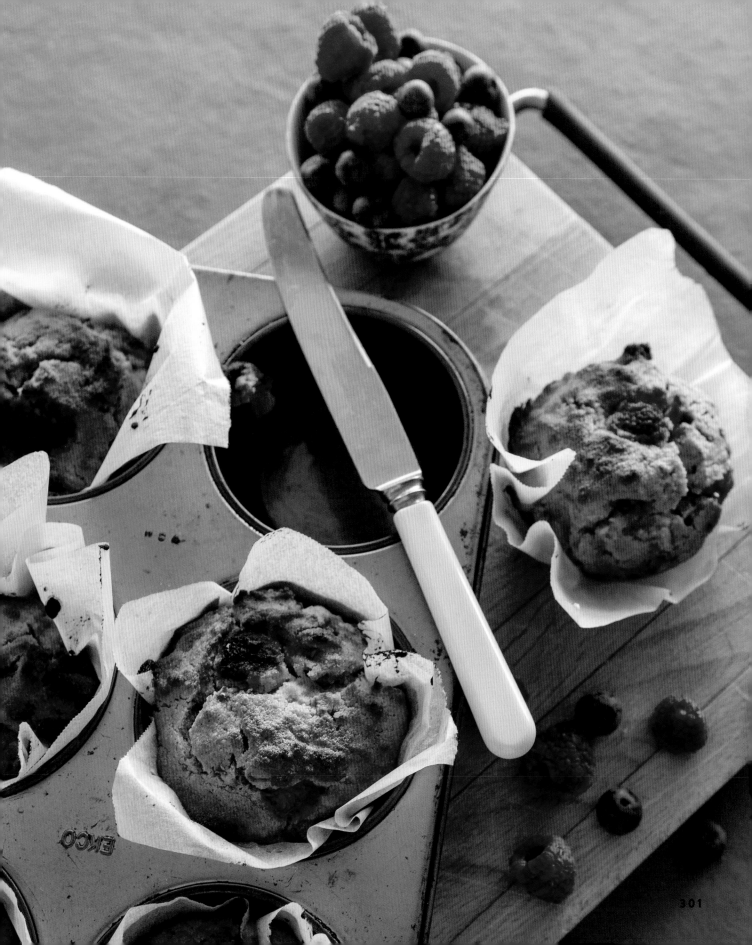

Choc Coconut Clusters

Ingredients

3/4 cup virgin coconut oil

1/4 cup rice malt syrup

1/2 cup almond butter

1 tsp natural vanilla essence or powder

1 tsp ground cinnamon or nutmeg

2 cups shredded coconut

1/4 cup pepitas

1 tbsp chia seeds

1/4 cup raw cacao powder

1/4 cup walnuts, crushed

1/4 cup flaked or slivered almonds

If you grew up in Australia, this recipe might bring back memories of eating coconut rough chocolates as a kid, only this is the healthy version! Thanks to the goodness of virgin coconut oil, nuts and fructose-free rice malt syrup, you can afford to indulge without the guilt trip. Remember though that treats are treats, so stick to one or two per serving. Enjoy with a cup of fresh herbal tea (my personal favourite is fresh ginger and lemongrass) served hot, or iced on a hot summers day.

Method

Line a baking tray with greaseproof/ parchment paper. Place the coconut oil into a large saucepan and melt over low heat. Add the rice malt syrup and almond butter, and stir gently to combine. Add remaining ingredients and stir through. You may need to add a little extra shredded coconut if your mixture is too runny, so it will bind together. Place mix in refrigerator for about 15-20 minutes to set otherwise the mix will flatten out like a pancake.

Drop tablespoons of the mixture onto the prepared tray, to form small clumps. Place into the fridge (or freezer if you are in a hurry) to set. Keep refrigerated in an airtight container for up to 2 weeks.

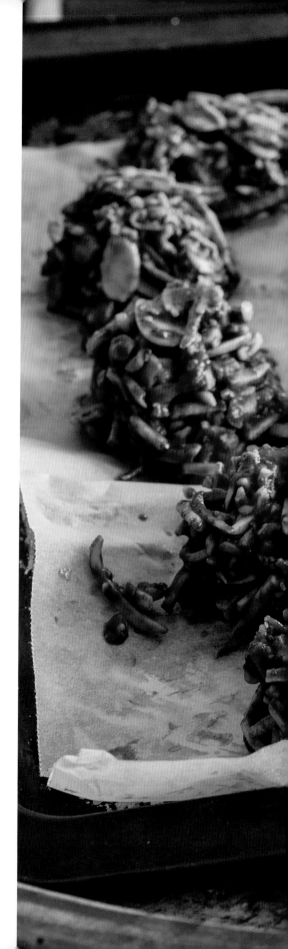

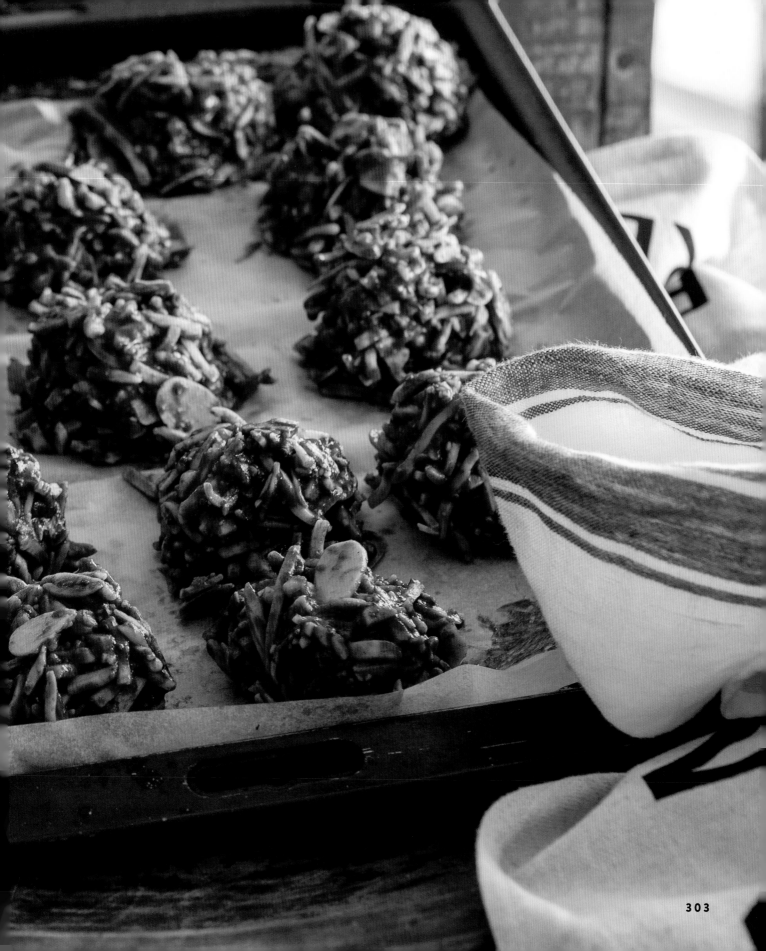

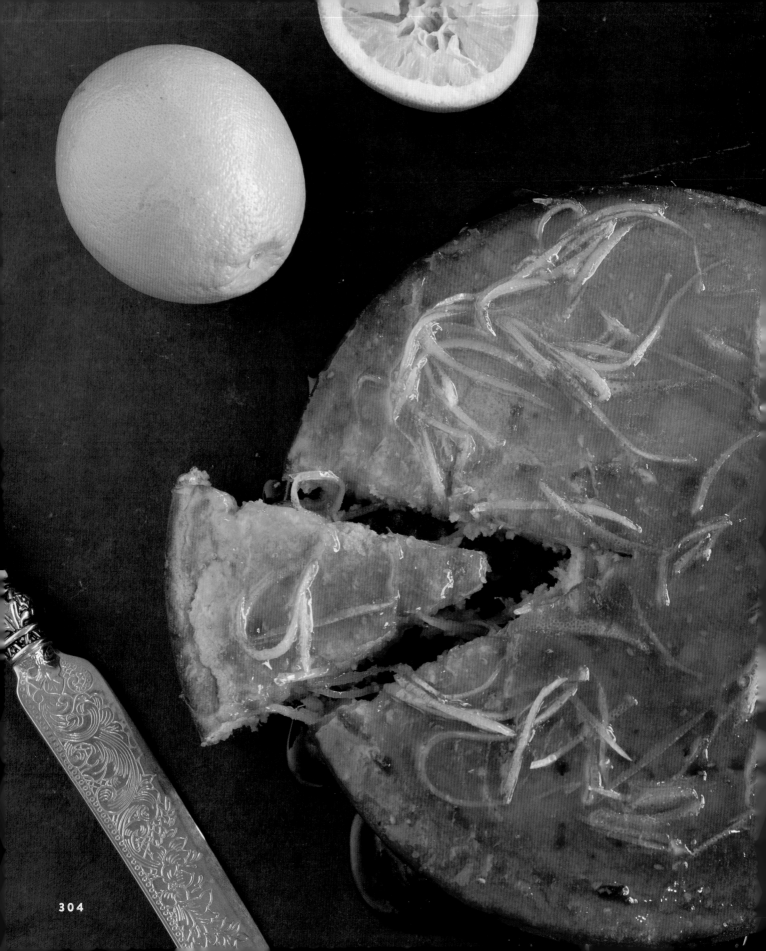

Flourless Orange & Chia Seed Cake

When you're looking for a recipe for a deliciously decadent cake, this 'Nothing Naughty Treat' does the trick! Although, like all my 'Nothing Naughty Treats', this recipe is only to be enjoyed occasionally. Despite containing 'healthier' sweeteners like xylitol, it's important to remember the aim of my program is to rebalance your appetite hormones and switch off your cravings for sweet foods. If you introduce this recipe too early in the program, you risk feeding those sweet cravings.

Method

Preheat the oven to 180°C/350°F. Grease a 20 cm springform cake tin and line with baking/parchment paper.

Trim the top and bottom from each orange, and score a 3cm deep cross in each end.

Place the whole oranges in a saucepan and cover with cold water. Bring to a boil and cook for 15 minutes.

Drain the oranges and cover with fresh cold water (this helps to reduce any bitterness). Bring to boil and cook, partially covered, for 45 minutes. Drain and refresh under cold water.

Cut the oranges into quarters and place into a food processor. Process until smooth. Add the eggs and xylitol and process until the mixture is thick and pale.

Add the almond meal, baking powder, and chia seeds, and process to combine. Pour into the prepared tin and bake for 1 hour until set when tested with a gentle touch in the centre.

Set aside in the tin for 15 minutes

To make the Orange Syrup, combine the orange rind and juice in a saucepan with the xylitol. Stir over low heat to dissolve the xylitol, then bring to a simmer and cook until the syrup thickens.

Take the cake from the tin and put onto a serving plate. Use a skewer to prick a few holes in the top of the cake, and drizzle the syrup over

SALLY'S TIPS

This is best served warm with a dollop of plain sheep or coconut yoghurt.

If you think you will be too tempted to overindulge in this delicious treat, then I suggest freezing in portions.

Ingredients

2 oranges

3 eggs

1 cup xylitol

3 cups almond meal

1 tsp gluten-free baking powder

2 tbsp chia seeds

Shredded rind and juice of 3 oranges

3/4 cup xylitol

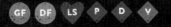

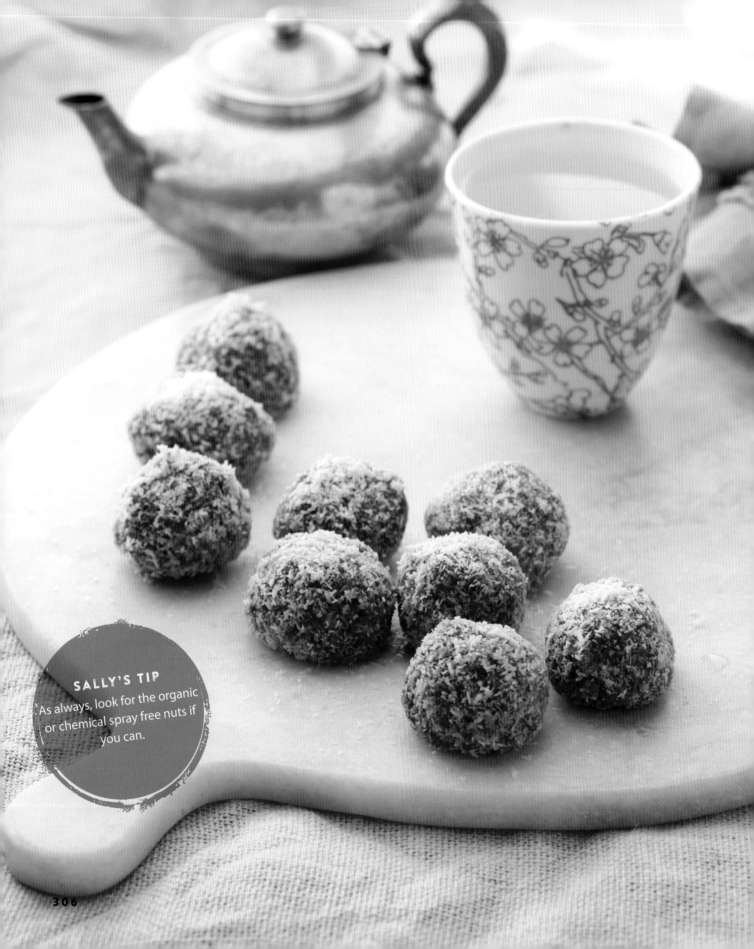

Bellissimo Balls

If you're looking for a fructose-free, high-protein snack, packed with good fats to leave you feeling totally satisfied when those hunger pangs or sugar cravings hit, then look no further than these delicious morsels, perfect in a lunch box, or as an afternoon pick-me-up. The exact measurements are fairly loose, so feel free to add or subtract, but just ensure they are moist enough to roll into little balls.

Ingredients

1/2 cup cashews

1/2 cup almonds

1/2 cup macadamias or walnuts

1/2 cup pepitas

1/2 cup sunflower seeds

1/2 cup chia seeds

1/2 cup goji berries (optional)

1/2 cup brown rice malt syrup

2 tbsp tahini

2 heaped tbsp raw cacao powder

3/4 cup virgin coconut oil, melted, plus extra if needed

1/2 cup desiccated coconut, add extra if needed

1 extra cup desiccated coconut, chia or sesame seeds to roll the balls in

Method

Place the nuts, seeds and goji berries (if using) into a food processor and process until finely chopped.

Add the rice malt syrup, tahini, cacao powder, coconut oil and desiccated coconut and process until well combined.

Pinch a little mixture between your fingers. If it seems too dry or crumbly to form into balls, add a little melted coconut oil until it is moist enough to stick together. If your mix is too wet, add desiccated coconut a little at a time, and process to combine.

Scoop a tablespoon of mixture and roll into balls about the size of a 20 cent coin. Spread desiccated coconut, chia seeds or sesame seeds onto a plate and roll the balls until well coated.

Serve with a cup of your favourite herbal or chai tea.

Store in an airtight container in the fridge for up to 2 weeks, if they last that long!

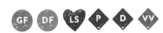

DATE-LESS (NOT DESPERATE!)

This has become another of my super-popular recipes. Because they don't contain high-fructose Medjool dates like similar balls do, they are much lower in sugar and won't go to your hips if you indulge in one too many. They are also high in anti-oxidants and magnesium.

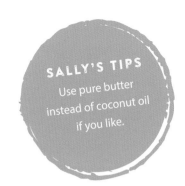

SALLY'S TIPS

Use pure butter instead of coconut oil if you like.

SERVES 8-10 (SERVING SIZE 1 SLICE)

Flourless Chocolate Cake

This decadent and delicious flourless chocolate cake is a real treat. Sit down and enjoy with a nice cup of herbal tea whenever you feel like you need spoiling, or want to spoil someone you love.

Method

Preheat the oven to 180°C Grease a 20cm cake tin and line with baking paper.

Place coconut oil and chocolate in a saucepan and heat gently until melted. Remove from the heat and allow to cool to room temperature.

Separate the eggs, taking care not to get any yolk in the whites as this will prevent the whites from whipping properly. Beat the yolks with half the xylitol until thick and creamy. Add the vanilla, almond meal and cooled chocolate mixture. Fold together until evenly combined.

Using clean beaters, beat the egg whites with the remaining xylitol until soft peaks form. Fold 1/3 of the egg white into the chocolate mixture to loosen it. Fold in the remaining egg white until just combined, so that you do not lose the volume. Spoon into the prepared tin.

Bake for 40 minutes, until set when tested with a gentle touch in the centre. Remove from the oven and allow to cool in the tin, covered with a clean tea towel. Serve with a dollop of plain sheep or coconut yoghurt and fresh raspberries.

Store leftovers in the fridge in an airtight container for up to 5 days, or freeze for up to 3 months.

Try this cake towards the end of the program.

Ingredients

100g virgin coconut oil

150g 85% dark chocolate, chopped

4 eggs, at room temperature

170g xylitol (or same weight of stevia powder)

1/2 tsp natural vanilla essence or vanilla bean powder

200g almond meal

Coconut Ice Cream

Method

Empty the contents of the room-temperature can of coconut milk into a large, heavy-bottom saucepan. Add the vanilla and sweetener if using and use a whisk to combine well. Cook over medium-high heat, for about 10 minutes, stirring frequently to prevent it from splattering, until the mix has reduced by at least half and thickened. Alternatively cook the mixture over low heat for about 35 minutes, and stir every 5 minutes, but be careful not to burn the milk, or you will have to start again.

Remove from the heat and set aside to allow to cool completely.

Remove the can of coconut cream from the refrigerator and empty into a bowl. Use a hand mixer to whisk the coconut cream on high speed for about 2 minutes, or until light and fluffy and nearly doubled in volume. Place the whipped coconut cream in the refrigerator to cool for about 10 minutes.

Add the gelatin to a small heatproof bowl, and mix well with 2 tablespoons of the cooled coconut milk mix. Allow to sit for 5 minutes until the gelatin dissolves. The mixture will swell. Heat a saucepan of water until boiling. Place the bowl containing the coconut milk and gelatin into the pot of boiling water, ensuring that it sits above the water line and melt the gelatin. Remove and allow to cool slightly, before adding the mixture to the remaining coconut milk.

Remove the whipped coconut cream from the refrigerator and add to the coconut milk mixture, along with the toasted coconut. Whip once more until light and creamy, and well combined (another 1 to 2 minutes). Use a spatula to add the mixture into a freezer-safe container or dish and cover tightly and freeze until firm (about 6 hours). Serve frozen. If the ice cream is difficult to scoop before serving, allow to sit in the refrigerator for 15 minutes to soften slightly

Ingredients

1 can (400ml/14 ounces) full fat coconut milk room temperature

1 can ((400ml/14 ounces) full fat coconut cream refrigerated

1/4–1/2 cup rice malt syrup, xylitol or stevia drops to taste

1-2 tsp. natural vanilla paste or extract

1 teaspoon unflavored powdered gelatin (I recommend the Great Lakes brand)

2 tbsp. shredded coconut, toasted (optional)

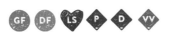

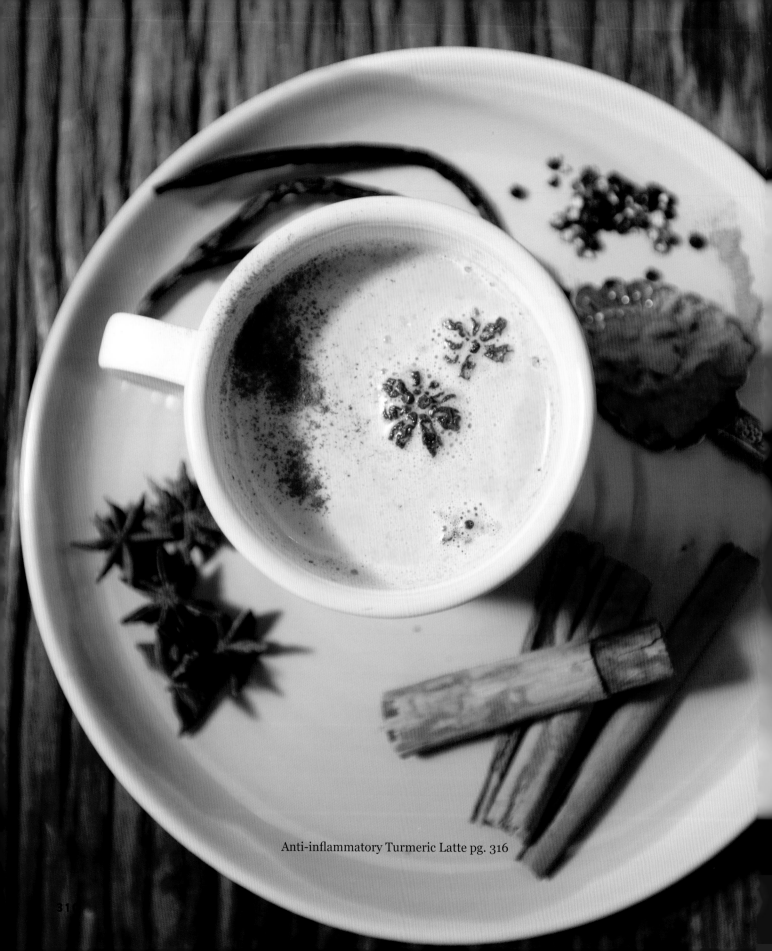

Anti-inflammatory Turmeric Latte pg. 316

Gut Healing Teas

I have included some recipes for fresh herbal teas and a delicious milk-based latte for when those coffee cravings hit, or you feel you need a little more nourishment.

Teas will become an important part of your daily food ritual and, if you're like me, your pantry will soon become adorned with a wide variety of quality herbal teas to suit any mood or your therapeutic needs.

Herbs possess incredibly powerful therapeutic benefits for your health, so relax and enjoy, knowing that your body is benefitting as well as your mind.

MY TOP 6 HEALING TEAS

recommended for regular consumption are:

- Green tea – for cardiovascular health
- Lemongrass – anti microbial and anti fungal actions
- Ginger/turmeric – to combat inflammation
- Licorice root – to nourish your adrenals and combat stress
- Dandelion – for improving liver function
- Peppermint/mint – to relieve tummy upset and gas

Just be sure to avoid any commercial brands of tea that use artificial ingredients or flavors and always use fresh herbs where you can.

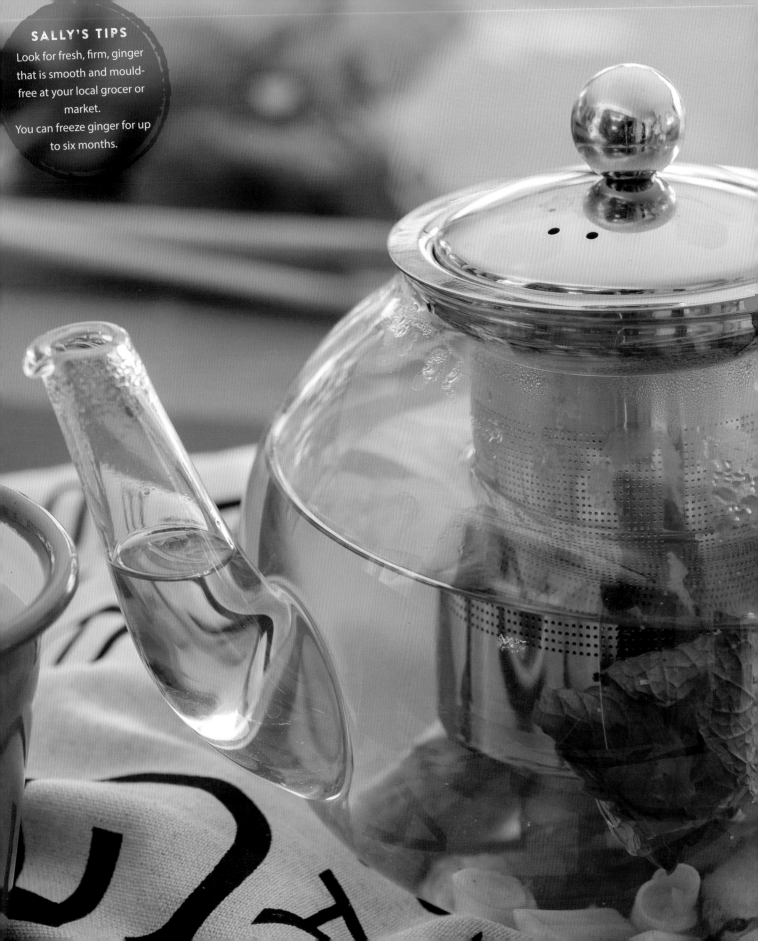

SALLY'S TIPS
Look for fresh, firm, ginger
that is smooth and mould-
free at your local grocer or
market.
You can freeze ginger for up
to six months.

Fresh Lemon Grass, Ginger & Mint Tea

Method

Place ingredients into a teapot or glass coffee plunger and cover with 2 cups boiling water. Allow to infuse for 5-10 minutes, depending how much zing you like in your tea.

COOL LEMONGRASS

Lemongrass tea is consumed in many SouthEast Asian countries, where the climate is often hot, because it has a cooling effect on the body. It also contains a compound, Citral, that has anti-microbial and anti-fungal properties which makes it effective in destroying or inhibiting some pathogens.

MINT

Mint adds a wonderful taste and aroma to tea and is naturally calming to the digestive system, helping to relieve abdominal upset and gas. Peppermint oil capsules work well to alleviate IBS symptoms and help clear the bowel. If you don't find the fresh mint tea strong enough, then add a few drops of fresh peppermint oil to warm water to relieve an upset stomach.

Ingredients

2 tbsp grated fresh ginger

1 stem fresh lemon grass

2 tbsp fresh mint.

AMAZING GINGER

Like turmeric, ginger is a powerful anti-inflammatory which has a warming and calming effect on the digestive system, helping to relieve the build-up of gas. It is an intestinal anti-spasmodic as well as a stimulant of saliva production, so it helps to soothe the intestinal tract, relieve vomiting and ease discomfort from gas and diarrhoea. It's a great natural remedy for morning and motion sickness. Ginger is also packed full of goodness, providing great natural stocks of vitamin C, magnesium, potassium, copper, and manganese.

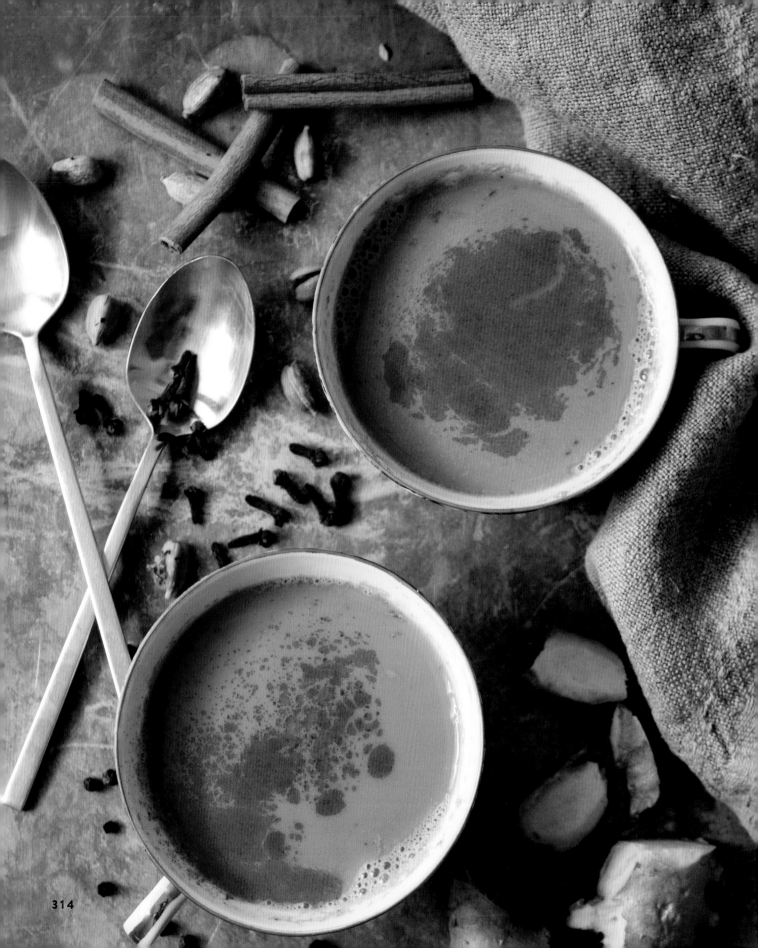

Ayurvedic Chai Latte

Ayurveda is the traditional medicine of India, dating back over 5000 years. The concept of using 'food as medicine' forms the basis of this ancient practice, meaning if you're going to put food in your mouth, you may as well make choices that have a medicinal and healing effect on the body, rather than a potentially damaging one. The spices in this tea have been chosen because they have a soothing and calming effect on the digestive and nervous system. I love this tea when I feel like something creamy and slightly sweet and spicy. I tend to avoid store bought chai lattes, because they are often made on a chai paste which is high in sugar! This tea makes a delicious alternative to coffee and, although it does contain black tea, the naturally occurring theanine should counteract any stimulating effects. Alternatively feel free to leave this out if you prefer. Look for these ingredients at your local health food store, or specialty spice store.

Method

In a large pot add water, cinnamon, cardamon pods, black tea, ginger, cloves and/or star anise, and peppercorns. Cover and bring to a boil. Turn down heat and let simmer for 5 minutes. Add black tea and stir into spice blend. Cover and let simmer for another 2-3 minutes. Remove from heat and strain tea and spices through a mesh strainer. Pour hot tea back into pot and add almond milk. Turn up heat and bring to a boil. Immediately, turn off heat and stir in liquid stevia. Pour into serving cups. Dust with cinnamon and serve hot.

Ingredients

3 cups purified water

4 cups almond milk

4 cinnamon sticks

35-30 whole green cardamon pods

2 tbsp loose leaf organic black tea

2 tbsp fresh ginger, grated

2 tsp whole cloves

1 tsp whole black peppercorns

1-2 star anise, to taste

1-2 tsp rice malt syrup or a few drops liquid stevia to taste

NICE SPICE

Cinnamon is used as a remedy for diabetes, indigestion and colds, and has a calming effect on the body. Ginger is a natural anti-inflammatory and improves circulation and digestion. Star anise is traditionally used to relieve colic, gas, headache, flatulence, nausea and vomiting and has antibacterial and antifungal properties.

Anti-inflammatory Turmeric Latte

The key ingredient to this healing drink is turmeric, which contains the active compound curcurim. The addition of black pepper works to activate the therapeutic compounds in the turmeric.

Ingredients

1 tsp ground or 2 tsp freshly grated turmeric

1/4 tsp ground ginger or 1teaspoon freshly grated

1/2 tsp ground black pepper

1/2 cup filtered water

1 cup unsweetened almond milk or coconut milk

1 tsp virgin coconut oil

1-2 tsp rice malt syrup, or 2-4 drops stevia

Method

To first make the turmeric paste, place the turmeric, ginger, pepper and water into a small saucepan and heat on medium-high heat. Stir to combine until a thick paste forms. Allow the mixture to cool then transfer to a small glass jar.

To make the turmeric latte combine the milk, coconut oil and 1/4 tsp of the turmeric paste in a small saucepan. Heat over medium heat, stirring, being careful not to boil the milk. Add the rice malt syrup or stevia. Use a stick blender to froth the milk to a latte consistency. If you have a coffee machine, transfer the mixture to a jug and use the milk steamer to froth the milk. Just be sure to wipe it down immediately as turmeric can stain easily!

Store the turmeric paste in the fridge for up to 3 weeks.

TURMERIC

Turmeric is renowned in traditional Indian medicine as one of the most powerful natural anti-inflammatory substances, which means it acts as a liver detoxifier and helps to regulate metabolism and digestive health. Conventional science is taking an interest nowadays too by investigating tumeric's amazing healing properties, including the potential positive effect on cancer and inflammatory-based diseases.

Metabolism Booster

I love to begin my day with this super charged elixer if I feel my metabolism needs a bit of a kick start. I won't deny it certainly packs a punch when you first try it, so add plenty of water and halve the ingredients if it is too hot to handle, until your palette adjusts.

Method

Add all ingredients to a large mug and stir to combine.

Drink on waking and follow with breakfast fifteen minutes or later.

Ingredients

1 cup hot water (or dilute to preferred strength)

Juice of 1/2 to one lemon

2 tsp extra virgin coconut oil

1 tbsp apple cider vinegar

1/8 tsp ground or freshly grated ginger and or turmeric

1/8 tsp cayenne pepper (I prefer to use drops as it dissolves better)

1 tsp brown rice malt syrup (optional)

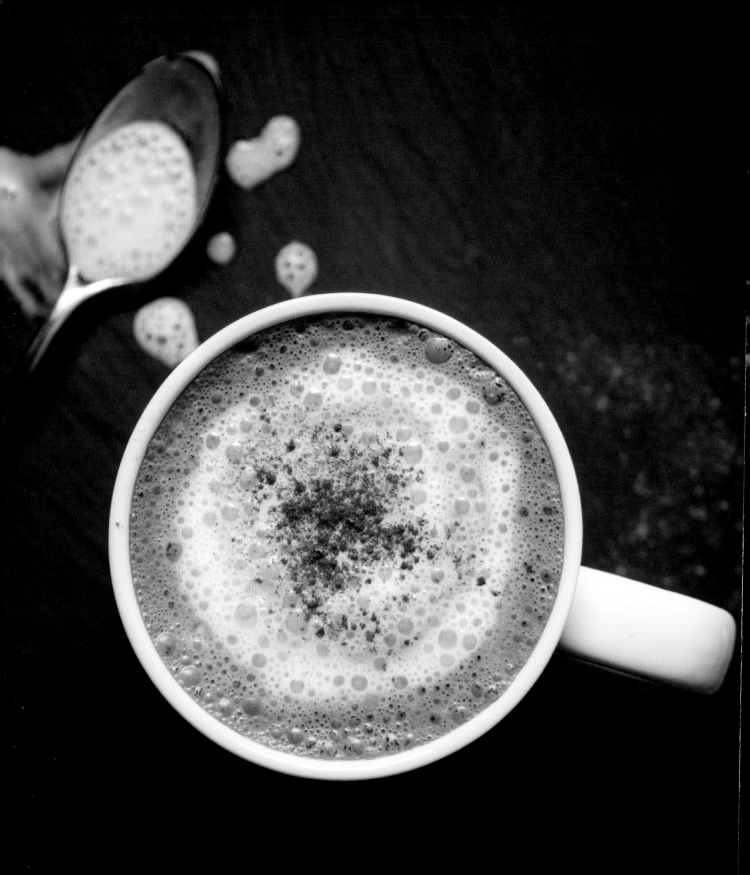

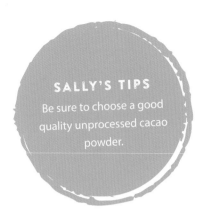

SERVES 1

Dande Mocha

If you're trying to give up coffee and can't quite go without yet, then let me introduce you to this healthy alternative that I think you may just end up growing to love! Dande Mocha combines the goodness of antioxidants and magnesium from raw cacao powder with the natural liver cleansing properties of dandelion.

Coffee is physically addictive, so giving it up is tough and requires changes to your mindset and routine. To help the process along, experiment with this or any of my fresh herbal tea recipes until you find something that you enjoy and makes you feel good. You'll be addicted to the healthy alternative in no time, I promise.

Ingredients

1 tbsp dandelion root

200ml unsweetened almond milk (see page 148) or coconut milk (see page 138)

1 tbsp raw cacao powder

1 tsp rice malt syrup

1/2 tsp ground cinnamon

Ingredients

Place the dandelion root into a teapot or glass coffee plunger with 150ml of boiling water and allow to infuse for 3-6 minutes, depending how strong you like your tea.

Heat the milk in a small saucepan, and use a stick blender to froth (if you have a coffee machine, use the milk steamer).

Place the cacao powder into a large mug and add the infused dandelion tea. Stir until well combined.

Add the milk and sweeten with the rice malt syrup. Serve sprinkled with cinnamon.

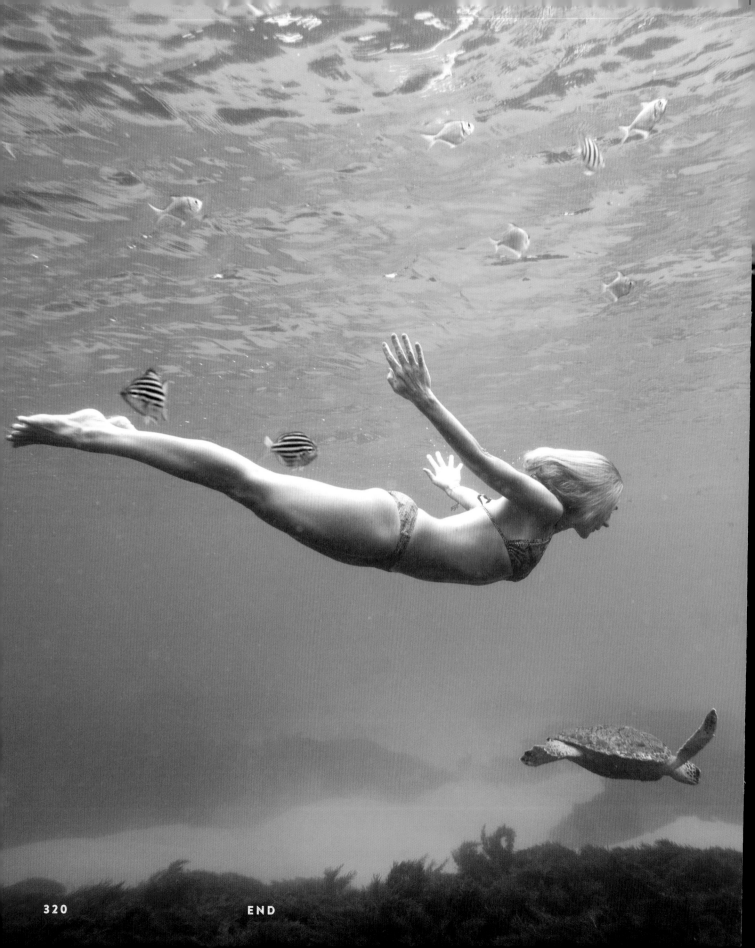

END

TAKE TIME OUT EACH DAY

It's funny how rarely we give ourselves permission to take time out and truly connect with ourselves. Instead choosing to live life on the surface - claiming we're 'too busy' and prioritising what we think is urgent, over what is actually important.

By making time to be with yourself each day in a quiet and peaceful environment, you are choosing to value yourself in a way that will help you to experience a greater sense of inner contentment and peace.

When you embark on a journey to improve your health, it's just as important to learn skills to help you enjoy a healthy mind, as well as body. One of the ways you can achieve this, is to remove any undue pressure or expectations you may have placed on yourself. Learning to be kinder and gentler with yourself, and forgiving any personal short-comings, will help set your mind free from constant self criticism.

As long as you choose to make positive changes through healthier choices, no matter how big or small - whether it's getting more sleep each night, spending less time sitting, starting your day with an alkalising vegetable juice, or learning how to meditate – these little changes will soon lead to big shifts in your long term health and happiness.

One of the best things you can do for yourself is to take time out for YOU each day. I make a point to do this, even if it's just to sit in the sun with a cup of my favourite herbal tea for ten minutes of nothing and no one else, no phones, no distractions, no matter how busy I am. If I don't do this each day, I feel restless, I may not sleep as well at night, little things can take on too much meaning, and I develop 'busy brain' and become less productive.

My favourite place to take time out, is in or by the ocean. This is the place where time stops for me and everything is still. It's where I am the most present and the most connected. It reminds me to keep life simple and uncomplicated. I also like to combine my exercise with my 'time out' whether it be stand up paddle boarding, taking long walks in the bush, or doing pilates or yoga.

Find your 'happy time out place' and be sure to visit it each and every day and I guarantee by giving more to yourself in ways that matter, you'll feel far more connected and content within.

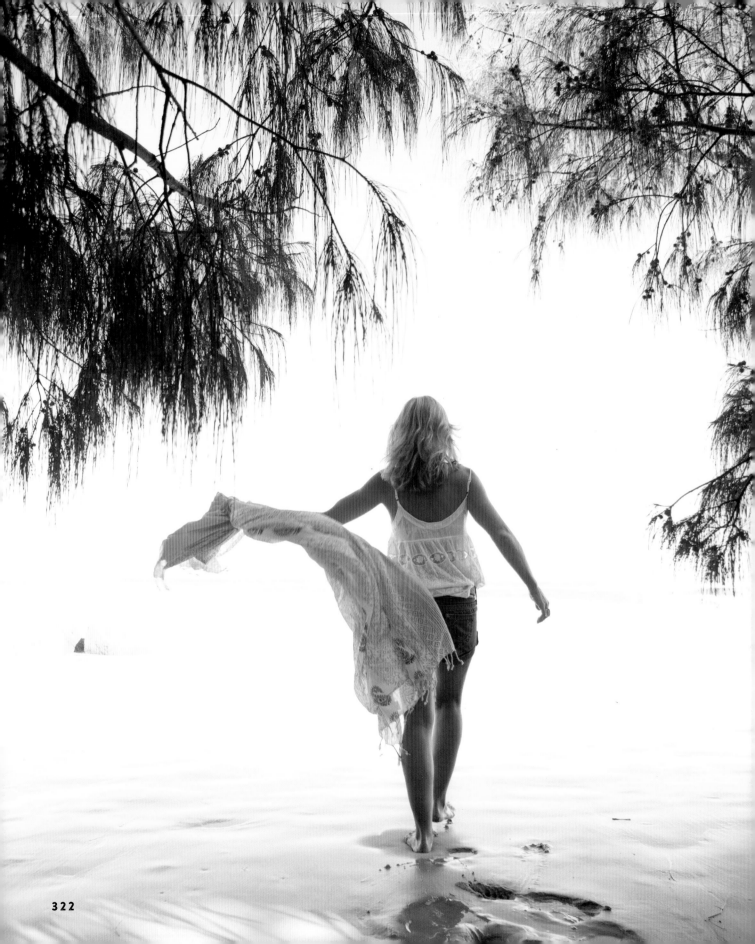

A Final Word

We are all unique in our own special way — what one person's body needs is different to another's when it comes to exercise, how much sleep we need and the amount and type of food we should eat. But we are all connected by one common denominator, the function of our gut and what lives inside it. So no matter what you desire to achieve with your health, remember good health always starts in your gut and its ongoing vitality is very much dependent on how well you maintain the colonies of good gut bacteria within it — without doubt, this is the most important thing you can do to achieve and maintain optimal health and wellbeing, and prevent chronic illness and disease in the future.

The information in this book should help to lay the foundations for you to achieve your healthiest, and I hope, happiest, self.

Modern science is only just beginning to understand the human microbiome contained within the gut and the power and influence it has on our health, but I hope as we begin to explore and learn more in this field of medicine, we will find the answers we have been searching for to resolve and even cure diseases, so we can all enjoy longer and, most importantly, healthier lives.

Remember, nature in its untouched state is able to maintain perfect equilibrium. It's only when man goes against nature's way that we see a disruption to the natural eco system, including the one living within our gut. So if you want to enjoy the best in health and all that comes with it, then whatever you do, love your gut and it will love you back.

References

- Kostic, A, Gevers D. (2012). Genomic analysis identifies association of Fusobacterium with colorectal carcinoma; Genome Res. Volume 22(2),p. 292–298;

- Lorscheider FL, Vimy MJ. (1995). Mercury exposure from silver tooth fillings: emerging evidence questions a traditional dental paradigm. The FASEB Journal; vol. 9(7). p.504-508.

- Guzzi,G, Grandi. (2006). Dental Amalgam and Mercury Levels in Autopsy Tissues: Food for Thought. American Journal of Forensic Medicine & Pathology. Volume 27(1). p 42-45.

- Lydiard R. (2001). Irritable bowel syndrome, anxiety, and depression: what are the links?'. J Clin Psychiatry.62 Suppl 8:38-45; discussion 46-7

- Padhy SK, Sahoo S. (2015). Irritable bowel syndrome: Is it "irritable brain" or "irritable bowel"?

  J Neurosci Rural Pract. Volume 6 (4), p.568-77.

- Fasano A. Ann N. (2012). Zonulin, regulation of tight junctions, and autoimmune diseases. Acad Sci. Volume 1258(1): p. 25–33.

- Hamed Khalili, Leslie M. (2013). Oral contraceptives, reproductive factors and risk of inflammatory bowel disease. Gut. Volume 62; p.1153–1159.

- Boorom K. Smith H. (2008), Oh my aching gut: irritable bowel syndrome, blastocystis and asymptomatic infection. Parasites & Vectors; 1:40. https://parasitesandvectors. biomedcentral.com/articles/10.1186/1756-3305-1-40

- Bested A. Logan A. (2013). Intestinal microbiota, probiotics and mental health: from Metchnikoff to modern advances: Gut Pathogens, Part II – contemporary contextual research. 5:3. http://gutpathogens.biomedcentral.com/articles/10.1186/1757-4749-5-3

- Sheldon Cohen. (2012). How stress influences disease; Journal of Applied Social Psychology. Volume 42(6). pages 1320–1334.

- Farrell R, Kelly C. (2002); Celiac Sprue. N Engl J Med. 346:180-188.

- Ludvigsson JF, Reutfors J. (2007). Coeliac disease and risk of mood disorders-a general population-based cohort study. J Affect Disord. Volume 99(1-3). p.117-26.

- Jackson J. Eaton W. (2012) Neurologic and Psychiatric Manifestations of Celiac Disease and Gluten Sensitivity; Psychiatric Quarterly, Volume 83, Issue 1, p. 91-102;

- Ventura A. Giuseppe A. (1999) Duration of exposure to gluten and risk for autoimmune disorders in patients with celiac disease Gastroenterology; Volume 117(2). P. 297–303.

- Millward C. Ferriter M. (2004). Gluten- and casein-free diets for autistic spectrum disorder;. Cochrane Database Syst Rev. Volume (2).

- Barrett J. (2006). The Science of Soy: What Do We Really Know? Environ Health Perspect. 114(6): A352–A358;.

- Lau K. McLean G.(2005). Synergistic Interactions between Commonly used food additives in a developmental neurotoxicity test; Oxford Journals, Toxicological Sciences. Volume 90(1) p. 178-187.

- Qing Yang (2010). Gain weight by "going diet?" Artificial sweeteners and the neurobiology of sugar cravings; Yale J Biol Med. Neuroscience Volume 83(2): 101–108.

- Feijó Fde M. Ballard CR (2013) 'Saccharin and aspartame, compared with sucrose, induce greater weight gain in adult Wistar rats, at similar total caloric intake levels'. Appetite. Volume.60(1) p. 203-7.

- Soffritti M, Padovani M. (2014) The carcinogenic effects of aspartame: The urgent need for regulatory re-evaluation. Am J Ind Med. Volume. 57(4) p.383-97.

- David S. Ludwig. Willett W (2013) Three Daily Servings of Reduced-Fat Milk An Evidence-Based Recommendation? JAMA Pediatr. Volume.167(9) p.788-789.

- Adebamowo CA, Spiegelman D. (2005). 'High school dietary dairy intake and teenage acne'. J Am Acad. Volume.52(2). p.207-14.

- Kamiński S, Cieslińska A. (2007). Polymorphism of bovine beta-casein and its potential effect on human health. J Appl Genet. Volume 48(3) p.189-98.

- Melnik B. (2011) Milk signaling in the pathogenesis of type 2 diabetes.. Med Hypotheses. Volume.76(4) p.553-9.

- AS Truswell. (2005). The A2 milk case: a critical review; European Journal of Clinical Nutrition. Volume.59. p.623–631.

- Bonthuis M, Hughes M. (2007) Dairy consumption and patterns of mortality of Australian adults. Mucosal reactivity to cow's milk protein in coeliac disease. Clin Exp Immunol. Volume. 147(3). p.449–455.

- Lidén M, Kristjánsson G. (2008). Cow's milk protein sensitivity assessed by the mucosal patch technique is related to irritable bowel syndrome in patients with primary Sjögren's syndrome; Clin Exp Allergy. Volume.38(6). p.929-35.

- Oranje A, Wolkerstorfer A.(2002). Natural course of cow's milk allergy in childhood atopic eczema/dermatitis syndrome. Ann Allergy Asthma Immunol. Volume.89(6 Suppl 1). p.52-5.

- (1997) Feskanich D, Willett WC. Milk, dietary calcium, and bone fractures in women: a 12-year prospective study. Am J Public Health. Volume.87(6) p.992-7.

- (2004). Bone Health and Osteoporosis: A Report of the Surgeon General. Rockville, MD: U.S. Department of Health and Human Services, Office of the Surgeon General.

- Feskanich D, Willett W. (2003). Calcium, vitamin D, milk consumption, and hip fractures: a prospective study among postmenopausal women. Am J Clin Nutr. Volume.77. p.504-511.

- Ross C, Taylor C. Food and Nutrition Board Institute of Medicine. (2010) Dietary Reference Intakes for Vitamin D and Calcium. National Academy Press.

- Holick M, Garabedian M.(2006) Vitamin D: photobiology, metabolism, mechanism of action, and clinical applications. In Primer on the metabolic bone diseases and disorders of mineral metabolism. American Society for Bone and Mineral Research. 6th edition. P.129-137.

- Bischoff-Ferrari H, Willett W. (2005). Fracture prevention with vitamin D supplementation: a meta-analysis of randomized controlled trials. JAMA Volume.293 p.2257-2264.

- Nordin B, Need A. (1993) The nature and significance of the relationship between urinary sodium and urinary calcium in women. J Nutr. Vol123. p.1615-1622.

- Teucher B, Dainty J. (2008) Sodium and bone health: impact of moderately high and low salt intakes on calcium metabolism in postmenopausal women. J Bone Miner Res. Volume. 23 p.1477-1485.

- Barański M, Srednicka-Tober D. (2014). Higher antioxidant and lower cadmium concentrations and lower incidence of pesticide residues in organically grown crops: a systematic literature review and meta-analyses. Br J Nutr.Volume.112.(5). p.794-811

- Oates L, Cohen M.(2014) Reduction in urinary organophosphate pesticide metabolites in adults after a week-long organic diet. Environmental Research. Volume 132. p105–111.

- Séralini G, Clair E. (2012). Long term toxicity of a Roundup herbicide and a Roundup-tolerant genetically modified maize; Food and Chemical Toxicology Volume 50.(11), p.4221-4231.

- Clark B. (2012). Pesticide Use Rises as Herbicide-resistant Weeds Undermine Performance of Major GE Crops, New WSU Study Shows. Washington State University https://cahnrs.wsu.edu/news-release/2012/10/01/pesticide-use-rises-as-herbicide-resistant-weeds-undermine-performance-of-major-ge-crops-new-wsu-study-shows/

- Aris A, Leblanc S. (2011) Maternal and fetal exposure to pesticides associated to genetically modified foods in Eastern Townships of Quebec, Canada. Reproductive Toxicology. Volume 31(4) p.528-33.

- Aristo Vojdani, (2014). The Prevalence of Antibodies against Wheat and Milk Proteins in Blood Donors and Their Contribution to Neuroimmune Reactivities; Nutrients. Volume 1(2), p. 15-36

- Susan Leech, (1998) Molecular mimicry in autoimmune disease; Arch Dis Child; Vol. 79 :p.448-451

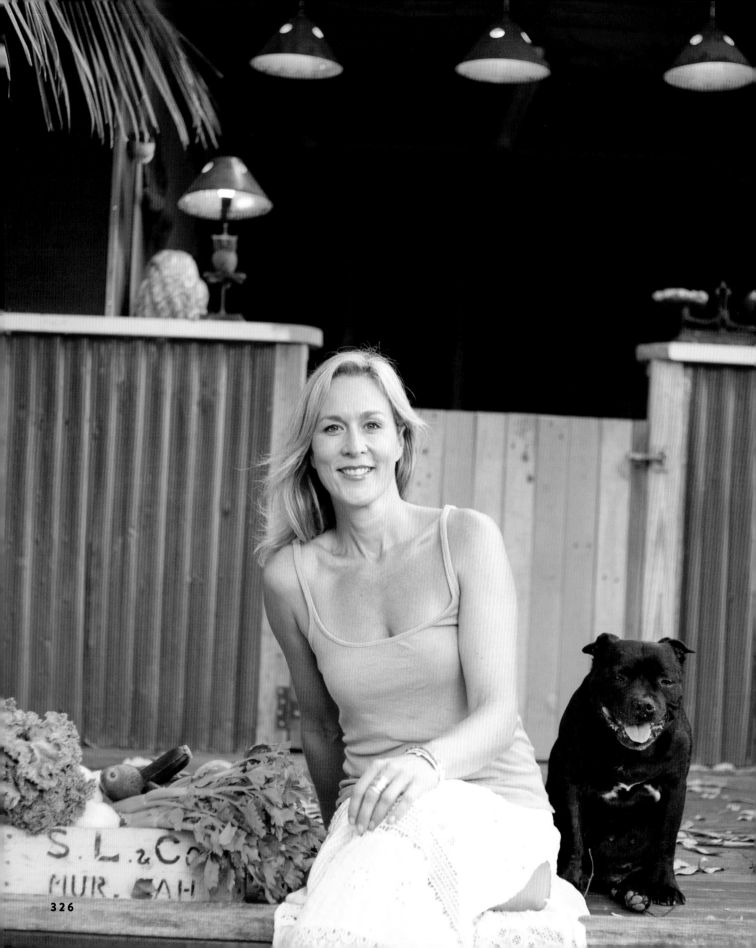

Special Thanks

Many people have helped make this book become a reality and supported me along the way, I owe special thanks to:

Daz - for your extraordinary talent with meal preparation and styling and Jaz (Jasmine Lord) - for your incredible photography talent; your hard work and dedication to the cause, makes you 'the A team'. I had so much fun working with you both.

Pam Le May - for helping with meal preparation and recipe testing.

Sebastian and Jonatan Lundmark - for your amazing creative talent behind the camera.

Laurel Anderson - for your creative assistance with the book design.

Charlotte Adams - for your beautiful and talented illustrations.

Veronica Crowther - for your editing.

Layne Beachley - for a fantastic foreword and your friendship over the years.

Katina Trout - thank you for your help with design and wonderful friendship and support.

Meggy, Annie & Elke – for being my three adorable nieces, I love you more than all the stars in the sky!

Mum and Dad - I owe you both so much, you have been incredible parents and mentors
and without your relentless and unconditional love, support and encouragement, this book would not have become a reality.

Index

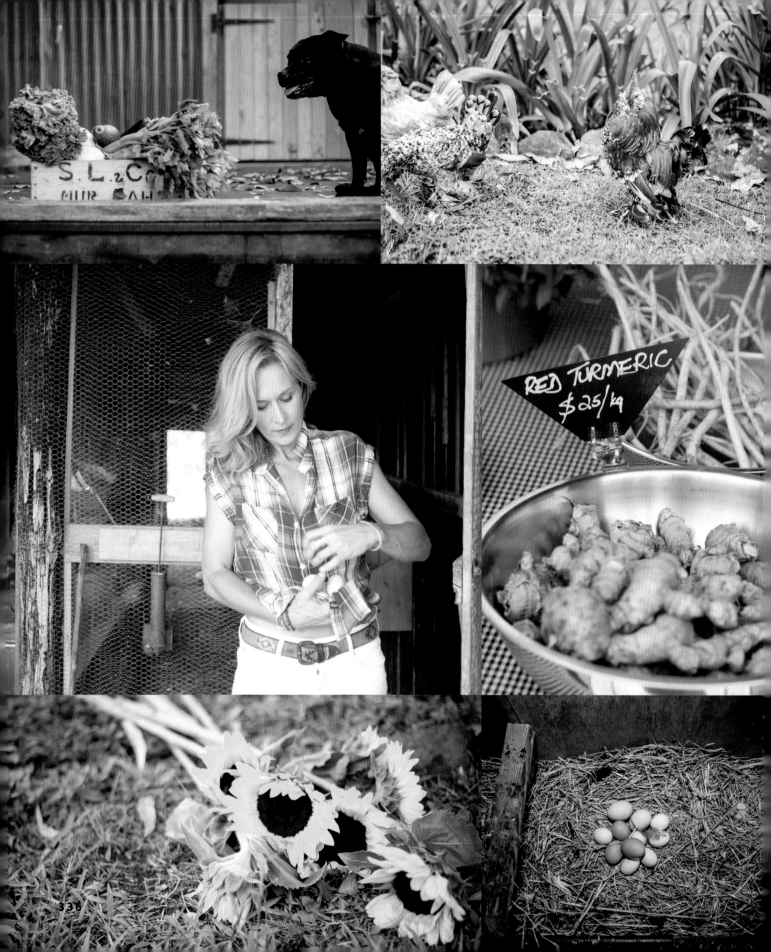

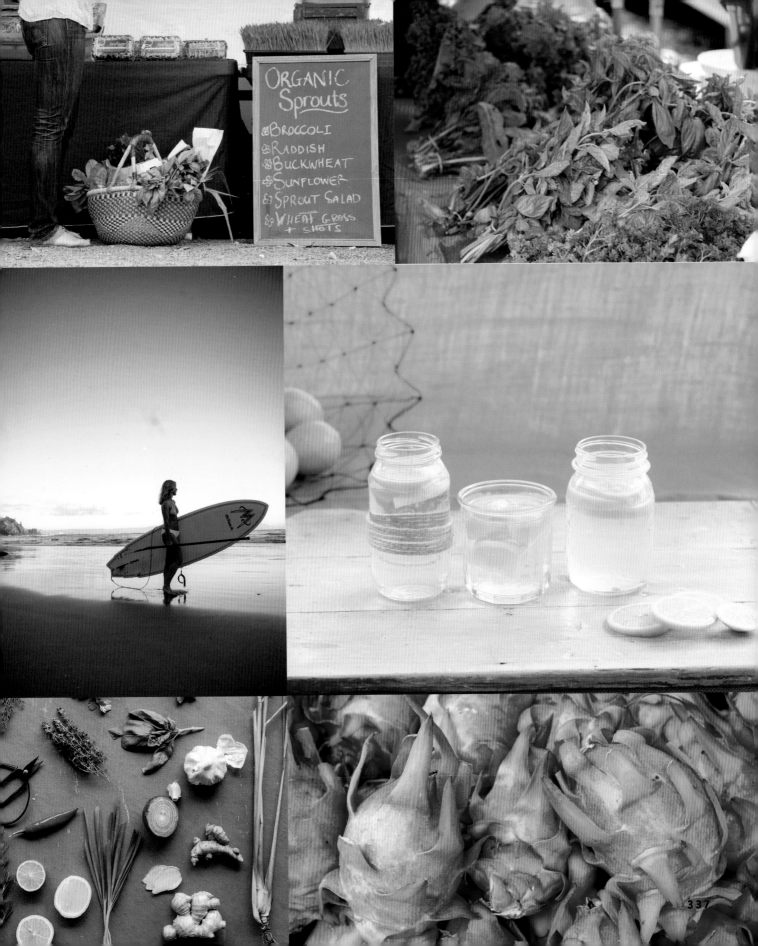

ORGANIC
Sprouts

✿ Broccoli
✿ Raddish
✿ Buckwheat
✿ Sunflower
✿ Sprout Salad
✿ Wheat Grass
      + Shots

Testimonials

"I see Sally Joseph for nutrition, She is amazing!" – MIRANDA KERR -INTERNATIONAL MODEL

"Sally's LYG program provided me with a thorough and simple understanding of why my body was failing to thrive and what I needed to do to get my health back on track. Through improving my digestion I was able to increase my energy and it felt amazing to have my whole body functioning at its best again. If you want to know what it's like to feel 100% fit and healthy, I thoroughly recommend Sally Joseph's Love Your Gut program."

– LAYNE BEACHLEY – 7 TIMES WORLD CHAMPION SURFER

"I've followed Sally's Love Your Gut Program for more than ten years and it has been such a gift to my life. I suffer Hashimoto's auto-immune disease and Sally's program has taught me the links between my body and mind and how stress affects my illness. I now feel armed with the knowledge I need to understand what it takes to be truly well and healthy. Sally is one of the most knowledgeable people I have met in this space and I trust her advice implicitly."

– MEGAN DALLA-CAMINA – AUTHOR, SPEAKER AND ENTREPRENEUR

"There are a lot of people who claim to be able to help you transform your life through diet, but Sally really does have the credentials on gut health and the results speak for themselves - I feel better than I've felt in years - my eyes are clearer, I sleep better, I'm not bloated and my skin conditions have cleared up. The best part is my mind is so much clearer and I feel on top of my game again, without the anxiety."

– FIONA R. MERMAID BEACH QLD.

"Sally's program taught me if I wanted to truly reach my goal weight, diet and exercise alone were not enough - I had to fix my gut! I learnt I wasn't absorbing my food properly and my bowel movements were never regular, but the LYG program solved that! Sally's program is so straightforward and I now apply the principles to my every day life with ease and have maintained my 18 kg weight loss to this day."

– GEORGIE. SINGAPORE

"After just a couple of months on Sally's LYG program I noticed an amazing improvement in the eczema I have suffered my whole life. Something I wasn't able to achieve with countless dollars spent on practitioners, creams and the latest "next best thing" in the fight against eczema."

– SHARON, SYDNEY

"I'm a personal trainer and have always eaten what I thought was a healthy diet and exercised regularly, but when I started to gain weight despite exercising more, I knew something wasn't working and if anything it was making me more fatigued. I had looked into the Paleo and raw food diets but neither of these worked entirely for me. Then I tried Sally's LYG program, which struck a perfect balance and taught me how different foods were affecting my body and how my gut health was influencing my symptoms. By day 4 my digestive system felt amazing! I now incorporate the program into my everyday life. I've lost weight and feel great and I was finally able to stop the contraceptive pill after struggling to come off it for 6 years without experiencing hormonal acne! I now have clear skin and my energy is back!"

– BELINDA G. SYDNEY

"I was overweight and tired all of the time despite, the fact I thought I had a reasonably healthy diet. I now realize I didn't! Since being on the on the LYG Program my husband lost 8kgs and I lost 6kgs and we both feel great! Goodbye 3pm slump! The change within myself amazed me. All sorts of symptoms I had put up with for years thinking they were just the norm, slowly but surely disappeared; sinus issues, dry skin and bronchial issues amongst other things. I have tried every other sort of 'diet' and have been a yo-yo dieter for years. I had a partial thyroidectomy 15 years ago and have struggled with weight ever since. The LYG program has become a 'way of life' for us and for the first time in a long time, I feel great! "

– S. FERGUSSON

"I suffered unbelievably debilitating menstrual pain for many years leaving me bedridden for at least a day a month, with severe cramping, vomiting & diarrhea. After having surgery for category 4 Endometriosis, I knew I had to radically rethink my diet which is when I discovered Sally's Love Your Gut Program. Sally's vast knowledge and experience set me on the path to good health like I have never experienced. LYG taught me about the changes I needed to make to my diet to heal my condition. My periods no longer take over my life each month – thanks to no pain and I have not been back to hospital for further surgery for over 8 years!"

– LOUISE, SYDNEY

"My main goal going on the LYG Program was to kick my sugar addiction, but what I achieved was so much more! By 41 I had twice suffered breast cancer and gone through endless rounds of chemo and radiotherapy, before experiencing premature menopause from a hysterectomy. I also suffered reoccurring depression. If there is one thing I have learnt about my health through Sally's program, it's how to fuel my body with the right foods and look after my gut. When it comes to getting healthy for life, it all comes down to getting the right knowledge, not going on a fad diet. The LYG Program shone through for me and a whole new way of living has opened up. I now know what I need to do to get healthy and stay healthy."

– ANNABELLE T. CENTRAL QLD

"I was diagnosed with Lupus in 2000 and was taking numerous pharmaceutical drugs to control the symptoms, but none of them targeted the underlying cause of my illness. I was desperate, depressed and my Lupus was spiraling out of control. Four years into following Sally's LYG program, and I am off all my Lupus medication and I no longer experience daily burning Lupus pain and I am back at full time work. My health will always be an ongoing journey, but I never thought I could feel this good. I now feel in control of my Lupus rather than it controlling me."

– EILEEN, SYDNEY

"The recipes and meal plans were so delicious and doable and Sally's smoothie recipes left my skin looking amazing! I was surprised at how delicious healthy food can be!"

– AMBER V. BRISBANE

"I thought I was a healthy eater and understood nutrition well – until I did Sally's LYG program. I discovered my diet was very high in hidden sugars. I loved the recipes on the program and so did my young family! I can still enjoy the foods I love, I've just learnt new ways to make healthier choices that are making a big difference. The extra baby weight I'd struggled to shift, despite hours of regular exercise, fell off me and now my entire way of eating has changed for the better."

– REBECCA, BRISBANE

"Since doing the LYG Program I have more energy, my skin is no longer dry and I notice that if I do occasionally eat sugar or bread now, it does not affect me the way it used to – oh and my allergies have gone! No more snuffly sinuses when I drink wine! On a whole I feel happier and so much healthier."

– NICK, GRAFTON

"I have been going to the gym and 'trying' to eat healthy for years. Whilst short-term weight loss came and went, I just couldn't get exercise & diet to 'click' together for me in a satisfactory way. It wasn't until I did Sally's LYG program that I became fully aware of what healthy eating meant. I think the greatest benefit of Sally's program is that it really gets results that last. I initially looked into this program out of vanity, specifically wanting to lose weight. What I came out with was so much more. I now literally spring out of bed in the mornings, feel more alert throughout the day and sleep much better than I have in years…oh, and losing 11kg's is also a welcome bonus towards my overall well- being!"

– IAN CZENZ, LANE COVE

Can't get enough of 'Love your Gut?'

Sign up to Sally's newsletter at www.sallyjoseph.com and stay in the loop to receive FREE regular health tips and the latest cutting edge health news and reviews, plus more delicious gut loving recipes!

LET'S CONNECT - FOLLOW ME

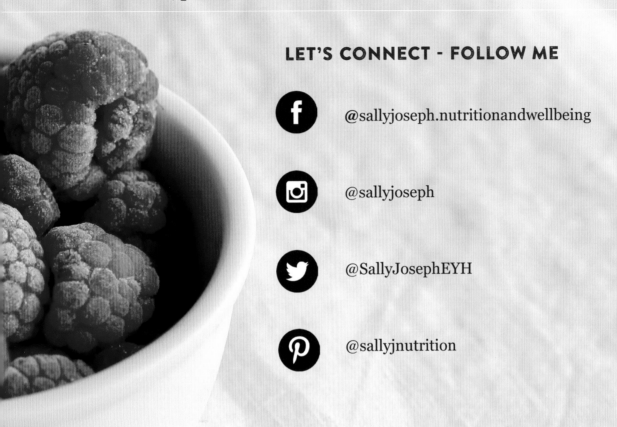

f @sallyjoseph.nutritionandwellbeing

@sallyjoseph

@SallyJosephEYH

@sallyjnutrition

Take your health to the next level

Need a little extra motivation and guidance? Join me for my next 6WK online nutrition program at eatyourselfhealthy.com to receive daily emails, educational videos and simple recipe demonstrations, delivered daily to your inbox!

You'll also get free access to my online community and support group! This is the perfect partner to 'Love Your Gut' and will be just like having me in your own home to step you through the program.

Design and type set by Laurel Anderson and Sally Joseph

Photography by Jasmine Lorde, Sebastian & Jonatan Lundmark, Demetre Minchev, Sally Joseph, Nelly Le Comte, Laurel Anderson

Food preparation by Daz Woodward, Pam LeMay, Sally Joseph and Angelica Arnott

Styling by Daz Woodward & Sally Joseph

Illustrations by Charlotte Adams & Leonie Berkenbosch

Editing by Veronica Crowther

Printed and bound in China

The recipe and photograph for Ayurvedic Chai (page 315) adapted with permission from Wild Plate by Laurel Anderson 2013.

ISBN# 978-0-692-73804-7

Disclaimer

This book is written as a source of information only. The information in this book is intended to supplement, not replace advice from a qualified health professional. If you are pregnant, or know or suspect you have a health condition, please consult with a health professional prior to making any changes to your diet. Whilst all effort has been made to ensure the accuracy of information at the time of publication, the author does not offer any guarantee that the information in this book is free from error or suitable for every individual and specifically disclaims any liability, loss or risk, personal or otherwise, that is incurred as a consequence, directly or indirectly, of the use and application of any of the contents of this book.

$AU 39.99

$US 29.99

About Author

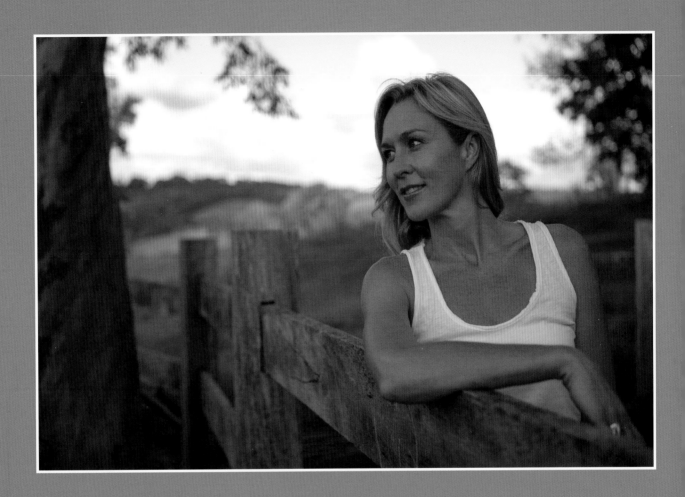

Sally Joseph is a leading Clinical Nutritionist, author, and speaker, with over 17 years experience in private practice. After using diet and nutritional medicine to overcome her own battle with Chronic Fatigue Syndrome, lupus, and autoimmune thyroid disease, Sally went on to qualify as a Nutritionist so she could help others achieve their full health potential. Sally is widely recognized as an expert in digestive health, as well as natural medicine approaches for managing autoimmune and thyroid disorders. Sally is also a regular contributor to the media and developer of the popular online nutrition program - Eat Yourself Healthy - available through her website sallyjoseph.com.

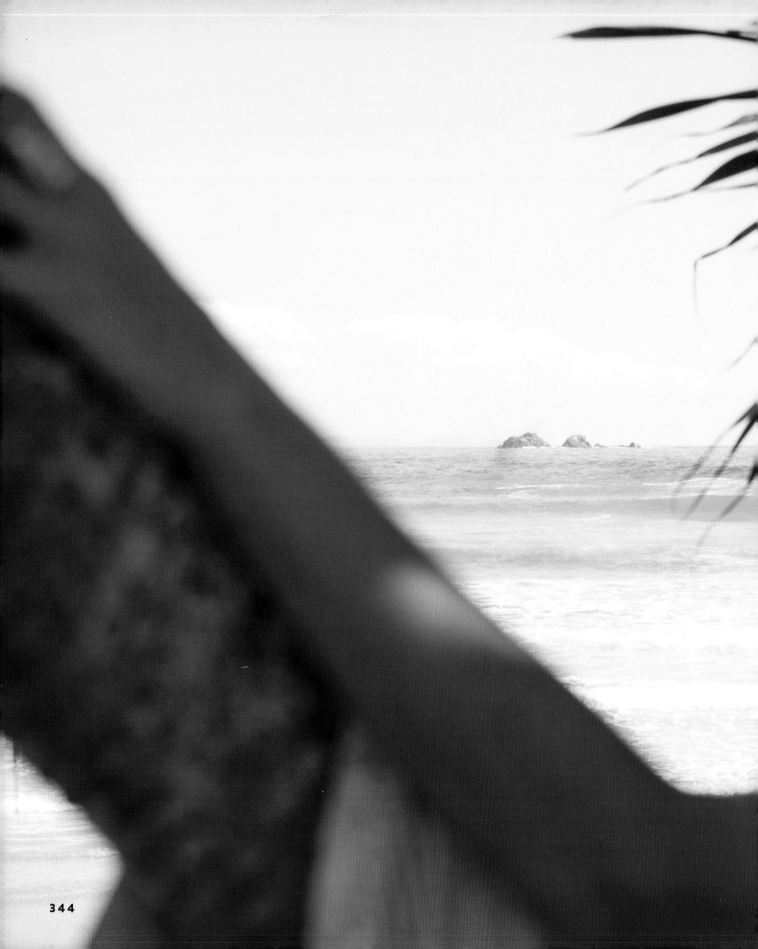

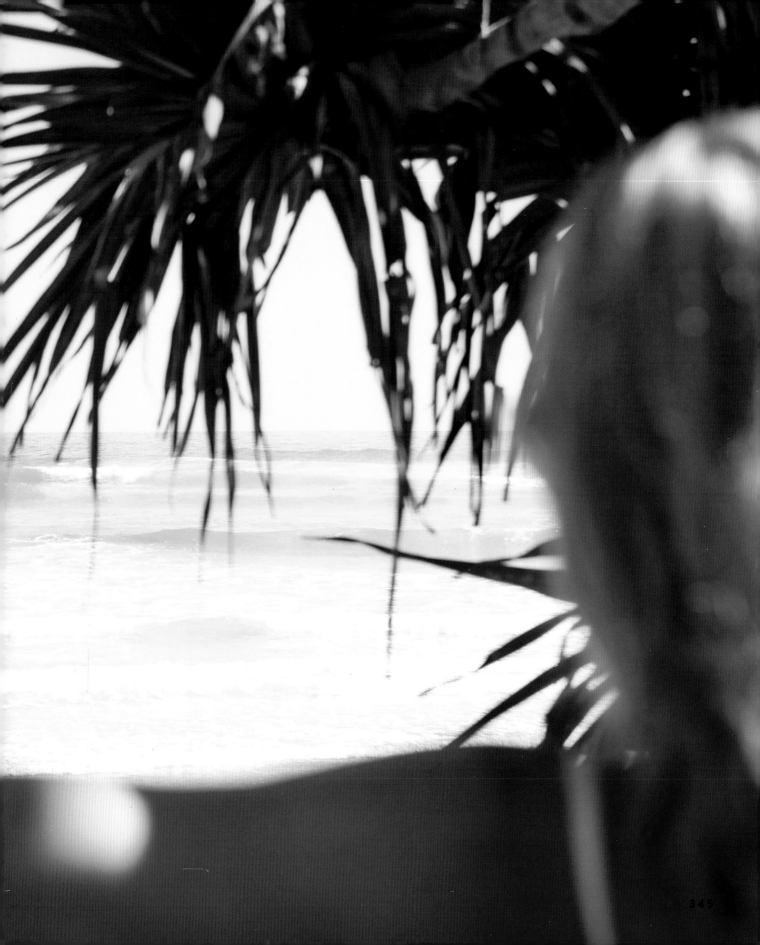